KU-222-214

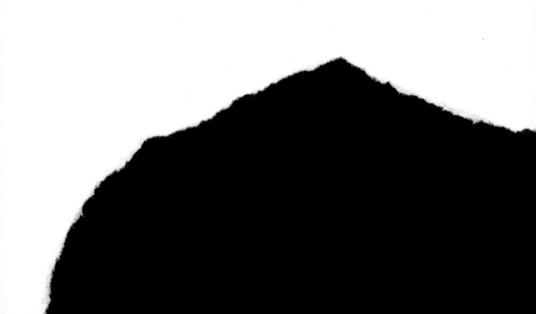

Praise for David Ludwig and

ALWAYS HUNGRY?

"Once in a generation a scientist comes along who tells a new story about why we are sick and how we can heal. Dr. David Ludwig is that scientist. *Always Hungry* is a powerful book that breaks apart every myth about weight loss, and explains for the first time why we get fat and why we are always hungry. If you want to end once and for all your struggles with weight, then read this book, and follow its guidance."

—Mark Hyman, MD, Director, Cleveland Clinic Center for
Functional Medicine, #1 New York Times bestselling
author of *The Blood Sugar Solution*

"Always Hungry? deftly explores the science underlying *why* we make our food choices. And this information, so well presented, is a game-changer. Dr. Ludwig's dietary plan let's you look upon food with passionate embrace as the fundamental key to changing your health destiny."

—David Perlmutter, MD, *New York Times*
bestselling author of *Brain Maker*

"For decades Dr. David Ludwig's research has formed the backbone of other diet programs. Now he has distilled his years of research into this fascinating and groundbreaking book. *Always Hungry?* will cause a much needed seismic shift in the way we think about weight loss. Prepare to change your health for the better."

—Andrew Weil, MD, Founder and Director of
the Arizona Center for Integrative Medicine,
University of Arizona

"David Ludwig is one of the very few voices of true authority in the world of obesity. As both a highly respected medical researcher as well as a practicing clinician, he understands the complexity of weight control and the difficulty in maintaining weight loss. This book goes to the heart of the underlying cause of weight gain—being constantly hungry. Based on the emerging science of satiety, this book offers a practical, lifetime approach to return to a state of improved wellness regardless of your weight. If you care about your health future, then this is the one book you should read and pay careful attention to."

—Dr. Barry Sears, author of the #1 New York
Times bestseller, *The Zone*

"Dr. Ludwig brings a fresh and welcome perspective, based on his extensive clinical and research experience, to the challenges facing millions of overweight Americans. Until now, most attempts at weight loss have focused primarily on calories consumed and burned, but what seems right in theory often fails in practice. Dr. Ludwig explains why throwing out our calorie-counters and paying more attention to the quality of our diets can result in a healthier weight, and to more enjoyment from eating at the same time. This is a must-read for anyone who has struggled to maintain a healthy weight."

—Professor Walter Willett, Harvard T.H. Chan
School of Public Health and author of
Eat, Drink, and Be Healthy

"Finally, an explanation for why so many people have failed in dieting, and a roadmap for how to improve metabolism, curb hunger, and lose weight successfully. Dr. Ludwig's book is not only instructive, it is life-transforming."

—Francine R. Kaufman, MD,
past president, American Diabetes Association and
author of *Diabesity*

"Starving yourself and over-exercising makes you weak, not thin. Learn from a leading voice in nutrition how to strategically use food to permanently end cravings. You'll never worry about calories again."
—Dave Asprey, *New York Times* bestselling author of
The Bulletproof Diet

"Finally, after decades of portion control, counting calories, and low-fat diets, a weight loss book based on modern science. Dr. Ludwig engagingly reveals why calorie counting is doomed to fail, and how we can harness the biologic power of different foods to regain control of our bodies, our health, and our joy of eating. All calories are not created equal, and all diet books are not the same: *Always Hungry?* sets a new standard for successful, healthy weight loss."
—Dariush Mozaffarian, MD, DrPH Dean,
Tufts Friedman School of Nutrition Science & Policy

"Ludwig's book is cutting-edge medicine wrapped with big doses of dietary advice and gentle explanations for why our appetite button may be permanently switched ON. It doesn't get better than this."
—Professor Jennie Brand-Miller, author of *The Low GI Handbook*

"This is NOT a diet book. Instead, it describes a way of eating that reprograms our fat cells to release excess fat for weight loss without hunger. Ludwig combines cutting-edge science and clinical experience into an achievable eating pattern that anyone could follow."
—Janet King, PhD, Executive Director,
Children's Hospital Oakland Research Institute and Chair,
2005 USDA Dietary Guidelines Advisory Committee

"David Ludwig is a leading thinker on nutrition and body weight control, and is one of the few who can harness the best of scientific information to help people in their everyday lives. This book is sound, helpful, and breaks new ground."
—Professor Kelly D. Brownell, PhD,
Dean, Sanford School of Public Policy, Duke University

"In *Always Hungry?*, world renowned endocrinologist and researcher David Ludwig explains in clear, accessible language what has made Americans so fat and what we can do to reverse the obesity epidemic for our ourselves, our children and our nation. This is a must-read!"

—Arthur Agatston, MD, *New York Times* bestselling author of *The South Beach Diet*

Testimonials from the Pilot Test

Weight and waist measurements reflect changes over the sixteen weeks of the pilot. See page 13 for details.

My husband said that he didn't think I was on a diet—he said diets are full of deprivation and, since I wasn't feeling deprived, I couldn't call it a diet anymore. It does feel good not to be driven by my stomach! I feel so different in such a good way.

—Donna A., 51, Selah, WA
Weight loss: 22 pounds. Decrease in waist: 5 inches

I've worked at the same hospital for fifteen years. I have people, two, three, five times a day coming up to me and saying, "Oh my God— you look fantastic." Which is truly a gratifying reward that I was not looking for. I was doing this purely for myself. And many, many, many people track me down and say, "Please, share it with me. I want to learn how to do this." Personally, I feel amazing.

—Eric F., 42, Needham, MA
Weight loss: 17 pounds. Decrease in waist: 3 inches

There is more to this program than just a number on the scale. I think they should call this "the change your brain diet" because I have a totally different outlook on food, my body, my personal journey, and wellness in general. Temptations are still there but I don't constantly feel hungry or deprived. I used to feel like there was something wrong with me, that I lacked willpower or fortitude. This program has shown me that I can do this—it has given me something very intangible that I have difficulty describing but hope others are feeling too. I feel like I can stick to this for the rest of my life.

—Lisa K., 52, Dedham, MA
Weight loss: 19 pounds. Decrease in waist: 6 inches

This program has proven to me that diet does matter...a lot! I have lost this weight without exercise. I never thought I could learn to eat differently, lose weight, and actually enjoy the food I'm eating.

—Deborah W., 52, Tewksberry, MA
Weight loss: 21 pounds. Decrease in waist: 4 inches

I have followed the program heart and soul. I have *never ever* been able to do that on a weight loss or health program before. I physically was not able to. I would cave and binge or would slowly trickle foods in and then feel bad and give up altogether. Life offers so many tasty ways to satisfy yourself—if you are not educated on what your body needs and limits are, you are eating blind!

—Dominique R., 40, St. Paul, MN
Weight loss: 28 pounds. Decrease in waist: 6.5 inches

Food no longer controls every waking moment of my life. Before doing the program, I was always thinking about the next meal or snack. I never felt full or satisfied. But now, I often have to remind myself that it is time to eat again. I feel so good, so much better than I have felt in a very long time. I cannot remember the last time I looked so good—my face is defined, I have a neck again, and now I have shoulders that do not look like they belong to a football player! I look in the mirror and like what I see now.

—Angelica G., 50, Sacramento, CA
Weight loss: 11.5 pounds. Decrease in waist: 3 inches

I'm very impressed with my results. The recipes taste excellent—and this is from someone who never cooks.

—Mary L., 51, Quincy, MA
Weight loss: 18 pounds. Decrease in waist: 2 inches

I am wearing jeans that I have not been able to zip or button for more than two years! The difference is the 4 inches I lost from my middle! *Never* again will I eat that processed food! I am so motivated!

—Joyce D., 70, Roswell, GA
Weight loss: 8 pounds. Decrease in waist: 4.5 inches

I chose this program because I was tired of not being able to keep up with my active lifestyle—I felt fatigued before my day started and lacked the motivation to do activities after work. Because I had such a busy schedule, I often binge ate, which would leave me feeling bloated and tired. After beginning the program, I immediately began to feel increases in energy along with restful sleep. For me, the most rewarding part of the program is being able to wake up refreshed and having the energy to conquer an eighteen-hour day. I've also learned to make healthy choices and listen to my body— why didn't I do this sooner?!

—*Amanda N., 28, Pepperell, MA*
Weight loss: 8 pounds. Decrease in waist: 5 inches

This program to me is about getting healthy. Losing weight will be a happy side effect. You can do fad diets where you lose 24 pounds in 24 days but then jump right back into old eating habits. Or you could lose a few pounds a month for a year and maintain that weight for the rest of your life while still enjoying eating.

—*Matthew F., 36, Roslindale, MA*
Weight loss: 31 pounds. Decrease in waist: 5.5 inches

Initially, giving up sweets was hard. But the program was perfect for me because you just ate what you like, but in smarter ways. Then, when I would eat pizza, soda, or popcorn, I would feel really gross. The program helped me obtain a much healthier and smarter relationship with food. I feel more mentally clear and just happier. I would recommend this program to anybody.

—*Kristin Z., 24, Dorchester, MA*
Weight loss: 20 pounds. Decrease in waist: n/a

Last winter was one of the most difficult I have ever experienced. I could have easily gained lots of weight from lack of exercise, carb cravings due to the cold and from being more housebound than usual. But the program has been a godsend and the easiest I have followed!

—*Katherine L., 56, Stoneham, MA*
Weight loss: 7 pounds. Decrease in waist: 2 inches

There have been many changes, and I love them! My weight is down. My waist size is down. My energy is up. My attitude is up. And what's really awesome about it all is that I believe that I can sustain this lifestyle. The food I have learned to prepare is delicious. I feel very sated after eating. And I am beginning to not feel deprived. This plan is really working for me (and my wife too!). I don't want this just to be a diet that ends when I reach my ideal weight. I am more healthy than ever and I don't want to revert to my old self. I am gaining confidence every week.

—Dan B., 45, Lehi, UT
Weight loss: 15 pounds. Decrease in waist: 1 inch

I have increased energy throughout the day, especially in the late afternoon when I would usually feel sluggish and need coffee. The recipes are easy to follow and I had a really good time learning to cook all of those tasty meals. And I've continued losing weight after the 16-week pilot ended!

—Benjamin P., 26, Natick, MA
Weight loss: 14 pounds. Decrease in waist: 2 inches

The biggest change has been my ability to make choices around food. I no longer feel victimized by food, or deprived. I look forward to ripe berries in the same way I used to think about cookies. The ability to choose food has given me freedom and has empowered me in other ways. Last year at this time, I had no hope that my body could change. But if I can do this, I can do anything.

—Kim S., 47, South Jordan, UT
Weight loss: 25 pounds. Decrease in waist: 3.5 inches

Because I no longer have the "craving crazies" drowning out thoughts and physical sensations, I am able to calmly notice what's going on with my mind and body. I know what feeling good feels like (mentally and physically), and it has less to do with a number on the scale than I expected it to. I feel hopeful—that's *huge*.

—Nancy F., 64, Eden Prairie, MN
Weight loss: 14.5 pounds. Decrease in waist: 7 inches

After years of hating my body—and thinking, "Oh, I don't look that bad," until I see myself in pictures—a guilt-free eating plan seemed awesome. As time goes on, it seems to be easier to say no to some of the foods I would overeat in the past. I have to admit, it does feel good to be able to say no and not feel deprived.

—*Ruth S., 65, Stillwater, MN*
Weight loss: 15 pounds. Decrease in waist: 2.5 inches

I actually have found this program to be life altering, quite frankly. I went into it with a goal of weight loss, but I came out with so much more in terms of the benefits. Not only for my own health and well-being, but for my family as well.

—*Lauren S., 52, North Andover, MA*
Weight loss: 28 pounds. Decrease in waist: 4.5 inches

I often experience a rut when it comes to food selections for meal preparations. When in those ruts, it is easy to turn to fast and unhealthy options, such as processed foods and fast foods. The recipes renewed my love of cooking. A big surprise was how much my children, ages eight and ten, enjoyed the recipes. I assumed they would turn up their noses at these new foods, but instead their palates were expanded. Another encouraging part of this process was the knowledge that if I were to derail from the program, all was not lost and I could get back on track to becoming a healthier version of myself.

—*Esther K., 38, Flower Mound, TX*
Weight loss: 11 pounds. Decrease in waist: 3.5 inches

It's like night and day! I used to be on antidepressants due to acute body aches, mild depression, and foggy head, and all of that has disappeared like magic! My tiredness and fibromyalgia have disappeared, and every day I wake up with a beaming smile on my face. My husband is shocked to see me not reaching out for Tylenol for my frequent headaches. What is this? I call it a miracle.

—*Jyoti A., 59, Muskogee, OK*
Weight loss: 7 pounds. Decrease in waist: 4 inches

This program really helped me understand the connection between my cravings and my blood sugar levels. My cravings seemed to disappear and I very rarely felt hungry—which has been a challenge for me in the past, especially with how active I am with CrossFit and triathlon. I learned a lot more about how to eat to live rather than the other way around. I sleep and train better now than I ever have. The recipes were shockingly delicious!

—*Amanda B., 35, Roslindale, MA*
Weight loss: 8 pounds. Decrease in waist: 2.5 inches

ALWAYS HUNGRY?

ALWAYS HUNGRY?

Conquer Cravings, Retrain Your Fat Cells,
and Lose Weight Permanently

DAVID LUDWIG, MD, PHD

This edition first published in Great Britain in 2016 by
Orion
an imprint of the Orion Publishing Group Ltd
Carmelite House, 50 Victoria Embankment,
London, EC4Y 0DZ
An Hachette UK Company

1 3 5 7 9 10 8 6 4 2

A CIP catalogue record for this book is available
from the British Library.

Hardback ISBN: 978 1 4091 5883 7
Trade Paperback ISBN: 978 1 4091 5884 4

Printed and bound by CPI Group (UK) Ltd, Croydon, CR0 4 YY

The Orion Publishing Group's policy is to use papers that are natural,
renewable and recyclable and made from wood grown in sustainable forests.
The logging and manufacturing processes are expected to conform to
the environmental regulations of the country of origin.

*Every effort has been made to ensure that the information in this book is accurate.
The information will be relevant to the majority of people but may not be applicable
in each individual case, so it is advised that professional medical advice is obtained for
specific health matters. Neither the publisher nor author accept any legal responsibility
for any personal injury or other damage or loss arising from the use or misuse
of the information in this book. Anyone making a change in their diet should
consult their GP, especially if pregnant, infirm, elderly or under 16.*

www.orionbooks.co.uk

To Benji, Joy, Dawn, and "Grandma Bettie"
—with whom I have shared many wonderful meals.

Note to Readers

All personal stories in this book are real and represent the authentic experience of pilot program participants. Each of these participants provided permission to include his or her actual first name, last initial, age, and location. Stories have been edited for grammar and brevity.

Contents

Prologue

A New Way to Think
About Weight Loss

Most weight loss programs require you to cut back calories. This one won't.

Many expect you to endure hunger. This one doesn't.

Some require grueling workouts. Not this one.

That's because the program in this book, the Always Hungry Solution, uses a radically different method of weight control, based on decades of groundbreaking, but little-known, research.

Conventional diets aim to shrink body fat by restricting calorie intake. But this approach is doomed to fail in the real world, because it targets the symptoms, not the root cause of the problem. After a few weeks of calorie restriction, the body fights back, and makes us feel hungry, tired, and deprived. Though we may be able to ignore these unpleasant feelings for a short while, they inevitably erode our motivation and willpower. Sooner or later, we succumb to temptation and the weight comes racing back—often leaving us heavier than before we started the diet.

The Always Hungry Solution turns dieting on its head, by ignoring calories and targeting fat tissue directly. Using the right types and combinations of foods (and other supportive techniques related to stress reduction, sleep, and enjoyable physical activities), this approach reprograms fat cells to release their stored calories. When this happens, the pent-up calories flood back into the body, shifting metabolism into weight loss mode. You'll experience a surge in energy levels and dramatically increased satiety—that pleasant sense of fullness after eating. You'll feel good, and begin to lose weight without hunger or cravings.

In our sixteen-week pilot program with 237 participants, some people like Donna A., Dominique R., and Matthew F. lost weight rapidly, right from the start (see pages v-vii). For others, weight loss was slower, but was accompanied by important health benefits like decreased waist size and reduced heart disease risk factors. In addition, participants consistently reported most or all of the following: reduced hunger, fewer cravings, long-lasting satiety after eating, increased enjoyment of food, better energy, and enhanced overall well-being. These positive experiences—the opposite of what typically occurs on a calorie-restricted diet—bode well for long-term success and an end to yo-yo dieting.

For sensational weight loss, starve yourself. But for sustainable weight loss, feed your fat cells well!

The Always Hungry Solution features savory proteins (with options for both meat-eaters and vegetarians), luscious sauces and spreads, filling nuts and nut butters, and a range of natural carbohydrates. This way of eating is so rich and satisfying that there will be little room left for the highly processed carbohydrates that have crept into our diets during the low-fat craze of the last few decades. You may notice that some of the recipes have a "retro," feel, harking back to those hearty meals of the 1950s, but each has been updated with modern flavors and fine-tuned to reflect the latest scientific insights. Getting the science exactly right lets us achieve maximum weight loss and overall health benefits with minimum effort. It's *diet without deprivation*.

This is not a typical low-carbohydrate diet. In Phase 1: Conquer Cravings, you'll give up—for just two weeks—starches and added sugars. But in Phase 2: Retrain Your Fat Cells, you'll add back moderate amounts of whole-kernel grains, starchy vegetables (except white potato), and a touch of sweetener. Then, in Phase 3: Lose Weight Permanently, you can mindfully reintroduce bread, potato products, and some other processed carbohydrates, depending on your body's ability to handle them—creating a customized diet that's right for you.

For anyone ready to get started right away, all of the key concepts are in Chapter 1: The Big Picture. Read it, then feel free to skip right to Part 2: The Always Hungry Solution. For others, chapters 2 through 4 provide a more in-depth exploration of the problem with conventional diets and the new science of weight loss without hunger. The program in part 2 has everything you'll need to put this plan into action, including recipes, meal plans, tracking tools, shopping lists, food preparation guides, and more. Finally, the epilogue offers ideas to make society a healthier place for all of us to live.

I hope you enjoy the many delicious and nutritious recipes in these pages. I'm confident that *Always Hungry?* will help you achieve lasting weight loss, experience increased vitality, and enjoy a healthy life.

And please write to me at drludwig@alwayshungrybook.com about your experiences.

David S. Ludwig, MD, PhD
Brookline, Massachusetts
June 2015

Part One

ALWAYS HUNGRY, NEVER LOSING WEIGHT

In 1905, during his term as secretary of war, William Taft weighed 314 pounds. On his doctor's advice, Taft began a low-calorie/low-fat diet and exercise program bearing striking similarity to standard weight loss treatment today. Soon, he reported feeling "continuously hungry." At his presidential inauguration three years later, Taft weighed 354 pounds.[1]

CHAPTER 1

The Big Picture

I completed my medical training in the 1990s, as the obesity epidemic approached crisis proportions. Incredibly, two out of three American adults had become excessively heavy. For the first time in medical history, type 2 diabetes (previously termed "adult onset diabetes") had begun striking children as young as ten years old. And economic forecasts predicted that the annual medical costs of obesity would soon exceed $100 billion. Amid these disturbing developments, I decided to specialize in obesity prevention and treatment.

Like many young doctors, I had received virtually no instruction in nutrition. Then, as now, medical schools focused almost exclusively on drugs and surgery, even though lifestyle causes most cases of heart disease and other chronic disabling conditions. In retrospect, my lack of formal knowledge of nutrition was a blessing in disguise.

The 1990s were the height of the low-fat diet craze, exemplified by the original Food Guide Pyramid, published in 1992 (see figure on page 4). Based on the notion that all calories are alike, the pyramid advised us to avoid all types of fat because they contain twice the calories of other major nutrients. Instead, we were told to load up on carbohydrates, including six to eleven servings each day of bread, cereal, crackers, pasta, and other grain products. Luckily, I hadn't been indoctrinated in these conventional teachings and began my career in research and patient care with an open (and mostly empty) mind when it came to nutrition.

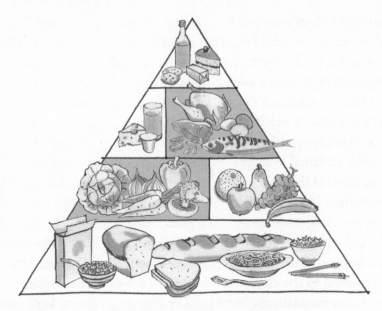

The Food Guide Pyramid of 1992

My first professional research position was in a basic science laboratory conducting experiments with mice. Soon after starting this work, I became amazed by the beauty and complexity of the systems that control body weight. If we fasted a mouse for a few days, it would, of course, lose weight. Then, when given free access to food, the animal ate voraciously until it had regained all of the lost weight—no more, no less. The opposite was also true. Force-feeding could temporarily make a mouse fat, but afterward it would avoid food until its weight dropped back to normal. Based on these and other experiments, it seemed as if an animal's body knew precisely what weight it wanted to be, automatically altering food intake and metabolism to reach a sort of internal set point, like a thermostat that keeps a room at just the right temperature.

Our most interesting scientific experiments explored how this "body weight set point" could be manipulated. If we modified certain genes, administered drugs, or altered diet in particular ways, the mice predictably gained weight to a new stable level. Other changes caused permanent weight loss, without apparent signs of distress. These experiments demonstrated a fundamental principle of the body's weight-control systems: Impose a change in *behavior* (for example, by restricting food), and biology fights back (with increased hunger). Change *biology*, however, and behavior adapts naturally—suggesting a more effective approach to long-term weight management.

In the midst of my stint in basic research, I helped develop my hospital's newly established family-based weight management clinic, called the Optimal Weight for Life (OWL) program. Like virtually all specialists at the time (and many to this day), our team of doctors and dietitians focused at first on calorie balance, instructing patients to "eat less and move more." We prescribed a low-calorie/low-fat diet, regular physical activity, and behavioral methods to help people ignore hunger, resist cravings, and stick with the program. When they returned to the clinic, my patients usually claimed to have followed recommendations. But with few exceptions, they kept gaining weight—a depressing experience for everyone involved. Was it the patients' fault for not being honest with me (and perhaps themselves) about how much they ate and how little they exercised? Or was it my fault for lacking the skills to motivate patients to change? I felt ashamed of judging my patients negatively and felt like a failure as a physician. I dreaded going to the clinic, and I'm sure some of my patients felt the same way. I suspect many doctors and patients at weight loss clinics throughout the country can relate.

After about a year of this schizophrenic existence—fascinated with biology in the lab, frustrated with behavior change among my patients in the clinic—I began to wonder about the disconnect. Why did basic scientists think one way about obesity and practicing clinicians another? Why did we disregard decades of research into the biological determinants of body weight when treating patients? And why were we using an approach to weight loss based on a "calories in, calories out" model that hadn't changed since the late 1800s, when bloodletting was still in vogue?

So I launched into an intensive examination of the literature, from popular diet book authors like Barry Sears (*The Zone Diet*) and Robert Atkins (*Dr. Atkins' New Diet Revolution*) to George Cahill,

Jean Mayer, and other preeminent nutrition scientists of the last century. I spent hundreds of hours poring over musty volumes in Harvard's medical library, rediscovering provocative but neglected theories about diet and body weight. And I began to realize just how little evidence there was to support standard obesity treatment.

Soon, my entire perspective shifted. I came to see food as so much more than a delivery system for calories and nutrients. Although a bottle of cola and a handful of nuts may have the same calories, they certainly don't have the same effects on metabolism. After every meal, hormones, chemical reactions, and even the activity of genes throughout the body change in radically different ways, all according to what we eat. These biological effects of food, quite apart from calorie content, could make all the difference between feeling persistently hungry or satisfied, between having low or robust energy, between weight gain or loss, and between a lifetime of chronic disease or one of good health. Instead of calorie counting, I began to think of diet in an entirely different way—*according to how food affects our bodies and, ultimately, our fat cells.*

MY PERSONAL TESTIMONIAL

At that time, I was in my thirties and, like so many Americans, had gained an extra pound or two each year since high school. For most of my life, I was fit and lean, and ate reasonably well, at least according to conventional standards: not too much fat, lots of whole-grain products, several servings a day of vegetables and fruits, and relatively little sugar. But after several years of steady weight gain, I had approached the threshold for becoming overweight, a body mass index (BMI) of 25.*

For my first clinical research study, I experimented on myself, guided by my rapidly evolving understanding of nutrition. I doubled

---

* BMI measures weight relative to height. For adults, a normal BMI is 18.5 to 24.9; overweight is 25 to 29.9; and obesity is 30 or greater. BMI is calculated as weight (in kilograms) divided by the square of height (in meters). See always hungrybook.com for a BMI calculator.

my intake of fat, with generous servings of nuts and nut butters, full-fat dairy products, avocado, and dark chocolate, and ate vegetables drenched in olive oil. I increased protein just a bit and cut back on my starchy staples, including bread, cereal, pasta, and pastries. I made a few other changes, none especially difficult, but no attempt to reduce calories, eliminate all carbohydrates, or deprive myself in any way.

Within a week, I felt an astonishing improvement in energy and vitality, and a robust sense of well-being that lasted throughout the day—as if some previously unknown but important metabolic switch had finally been flipped on. Four months later, I had lost 20 pounds and needed a new wardrobe two pants sizes smaller. Most remarkably, all this had occurred with no hunger and no carbohydrate cravings. Previously, I would be famished by late afternoon, and usually staved off hunger in the lab with a four p.m. break for a carb-laden vanilla scone from the local bakery. But with my new diet, I felt full for hours after eating. For the first time in my life, I completely lost interest in bread, which used to accompany my every breakfast, lunch, and dinner. And when it was time for a meal, I'd experience a pleasant, stimulating interest in food, entirely different from feeling starved and in desperate need of calories.

The successful outcome of this self-experiment, coupled with new insights into nutrition, renewed my enthusiasm for patient care, with the exciting prospect of something that might actually work in the clinic. Over the next few years, I transitioned out of the animal laboratory and into clinical research. I made it my mission to explore alternative diets under scientifically controlled conditions and have continued that line of research to this day.

FORGET CALORIES

Virtually all weight loss recommendations from the U.S. government and professional nutritional organizations rest on the notion that "a calorie is a calorie"[1]—a strategy with appealing simplicity.

"Just eat less and move more," they say. "Consume fewer calories than you burn off, and you'll lose weight." There's just one problem: This advice doesn't work—not for most people over the long term. Obesity rates remain at historic highs, despite an incessant focus on calorie balance by the government, professional health associations, and the food industry (witness the "100 calorie pack"). Furthermore, the customary method to reduce calorie consumption since the 1970s—a low-fat diet—has failed miserably.

Although the focus on calorie balance rarely produces weight loss, it regularly causes suffering. If all calories are alike, then there are no "bad foods," and the onus is on us to exert self-control. This view blames people with excess weight (who are presumed to lack knowledge, discipline, or willpower)—absolving the food industry of responsibility for aggressively marketing junk food and the government for ineffective dietary guidance.

All too often, people hear the message, "It's your fault that you're fat"—as if they could simply will away the extra weight. In a sense, being heavy has become prime evidence of a weakness of character, provoking prejudice and stigmatization. Overweight children commonly experience teasing, abuse, and bullying from peers, sometimes with tragic consequences.[2] Adults face endless indignities, from workplace discrimination to insensitive characterizations on television. Not surprisingly, high BMI is sometimes accompanied by major psychological distress, including anxiety, depression, and social isolation.[3]

The "calorie is a calorie" concept also has prompted development of some patently bizarre products, such as "low-fat" candy, cookies, and salad dressings, typically containing more sugar than the original full-fat versions. Are we really to believe that, for someone on a diet, a cup of cola with 100 calories would make a better snack than a 1-ounce serving of nuts containing almost 200 calories?

New research has revealed the flaws in this way of thinking. Recent studies show that highly processed carbohydrates adversely affect metabolism and body weight in ways that can't be explained by their calorie content alone. Conversely, nuts, olive oil, and dark chocolate—some of the most calorie-dense foods in existence—appear to prevent obesity, diabetes, and heart disease. In truth, the obesity epidemic is not about willpower or weakness of character. All this time, we've been diligently following the diet rules, but the rulebook was wrong!

In a recent study published in the *Journal of the American Medical Association* (*JAMA*),[4] my colleagues and I examined twenty-one young adults with high BMI after they had lost 10 to 15 percent of their weight on diets ranging from low fat to low carbohydrate. Despite consuming the same total calories on each diet, the participants burned about 325 calories a day more on the low-carbohydrate diet than on the low-fat diet, amounting to the energy expended in an hour of moderately vigorous physical activity. So the *type* of calories we eat can affect the *number* of calories we burn.

Over the last few years, we seem to have been moving toward the tipping point, with reputable scientists acknowledging the previously unthinkable possibility that all calories aren't alike. Even Weight Watchers, for decades the leading advocate of calorie counting, now assigns "0 Points" to fruit.[5] Meaning that if you had the fortitude, you could eat a 10-pound watermelon containing most of your daily calorie requirement "for free"—in flagrant defiance of the calorie-counting approach to weight loss. The entire concept of calorie balance seems to be tottering!

It's time for a new approach, but which way do we turn?

FOCUS ON THE FAT CELL

Just as food is much more than the calories and nutrients necessary for survival, so are fat cells much more than passive storage sites for excess calories. Fat cells take in or release calories only when instructed to do so by external signals—and the master control is insulin. Too much insulin causes weight gain, whereas too little causes weight loss. So if we think about obesity as a disorder involving fat cells, then a radically different view emerges:

Overeating doesn't make us fat. The process of becoming fat makes us overeat.

In other words, hunger and overeating are the consequences of an underlying problem.[6] Though this proposition sounds radical, consider what happens in pregnancy. The fetus doesn't grow because the mother eats more; she eats more because the fetus is growing. With pregnancy, this is normal and healthy. With obesity, it's not.

How and why does this happen? For many people, something has triggered fat cells to suck up and store too many calories from the blood. Consequently, fewer calories are available to fuel the energy needs of the body. Perceiving a problem, the brain unleashes the starvation response, including measures to increase calorie intake (hunger) and save energy (slower metabolism). Eating more solves this "energy crisis" but also accelerates weight gain. Cutting calories reverses the weight gain temporarily, but inevitably increases hunger and slows metabolism even more.

One obvious source of the problem is highly processed carbohydrates—the bread, breakfast cereals, crackers, chips, cakes, cookies, candy, and sugary drinks that flooded our diets during the low-fat era. Anything containing primarily refined grains, potato products, or concentrated sugar digests rapidly, raising insulin levels excessively and programming fat cells to hoard calories. But refined carbohydrates aren't the only problem. Other aspects of our highly processed diet and elements of our modern lifestyle—including stress, sleep deprivation, and sedentary habits—have forced fat cells into calorie-storage overdrive.

Fortunately, these negative effects are reversible.

TAKE BACK CONTROL

The conventional calorie balance approach fails because it's focused on the wrong target. The fundamental problem isn't having too many calories in the body; it's having too few in the right place, circulating in the bloodstream and available for our immediate needs. Highly processed carbohydrates overstimulate fat cells, driving them into a frenzy. They become greedy and consume more than their fair share of calories. While fat cells feast, the rest of the body starves. Like unruly children with indulgent parents, these cells run the show and wreak havoc on our metabolism. Under these conditions, we become quite powerless.

Sure, we can cut back our calories for a while. But further limiting the calories available to the body actually makes matters worse. Before long, our bodies rebel against enforced deprivation. It's not a matter of willpower so much as biology and time. Eventually, we succumb and overeat, typically on all the wrong foods, fueling a vicious cycle of weight gain.

The conventional approach, the calorie-restricted diet, aims to force calories out of the fat cells so that we lose weight—but in that battle fat has the upper hand. Before those cells will shrink, the body must suffer. Our mind may say "eat less," but our metabolism responds "NO!"—a battle that the mind rarely wins.

The solution is to make a truce with our fat cells, help them calm down, and convince them to cooperate with the rest of the body. The way to do this is by changing *what* we eat, not how much. Here's the basic strategy:

1. Turn off the starvation response by eating whenever you're hungry and until fully satisfied.
2. Tame your fat cells with a diet that lowers insulin levels, reduces inflammation (insulin's troublemaker twin), and redirects calories to the rest of your body.
3. Follow a simple lifestyle prescription focused on enjoyable physical activities, sleep, and stress relief to improve metabolism and support permanent behavior change.

Think of this plan as obedience training for your fat cells. I'll show you how to do it, step by step, in part 2.

GAIN WHILE LOSING

Many people associate the word "diet" with suffering, and for good reason. Most diets demand great sacrifice in the present (food deprivation, hunger) in exchange for the promise of an abstract benefit at some seemingly distant point in the future (being thin, avoiding diabetes). That's a recipe for failure. We may begin a diet with the best of intentions, but soon succumb to cravings if our sacrifice isn't rewarded. It's human nature.

The Always Hungry Solution in part 2 aims to put the science of metabolism on your side and by doing so, provide maximum benefit with minimum effort. When what we eat supports our body's metabolism, the benefits begin right away, even before the first pound is shed—less hunger, fewer cravings, longer-lasting satisfaction from food, improved energy, and more stable mood. It's like finally shifting your bicycle into the right gear. Suddenly, you move much faster and with less exertion. This way, enjoyment of life increases even as weight loss proceeds.

You might be wondering how anyone could enjoy a weight loss diet. Isn't the problem that we've given in to pleasure too often and can't resist tasty food? Why would we overeat if it weren't so enjoyable?

Of course, we do all sorts of things for a bit of pleasure now, at the cost of long-term suffering later. That's the nature of addiction. For many people, eating involves constant swings from unpleasantly hungry to uncomfortably full. On this roller-coaster ride, highly processed food may provide a few minutes of enjoyment, but it quickly sets us up for the next downward swing, with negative effects on our physical and mental well-being. Fortunately, unlike many classic addictions, we can quickly free ourselves from this vicious cycle and increase overall enjoyment, even as we lose weight. When we fill up on luscious, satisfying foods, there's little room left for the other stuff.

SENSATIONAL VERSUS SUSTAINABLE WEIGHT LOSS

All too often, popular diets today promise extreme weight loss. Most never live up to expectation. But even if they did, what's the benefit of losing 14 pounds in ten days, if you're starving, fatigued, and struggling to keep the weight off? These diets can also take a big psychological toll. Many of us are, in a sense, estranged from our bodies and have learned to disregard critically important feedback signals that provide information about our internal state. Calorie-restricted diets require you to ignore one such signal—hunger—providing an endless array of behavioral tricks to do so. Drink lots of water, call a friend, go for a walk—anything to take your mind off your hunger. Or serve meals on a small plate, so that you'll believe you've eaten more than you have. The problem is, this strategy makes the body-mind disconnect worse.

In reality, we've outsourced control of our bodies to the "experts." But no diet book author could possibly know what level of calorie intake is right for everyone. People's needs vary based on age, size, physical activity level, and individual metabolic differences. And some people, perhaps for genetic reasons, simply can't tolerate rapid weight loss.

The Always Hungry Solution is designed to work from the inside out, creating the internal conditions for weight loss to occur naturally. Follow the meal plan, eat when hungry, and stop when satisfied but before becoming uncomfortably full. This way, your body will find the rate of weight loss right for you—2 pounds a week or more for some people, perhaps just half a pound a week for others. But without deprivation or hunger, these results will be progressive and sustainable.

My team and I conducted a 16-week pilot test of the Always Hungry Solution with 237 women and men, including 137 employees of Boston Children's Hospital and 100 people who responded to a call for participants that appeared in a national health magazine. In addition to weight loss, participants consistently reported other benefits that predict long-term success, including:

- Decreased hunger
- Longer-lasting satiety after eating
- Great satisfaction with food

- Increased energy level
- More stable mood
- Improved overall well-being
- Reduced weight-related complications

You'll read about the experiences of these participants throughout the book and especially in part 2.

WINDING UP, GETTING STARTED

In full disclosure, this diet—like all other diets—hasn't been fully proven. The pilot project didn't include a control group and wasn't intended as scientific research. We can't be sure how these outcomes would apply to the general public. But the ideas presented in this book culminate a century of research questioning the calorie balance model of obesity, and represent a fundamentally different way to understand why we gain weight and what we can do about it.[7] For those of you with a scientific bent, I've included hundreds of supporting studies from many research teams among the references.

The central concept of *Always Hungry?* is that while cutting calories will decrease weight for a short while, the body resists by increasing hunger and slowing metabolism. Sooner or later we succumb, and weight tends to pop back up, like an air-filled balloon being pushed into a bucket of water. In contrast, improving the *quality* of what we eat will reprogram fat cells to store fewer calories, in effect reducing the "body weight set point." As a result, weight lowers naturally, as the balloon would if some water were drained from the bucket in which it floats.

I base this book on my twenty years of experience as a physician and researcher at Harvard Medical School. During that time, I have overseen dozens of diet studies, authored more than one hundred peer-reviewed scientific articles, and cared for thousands of patients struggling with their weight. I am convinced of the power of this approach and believe it will help you lose weight, feel better, avoid type 2 diabetes and other chronic diseases, and improve the overall quality of your life—without the struggle so common to conventional diets.

The stories you'll read about people following this program are real, and represent their authentic experience. Pilot participants provided their stories freely and received no financial compensation.

Now I invite you to forget calories, focus on the quality of your food, and judge for yourself if this program works for you.

My Always Hungry Story

I recently met my birthmother and full and half siblings. I guess I shouldn't have been surprised they were all overweight—one half-brother, only thirty-eight years old, was 600 pounds! I've always had to work extra hard to lose weight, but now I know why.

I've tried many diets in the past and was hungry all the time, looking for my next thing to eat. But the full-fat foods on this program sounded scary! For twenty years, we've heard, "You must eat low-fat this, low-fat that." I thought I'd balloon up another twenty pounds in the first ten days. Then, when everything tasted good and was satisfying, I wasn't starving between meals, and I was still losing weight—*that* was shocking to me. Went against everything that I had been taught about weight loss, and I'm a nurse practitioner.

After you get used to not having all the processed carbs, things like berries taste *so* sweet. I love fruit now. I ate a cookie, and it was too sweet, didn't even taste good. And I'm glad this isn't one of those stressful, cookie-cutter type programs that everybody does exactly the same way.

My face and body shape changed really quickly. I feel more mentally clear and energetic. Being lighter helps, but I've lost weight in the past and haven't felt this much energy. I feel so much better. I'm kinder to myself, definitely more relaxed. I feel like I've been given a gift. This is my "plan for life."

—Lisa K., 52, Dedham, MA
Weight loss: 19 pounds. Decrease in waist: 6 inches

CHAPTER 2

The Problem

To lose weight, simply eat less and move more.
In the textbooks, it's: calories in – calories out = calories
stored.

For more than a century, experts have embraced this concept with reverential regard.

Every day, millions of Americans meditate on calories, wishing for weight loss.

Sadly, for most of us, lasting weight loss is little more than a prayer.

―――――――

The science of nutrition seems to be stuck in the Dark Ages. While we've made many advances in the last few decades, in practice, very little has changed. We've discovered hormones that dramatically affect body weight. We've developed sophisticated psychological theories about eating behavior. Machines can measure calories entering and leaving the body with precision. Yet we struggle to explain the ongoing obesity epidemic and suffer enormously from diet-related diseases.

Perhaps the problem is our genes, which evolved during times of scarcity.

Or the modern environment, with too many tasty foods.

Or our lack of discipline and willpower.

Out of this uncertainty has emerged a dizzying array of diets: low-fat, low-carbohydrate, high protein, no sugar, gluten-free, paleo…each extolled by its disciples with near religious fervor.

Unfortunately, weak research all too often contributes to the confusion. Unlike modern clinical trials involving drugs, diet studies typically involve just a few dozen, or occasionally a few hundred, participants, who are followed for a year or less. In addition, these studies characteristically rely on ineffective counseling methods, with most participants reporting few lasting changes in diet. Not surprisingly, research like this yields conflicting and discouraging findings. And without any one diet showing consistent success, many experts cling to the concept of calorie balance as ultimate nutritional truth.

"All calories are alike."
"There are no bad foods."
"Just eat less, and move more."

According to the USDA's Choose MyPlate website, "Reaching a healthier weight is a balancing act. The secret is learning how to balance your 'energy in' and 'energy out'…." A secret, indeed![1] In reality, no one, not even nutrition experts, can accurately "practice" calorie balance. Without elaborate technology, it's virtually impossible to estimate to within 350 calories a day how much we eat and burn off. A calorie gap of that magnitude can mean the difference between remaining thin and developing morbid obesity in just a few years.[2] For that matter, if counting calories were key to weight control, how did humans manage to avoid massive swings in body weight before the very concept of the calorie was invented?

My Always Hungry Story

I try and tell myself it is only a number and doesn't change the person I am, but, gosh, it affects me daily. Is the number up? I failed again. Is the number down? OK, I am on my way. Yay! Back up? Shoot! I messed up again. And so the cycle continues. My weight has caused frustration, discouragement, shame, and general fatigue. It has cost me money as I have bought magazines, books, programs that promise me success, but didn't deliver.

—Yvonne N., 63, St. Paul, MN
Weight loss: 12.5 pounds. Decrease in waist: 0.5 inch

THE FORTY-YEAR LOW-FAT FOLLY

It seemed to make sense: If you don't want fat *on* your body, don't put fat *into* your body. Fat has 9 calories per gram (about 120 calories in a tablespoon), compared to just 4 calories per gram for carbohydrates or protein. So, in the 1970s, prominent nutrition experts began recommending that everyone follow a low-fat diet, in the belief that eating less fat would automatically help lower calorie intake and prevent obesity.

Thus began the biggest public health experiment in history. Over the next few decades, the U.S. government spent many millions of dollars in a campaign to convince Americans to cut back on fat, culminating in the creation of the original Food Guide Pyramid (see the figure on page 4). Published in 1992, the Pyramid advised us to eat all types of fat sparingly, and instead load up on grain products—up to eleven servings a day! The food industry joined this campaign with a vengeance, realizing that they could replace the fat in their standard products with cheaper refined carbohydrates, label them as health food, and sell them at a premium price. Since then, food aisles have overflowed with packaged products like fat-free cookies, low-fat salad dressings, reduced-fat peanut butter, and countless other variations. At the same time, high-fat natural foods like nuts, olive oil, avocado, and cheese were given a bad reputation. Today, a typical dairy section might have fifty kinds of low-fat and nonfat yogurt (almost all highly sweetened), but try finding the plain, whole-milk variety. Until recently, sugar was even promoted as a good way to displace fat from the diet,[3] and sugary beverages were touted as fat-free.

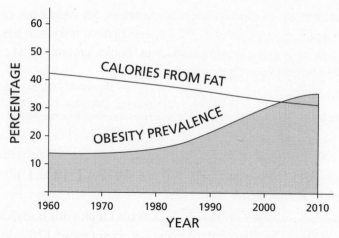

Opposite Trends in Fat Consumption and Obesity Prevalence

Unfortunately, this experiment didn't turn out well. In the 1960s, Americans ate more than 40 percent of calories as fat. Today, fat intake approaches the government-recommended limit of 30 percent, but rates of obesity have skyrocketed, as shown in the figure above. These opposite trends are probably not coincidental.[4]

My Always Hungry Story

I think for most people, the idea is that the less fat you eat, the better. Recently I was in the grocery store and saw there were more calories in the sweetened nonfat yogurt than the plain full-fat one. It's stunning to realize just how much sugar is in there. I think that we don't appreciate the fact that fat has significant benefits to us feeling less hungry for longer.

—Eric F., 42, Needham, MA
Weight loss: 17 pounds. Decrease in waist: 3 inches

With enthusiasm for the low-fat diet reaching a crescendo in the 1990s, the government launched the world's largest clinical diet trial as part of the Women's Health Initiative (WHI).[5] At a total cost of $700 million, the WHI randomly assigned about fifty thousand postmenopausal women throughout the United States to a low-fat diet or a control group for eight years. However, the study had a fundamental flaw, with a clear bias in favor of the low-fat diet built into the design. Women in that group received intensive nutritional and lifestyle support—not only to reduce dietary fat, but also to increase vegetables, fruit, grains, and fiber—including eighteen group counseling sessions and an individual session during the first year alone. Thereafter, they had quarterly maintenance sessions and optional monthly peer group meetings. In striking contrast, women in the control group received only written educational materials. Considering the dramatically different amounts of attention paid to the two groups, you'd expect the low-fat group to fare much better than the control group. And yet, the results show anything but.

According to a well-recognized principle in clinical research known as the Hawthorne effect,[6] people typically change behavior for a short while when they are aware of being observed. In diet studies, participants often lose weight when they receive the attention of investigators, regardless of what nutritional advice is given. Once the intensity of attention decreases and the novelty of the study wears off, the weight is regained.

The main results of the WHI trial were released in 2006, generating a media firestorm. Women in the low-fat group lost a maximum of only 5 pounds compared to the control group, and this small difference decreased to 1 pound by the end of the study.[7] Furthermore, there was no reduction in rates of cancer, diabetes, or heart disease.[8] From any perspective, this was a resounding failure for the low-fat diet.

Many smaller but better-designed studies, in which all participants received similar intensity of treatment, have since been conducted. This way, the effects of different diets can be compared directly, in a fair and meaningful way. Several systematic reviews of such studies (called meta-analysis) have been published, and the results are sobering. Low-fat diets produced less weight loss than higher-fat diets, including Mediterranean and low carbohydrate[9]— raising the possibility that the most widely recommended method for four decades to reduce calorie intake has done more harm than good.

My Always Hungry Story

I think it will take some time to get my head around the concept of a higher-fat diet. Too long I've been told that to lose weight I need to cut the fat out of my diet. But it never worked for me, at least not for the long term. I have a little bit of disbelief that eating fats will help me lose fat. I think for a while I am going to feel guilty for eating foods that I so long have thought of as bad for weight loss.

—*Donna A., 51, Selah, WA*
Weight loss: 22 pounds. Decrease in waist: 5 inches

TOO LITTLE PHYSICAL ACTIVITY?

Perhaps the problem isn't consuming too many calories, but rather not burning off enough of them. A century ago, most people obtained regular physical activity at work, while traveling, and in recreation. Today, many of us have sedentary jobs, use cars for transportation, and spend much of our spare time in front of screens. Is exercise the answer?

Hundreds of studies have asked this question, employing almost every imaginable approach to increase physical activity: aerobic training, resistance training, or aerobic plus resistance training; based at school or at work; high or low intensity; in little bouts throughout the day or during specially dedicated times; and accompanied by various types of diets. These studies involved thousands of participants, from children to the elderly, and taken together, they paint a clear picture. Some people lose a few pounds, others gain a few pounds, but most experience no meaningful weight change at all.[10]

Why doesn't exercise produce much weight loss? A simple explanation is that physical activity makes us hungrier, so we "compensate" by eating more.[11] For instance, a brisk walk before dinner stimulates appetite and enhances the enjoyment of eating. And (unfortunately for dieters) calories enter the body more easily than they leave. A jogger might burn off 200 calories in 30 minutes and then replace them with a sports drink a minute later.

My Always Hungry Story

I've always tried to lose weight with exercise. But I'd tell myself, "I ran four miles this morning, so I can have this or this." Then all the work I was doing with running got swallowed up by me eating poorly.
—Eric D., 44, Catonsville, MD
Weight loss: 21 pounds. Decrease in waist: 3 inches

We may also compensate by being less active at other times.[12] In a cleverly designed study,[13] thirty-seven adolescents with obesity engaged in varying levels of exercise—high intensity, low intensity, or rest—on three different mornings. As expected, the teens burned off more calories during exercise than at rest. But calorie expenditure plummeted in the afternoon following the high-intensity exercise. As a result, total calories burned throughout the day remained the same, regardless of how vigorously the teens exercised. The more active we are at one time, the less active we may later be.

What about prevention? Observational studies show that lean people tend to be more active than their heavier counterparts. If physical activity doesn't produce much weight loss, wouldn't a diligent daily exercise routine at least help avoid weight gain in the first place? Here again, the answer may be surprising. Two recent studies with a combined total of five thousand European children used sophisticated statistical calculations to disentangle cause and effect.[14] Together, they suggest that sedentary habits may not lead to increased body fat in the way we tend to think. Instead, the process of gaining fat may cause people to become less active.

None of this is to endorse a sedentary lifestyle. Physical activity has many benefits (as we'll discuss in part 2). But short of marathon-level intensity, lower body weight isn't usually one of them.

My Always Hungry Story

Last year, I did a program that required me to go to the gym five days a week and reduce my portion size. I lost 10 pounds, but as soon as I cut down on the gym and started eating normally, my body completely did a one-eighty—I ended up regaining about 25 pounds.
—Kristin Z., 24, Dorcester, MA
Weight loss: 20 pounds. Decrease in waist: n/a

GENETIC DESTINY?

Some people can eat whatever they want, whenever they want, and never gain an ounce. Others seem to put on weight just walking past a bakery. If you're in the second category, life may feel a bit unfair.

Of course, many physical characteristics differ widely according to the genes we've inherited from our parents, including weight. Recent research indicates that dozens of genes affect body weight to some degree,[15] most by only a tiny amount. Together, however, they significantly influence how likely you are to gain weight.

Rarely, mutations in certain genes cause massive obesity, typically from early in childhood. One such gene makes leptin, a critical fat cell hormone discovered in the 1990s that tells the brain and other organs when enough body fat has been stored. People without leptin act as if they're in a state of perpetual starvation, with insatiable hunger, no matter how heavy they become. Leptin treatment in this genetic syndrome produces a dramatic transformation. Almost immediately, hunger subsides and metabolism improves, leading to effortless weight loss, sometimes totaling several hundred pounds.[16]

Unfortunately, this is the only example of a miracle drug cure for obesity, and it would only work for the few dozen people worldwide with this genetic form of leptin deficiency. Leptin treatment has minimal effect on other causes of obesity. All other available drugs produce modest weight loss at best, and carry risk of serious side effects. Fortunately, for the vast majority of us, genetic tendency isn't destiny.

In any event, genes can't explain the epidemic of obesity. Since the end of World War II, most people in developed nations have had access to an abundance of food, but obesity prevalence didn't begin rising significantly until the 1970s in the United States, the 1980s in Europe, and the 1990s in Japan. The obesity epidemic developed far too fast to be attributable to genetic changes. Although genes haven't changed rapidly, the environment has.*

TOO MUCH TASTY FOOD?

Some notable public health experts and science writers have eloquently described how the food industry manipulates three basic flavors—sweet, fat, and salt—to make modern processed food irresistible.[17] These exceedingly tasty products, as the argument goes, overstimulate the pleasure circuits in the brain, leading to compulsive eating behaviors. Remember the Lays potato chip slogan, "Bet you can't eat just one"?

As we will later discuss in depth (see chapter 3), highly processed industrial food products are prime suspects in the obesity epidemic. But what's the evidence that too much tasty food is the actual problem? Must we restrict ourselves to bland fare—typical "diet" foods like baked chicken breast and steamed broccoli—to safeguard against overeating? If so, why do countries celebrated for delicious cuisine like France, Italy, and Japan have notably lower obesity rates than the United States and many other countries?

Although we tend not to realize it, tastiness (or palatability, to

---

* There is no simple way to determine what proportion of obesity is genetic compared to environmental in origin. And even if there were, that number would differ among populations and through time. For a society in which most people eat healthy diets, the few cases of obesity that did exist would be mostly related to genes. But for a society in which many eat poorly, the opposite would apply (and the United States is closer to this extreme).

use the technical term) is not an inherent characteristic of food. True, babies are born with an innate preference for sweet rather than bitter, an instinct that programs them to like breast milk and avoid ingesting toxic substances. However, with appropriate exposure, children outgrow this instinct and learn to appreciate an increasingly wide variety of tastes, such as savory, sour, spicy, and bitter. If this normal maturation process didn't occur, humans would have starved to death after weaning generations ago.

Food palatability varies greatly among individuals, between cultures and throughout time. Some people love liver, and others hate it. The same is true for blue cheese, oysters, coconut, Brussels sprouts, ketchup, and cilantro. Many Japanese prize aged fermented soybeans (called *natto*), with its powerful, ammonia-like smell and slimy texture. But some restaurants in Japan refuse to serve this delicacy to Westerners, knowing how they'll react. Some Asians and Africans used to consuming their traditional diets find American fast food repulsive at first.

Beyond infancy, most food is quite literally "an acquired taste," determined primarily by our biological responses. Remember the first time you tried black coffee or stole a sip of beer? They probably tasted awful. But with repeated exposure, the body comes to associate these tastes with the pleasurable effects of caffeine and alcohol. That's why many adults savor a cup of java in the morning and a brew in the evening. For cake, cookies, chips, and other highly processed carbohydrates, the rush of sugar into the body after ingestion provides the biological reward. The effects also work in the opposite direction. If you eat a favorite treat, say, strawberry cheesecake, and soon thereafter get sick from food poisoning, you might develop an intense aversion to similar foods for quite a while.

Perceptions of a food's palatability can change rapidly, based on the internal state of the body. Suppose you've skipped breakfast and lunch to leave room for a big Thanksgiving dinner. How would that first bite of buttery stuffing taste? But after turkey and all the trimmings, a bit too much alcohol, and much too much dessert, how would you feel about more stuffing?

In long-term studies with humans, the effects of palatability, or tastiness, can be difficult to distinguish from other aspects of diet, but animal studies have been informative. Like humans, rodents have a special fondness for sweetness, especially in liquid form. They dislike bitter-tasting foods and ordinarily avoid them. Rats given free access to solutions of sugar or other carbohydrate in water predictably overeat and become overweight. However, they become equally overweight when the carbohydrate solution is spiked with an intensely bitter chemical, evidently overcoming their instinctive aversion to bitterness. The biological responses to food dominate (and largely determine) perceptions of palatability.[18]

Leaving cost aside for the moment, many people would enjoy the taste of dinner at a fine Italian restaurant at least as much as a meal at McDonald's. Yet a Mediterranean eating pattern is consistently associated with lower body weight than a fast-food eating pattern.[19] It's hard to believe that America leads the world in obesity because we have the world's most delicious diet.

My Always Hungry Story

I went to a fast-food restaurant the other day because a friend of mine wanted to eat there. I ended up throwing most of my lunch away. It just did not taste as good as I had remembered. Felt good— no guilt for wasting food, but rather a feeling of relief for not forcing myself to eat my entire meal and not really liking the taste.
—*Carin M., 42, Parker, CO*
Weight loss: 4 pounds. Decrease in waist: 4.5 inches

LACK OF WILLPOWER?

Hippocrates, known as the father of Western medicine, said, "Obese people...should perform hard work...eat only once a day, take no baths, sleep on a hard bed and walk naked as long as possible."[20] The Seven Deadly Sins equate gluttony with anger, avarice, envy, lust, pride, and sloth.

For more than two thousand years, Western society has considered obesity a weakness of character, or at least evidence of poor self-control. Probably for that reason, people are subjected to abuse, discrimination, and stigma because of their weight, even though such prejudice directed at virtually any other physical characteristic or medical condition would be socially unacceptable today.

My Always Hungry Story

My weight affects me in every area of my life. I was embarrassed to spend Thanksgiving with my family because I felt so fat and depressed. I didn't book any speaking events in 2014 because I was uncomfortable with my weight. I see the world through this filter of less-than, that somehow my intelligence and my insights are not well received because I can't even control my weight—so how am I supposed to work with people to help them change their lives? That question haunts me. Feeling conspicuous because I'm fat has stopped me from doing the things that I love. I want to have the energy to shift my focus and get off the couch and get out and enjoy life again without that wicked voice in my head criticizing me for being fat.

—Kim S., 47, South Jordan, UT
Weight loss: 25 pounds. Decrease in waist: 3.5 inches

In one of the only studies to address this issue in a general population, researchers examined whether common stereotypes about people with obesity have any basis in reality. Using a nationally representative survey, the investigators compared body weight with personality traits among 3,176 adults living in the United States. They found negligible or no relationships between weight and measures of conscientiousness, agreeableness, emotional stability, or extraversion. In contrast, demographic factors like age and gender were significantly associated with each of these traits.[21] This and other research shows that a person's size has nothing to do with his or her inner qualities.

In fact, weight loss is difficult for almost everyone, regardless of

My Always Hungry Story

For guys, you're supposed to be just sort of casual and happy no matter what. Whether you're able to eat like Michael Phelps or you're like the late Chris Farley, you're supposed to just be sort of jolly about it. You're not supposed to look like you care. Women can comfortably talk about food; guys are supposed to be sort of covert about it, effortless, and even sort of derisive of the enterprise. Your struggle is supposed to be invisible.

—Jason F., 41, Boston, MA
Weight loss: 11 pounds. Decrease in waist: 5.5 inches

starting weight. Someone 5 feet 10 inches and 170 pounds (within the normal range for body weight) would probably have no less difficulty losing 20 pounds than a person of the same height weighing 100 pounds more.

So, we've looked at the effects of physical activity, genes, tasty food and willpower on body weight. Although each can have some influence, we seem to have missed a critical factor. We've spent decades counting calories, eating fat-free foods, sweating it out at the gym, and testing our willpower, and where has it gotten us? We are a nation of dieters, and the diet isn't working. Most current strategies to battle obesity appear doomed to fail. And this is a very big problem that's about to get worse.

THE APPROACHING TSUNAMI OF OBESITY-RELATED DISEASE

Stories about obesity appear regularly in the media, but what gets lost in all the attention is just how quickly this epidemic has emerged. Fifty years ago, 13 percent of adults in the United States had a BMI in the obese range.[22] Today, that figure is 35 percent. An additional

34 percent are overweight, leaving fewer than one in three adults in the normal weight range.[23] The epidemic has spared no segment of society or region of the country, although people in lower-income communities and belonging to some racial-ethnic groups have suffered most severely.

Recent national surveys report that the year-after-year increases in obesity rates observed since the 1970s may now be reaching a plateau, providing a first glimmer of hope. However, even without further increases in prevalence, the toll of obesity will continue to mount for decades, as successive stages of the epidemic arrive[24] (see the chart below). In Stage 1, obesity rates increased rapidly during the late twentieth century. But it may take years for complications like diabetes or fatty liver to develop in someone with obesity (Stage 2) and many additional years for those complications to cause a life-threatening event like a heart attack, stroke, cirrhosis, or kidney failure (Stage 3).

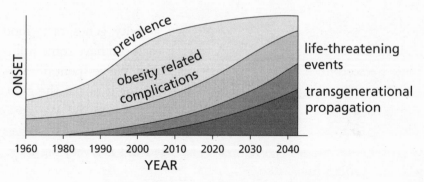

Four Stages of the Obesity Epidemic

Astoundingly, almost one in two American adults now have diabetes or prediabetes[25] and one in three have fatty liver,[26] providing evidence for just how rapidly the epidemic has progressed so far. By middle age, many people take a cocktail of powerful drugs to lower blood pressure, cholesterol, and blood sugar, attempting to stave off heart attack and stroke. As the first generation with epidemic obesity reaches old age, cases of neurodegenerative diseases like Alzheimer's are rising precipitously, placing even greater burdens on families and the health care system.

In Stage 4, the epidemic propagates from one generation to the next at an accelerating rate. Being heavy in childhood leads to obesity later in life for several reasons, as shown in the figure below. And obesity in a woman increases the risk for her children not only because of shared genes and environment, but also because of "fetal programming."

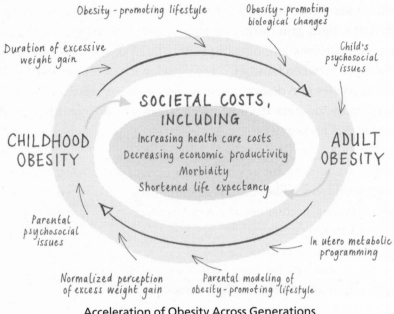

Acceleration of Obesity Across Generations
Adapted from JAMA 2012;307(5):498–508[27] with permission

Excessive weight affects virtually every organ system in the body, and that includes the womb. In a pregnancy complicated by obesity, the fetus may be exposed to an abnormal intrauterine environment—including higher blood glucose, altered hormone levels, and inflammation—at critical stages of development, producing potentially permanent changes in metabolism.

To examine the effects of prenatal exposure, researchers divided female rats from the same strain into two groups: One group was kept lean on a standard diet, the other made obese with a special diet. Then the animals were mated. Offspring of the obese mothers became fatter and had higher blood sugar than those of the lean mothers, even though both groups of offspring had the same genetic makeup and ate the same diet.[28] Such an experiment would be virtually impossible to do in humans for practical and ethical reasons, but carefully controlled observational studies affirm the existence of the same phenomenon in humans.

Working with colleagues at Princeton University and University of Arkansas a few years ago, I looked at the relationship between maternal weight gain during pregnancy and weight of the offspring, using comparisons among siblings to cancel out genetic and other differences between families.[29] For these analyses, we accessed state-based registries in Arkansas, New Jersey, and Pennsylvania providing population-wide data from many thousands of people. Our results were clear: The heavier a mother became in pregnancy, the heavier her offspring were likely to be, both at birth and in mid-childhood, possibly accounting for several hundred thousand annual cases of obesity worldwide. These findings show that excessive weight in one generation may predispose the next for higher lifetime risk of obesity, apart from genetic inheritance and the tendency of offspring to pick up their parents' lifestyle habits.

In short, many factors may conspire to create a vicious intergenerational cycle of obesity that will increase human suffering and have catastrophic consequences to the U.S. economy in the next few decades.

In 2005, my colleagues and I predicted that obesity would shorten life expectancy in the United States for the first time since the Civil War—by an amount equal to the effects of all cancers combined—unless something is done about it.[30] Fortunately, this prediction has not yet come to pass, but worrisome warning signs are already present. Between 1961 and 1983, prior to the brunt of the obesity epidemic, life expectancy increased in a relatively consistent fashion throughout the U.S., and no county had a significant decline. However, between 1983 and 1999, life expectancy decreased significantly in 11 counties for men and 180 counties for women.

Of particular concern, the counties that showed relative or absolute decreases correspond closely with those most severely affected by the obesity epidemic, located predominately in the South and Midwest. These trends have continued through the last decade.[31]

The medical costs for treating obesity-related disease in the United States are estimated at $190 billion per year (in 2005 dollars), or 20.5 percent of total spending on health care, a figure that does not include indirect costs arising from lower worker productivity.[32] By 2020, total annual costs for diabetes is projected to approach $500 billion.[33] Perhaps most frightening of all, a recent Brookings Institution report predicted that if all 12.7 million children in the United States with obesity remain obese as adults, the increased lifetime costs to society may exceed $1.1 trillion ($92,000 per individual).[34] These massive sums could mean the difference between the stability or bankruptcy of Medicare; expanding or contracting health care coverage; and investment in or neglect of the national infrastructure (including schools, the transportation system, the communication network, and research). All this has direct implications for the future international competitiveness of the U.S economy.

Without obesity, Democrats could conceivably have robust social spending, Republicans could have a balanced budget, and the two parties might find a way to cooperate. And that should make people of any political affiliation happy. But with so much money diverted to care for obesity-related diseases and lost to lower productivity, the pool of discretionary funds for everything else has shrunk, arguably contributing to the polarization and paralysis of our national politics.

But this dire scenario needn't continue to unfold. New research points the way to a paradigm shift in how we think about weight gain and its treatment.

My Always Hungry Story

I have seventeen-year-old twins who are going in a million different directions, and I work full-time. Sometimes making something out of a box was the only way we were going to eat dinner. Or so I thought at the time. During the first week of the program, I was faithful with food prep, but I did say to myself, "I don't have time to make salad dressing. How am I going to do this?"

And then my husband landed in the hospital for open-heart surgery. Talk about stress. I almost dropped out five times over the course of that weekend. Sheer stubbornness made me say, "Nope. He's going to get through this, and then you're still not going to have what you want in terms of your own health." He did, and now I'm on my way.

I started at a weight of well over 200 pounds, one of my highest weights ever. Most of the diets I've tried in the past focused on struggle and deprivation: "When can I eat again?" and "How do I deal with the cravings?" and "Why am I so hungry?" Removing the concept of counting calories was totally new to me. I couldn't believe I'd lose weight eating high-fat foods—even heavy cream and dark meat. My mother actually said, "You're never going to lose weight on that."

The initial structure helps you learn to make better choices. I'm thinking about dinner *this week* as opposed to *in two hours*. And my taste for sweets has changed completely. I can break a piece off a cookie as opposed to eating three cookies. I've also been able to impact my family. The first time I served the shepherd's pie from the recipes, I didn't say what was in it. My kids started eating and my husband looked at me and said, "You're not supposed to have mashed potatoes." And I said, "We're not eating mashed potatoes." Even after I told them it was made with white beans and cauliflower, they kept eating, and now it's become a staple. Fast-forward to two weeks ago: My seventeen-year-old son said to me, "I think I've had too many carbs today."

The program changed my whole philosophy about eating and exercising and health. For the first time, I actually see the potential to not be overweight. I'm a nurse, so you'd think I would've figured it out before now!

—*Lauren S., 52, North Andover, MA*
Weight loss: 28 pounds. Decrease in waist: 4.5 inches

CHAPTER 3

The Science

"When we read that 'the fat woman has the remedy in her own hands—or rather between her own teeth' ... there is an implication that obesity is usually merely the result of unsatisfactory dietary bookkeeping ... [Although logic suggests that body fat] may be decreased by altering the balance sheet through diminished intake, or increased output, or both ... [t]he problem is not really so simple and uncomplicated as it is pictured."

These words were written by the editors
of JAMA in 1924.[1]

For most of the last century, the usual way of thinking about body weight has been based on the law of physics that energy can neither be created nor destroyed. In other words, calorie intake minus calorie expenditure must equal calories stored. Surrounded by tempting foods, as this reasoning goes, we tend to consume more calories than we can burn off, and the excess is deposited as fat (see The Calorie Balance Theory of Obesity, on page 35). This view regards body fat as an inert object, like water in a bathtub. If you have too much, simply eat less (turn down the faucet) and exercise more (open up the drain). Since people unable to do so are presumed to lack knowledge or self-control, standard weight loss treatment involves instructing them about calories and counseling them to control behavior. The problem is, this approach has failed miserably in practice.

My Always Hungry Story

I have tried to lose weight with many programs and have initial success, but I eventually plateau out and then gain back most of what I have lost. I really need a program that will work for me.

—*Betty T., 76, Garland, TX*
Weight loss: 17 pounds. Decrease in waist: 3 inches

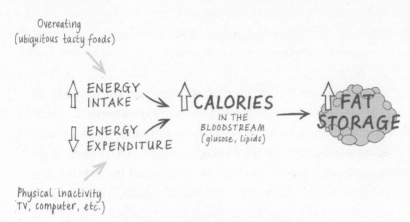

The Calorie Balance Theory of Obesity

In 1959, researchers in Philadelphia and New York conducted the first systematic review of medical weight loss programs, focusing on the highest-quality studies published during the preceding thirty years.[2] They came to a striking conclusion—these programs didn't work. Many participants dropped out. Of those people who remained, most didn't lose much weight. And of those who did lose weight, most regained it within two years. The authors emphasized that these results, "poor as they seem, are nevertheless [probably] better than those obtained by the average physician."

In the early 1990s, more than three decades later, the National Institutes of Health assembled an expert panel to evaluate contemporary methods for voluntary weight loss.[3] Their findings were remarkably similar to those from the first review. Participants who remained in weight loss programs attained a maximum weight loss of only about 10 percent. Most of this weight was regained in one year, and almost all was regained after five years. Unfortunately, current statistics don't offer much more hope. Only one in six American adults with a high BMI report ever having lost at least 10 percent of their weight for one year, according to a national survey.[4] And even that meager figure—representing just a fraction of the respondents' excess weight—is probably exaggerated, because people tend to overstate success in self-reports. Among children, the outcomes are no better, with most interventions "marked by small changes in relative weight or adiposity and substantial relapse."[5] Based on these data, conventional obesity treatment seems to have mostly failed.

The problem isn't with our calorie-counting abilities or self-control, but rather the current understanding of the cause of—and cure for—obesity. As eloquently argued by the editors of *JAMA*, the calorie balance view didn't work in the early twentieth century. There's no reason to think it will in the twenty-first, with ever-increasing opportunities to overeat.

BIOLOGY CONTROLS BODY WEIGHT

Cutting back on calories will cause weight loss for a while, which gives the illusion that we have conscious control of our weight over the long term. However, many bodily functions are within our temporary, but not permanent control. For example, many people can lower the amount of carbon dioxide in the blood for several minutes by breathing fast, but few can do so for much longer.

Researchers have actually known for decades why conventional diets don't work over the long term, although this knowledge has been generally disregarded. When we begin to cut calories, the body launches potent countermeasures designed to prevent additional weight loss. The more weight we lose, the more forcefully the body fights back.

In a classic series of studies dating to the 1980s, investigators at Rockefeller University in New York underfed volunteers to make them lose 10 to 20 percent of their weight, and then studied their metabolism during lengthy admissions to the research unit.[6] Regardless of whether the participants had normal or high body weight at the beginning of the study, they experienced a large drop in metabolic rate—far more than could be attributed to weight change alone. And of course, underfeeding made the participants hungrier.

These findings explain an experience all too familiar to anyone who has been on a diet. When you eat fewer calories, the body becomes more efficient and burns fewer calories, even as your desire for extra calories heightens. This combination of rising hunger and slowing metabolism is a recipe for failure. After a few weeks of calorie deprivation—long before our weight loss target is within sight—we become tired and tempted to quit our exercise routine, and collapse on the couch with a pint of ice cream. If we marshal a Herculean effort, stick to the diet, and stay active, metabolic rate will continue to fall, so we'll need to cut calories even more drastically to keep losing weight.

My Always Hungry Story

I have struggled with my weight for the last ten years. When I lose weight, I put most of it back on again. I am so unhappy with myself and can't seem to break through to a healthy weight. I walk approximately 6 miles a week, eat fairly healthy food, and keep gaining weight. I am always hungry.

—Pam A., 56, Vernon Hills, IL
Weight loss: 9 pounds. Decrease in waist: 1 inch

The body's weight control systems also work in the other direction. When volunteers are forced to gain weight by overfeeding under carefully monitored conditions, their metabolism speeds up and they tend to lose all interest in food. After the period of enforced feeding ends (to the relief of the volunteers), weight typically drops quickly back down to each individual's usual level.[7]

In fact, it's difficult for anyone to change body weight significantly in either direction. Just as a heavy person would struggle to lose 50 pounds, so would a lean person struggle to gain 50 pounds. For both over- and undereating, these biological responses push weight back to where it started—to a sort of "body weight set point" that seems largely predetermined by our genes (see The Body Weight Set Point below). If you inherited obesity genes from your parents, the biological responses that defend body weight will kick in for you at a higher range compared to someone who didn't inherit those genes.

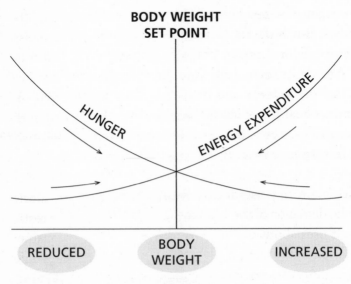

The Body Weight Set Point

Consider what would happen during a fever if you attempted to force your temperature down by taking a bath in ice water. Your body would resist—with severe shivering and blood vessel constriction to generate and conserve heat—and you'd soon experience an overwhelming desire to be someplace warm and dry. For these reasons, ice baths aren't a popular treatment option today. Aspirin is more effective because it lowers the "body temperature set point" during fever, allowing excess heat to dissipate more easily (and comfortably). In a sense, the calorie balance view of obesity is like considering fever a problem of heat balance. It's technically not wrong, but also not very helpful.

But if biology, not willpower, controls body weight over the long term, why have obesity rates risen so fast worldwide? Most important, what can we do about it? The answers can be found in our fat cells.[8]

THE PURPOSE OF BODY FAT

In our weight-obsessed culture, it's common to disparage the fat in our bodies. But body fat (scientifically termed "adipose tissue") is a highly specialized organ, critically important for health and longevity. Among its many functions, fat surrounds and cushions vital organs like the kidneys and insulates us against the cold. Body fat also signifies health, conferring beauty when distributed in the right amounts and locations. But critically, fat is our fuel tank—a strategic calorie reserve to protect against starvation.

Compared to other species our size, humans have an exceptionally large brain that requires an enormous amount of calories. The metabolic demands of the brain are so great that, under resting conditions, it uses about one of every three calories we consume. And this calorie requirement is absolute. Any interruption would cause immediate loss of consciousness, rapidly followed by seizure, coma, and death. That's a problem, because until very recently in human history, access to calories had always been unpredictable. Our ancestors faced extended periods of deprivation when a hunt or a staple food crop failed, during harsh winters, or when venturing out across an ocean. The key to their survival was body fat.

If we go for more than a few hours without eating, the body must rely on stored fuels for energy, and these come in three basic types, familiar to anyone who reads a nutrition label: carbohydrate, protein, and fat. The body stores accessible carbohydrate in the liver and protein in muscle, but these are in dilute forms, surrounded by lots of water. In contrast, stored fat is highly concentrated, since fat tissue contains very little water. In addition, pure carbohydrate and protein have less than half the calories of pure fat, making them relatively weak sources of energy. For these reasons, liver and muscle contain only a small fraction of the calories in fat tissue (less than 600 compared to about 3,500 per pound). In the absence of body fat, even a muscular man would waste away in days without eating, whereas all but the leanest adults have enough body fat to survive many weeks.

And these fat cells aren't just inert storage depots. Fat cells actively take up excess calories soon after meals and release them in a controlled fashion at other times, according to the body's needs. Fat tissue also responds to and emits a multitude of chemical signals and neural messages, helping fine-tune our metabolism and immune system. But when fat cells malfunction, big problems ensue.

HUNGRY FAT

We generally think that weight gain is the unavoidable consequence of consuming too many calories, with fat cells being the passive recipients of that excess (see The Calorie Balance Theory of Obesity on page 35). But fat cells do nothing of consequence without specific instructions—certainly not calorie storage and release, their most critical functions.

Insulin: The Fat Cell Fertilizer

Many substances produced in the body or contained in our diet directly affect fat cell behavior, chief among them the hormone insulin. Insulin, made in the pancreas, is widely known for its ability to lower blood sugar. Problems with the production or action of insulin lead to the common forms of diabetes, specifically type 1 (previously called juvenile diabetes) and type 2 (a frequent complication of obesity). But insulin's actions extend well beyond blood sugar control, to how all calories flow throughout the body.

Soon after the start of a meal, insulin level rises, directing incoming calories—glucose from carbohydrate, amino acids from protein, and free fatty acids from the fat in our diet—into body tissues for utilization or storage. A few hours later, decreasing insulin level allows stored fuels to reenter the blood, for use by the brain and the rest of the body. Although other hormones and biological inputs play supporting roles in this choreography, insulin is the undisputed star.

Insulin's effects on calorie storage are so potent that we can consider it the ultimate *fat cell fertilizer*. For example, rats given insulin infusions developed low blood glucose (hypoglycemia), ate more, and gained weight. Even when their food was restricted to that of the control animals, they still became fatter.[9] Conversely, mice genetically engineered to produce less insulin had healthier fat cells, burned off more calories, and resisted weight gain, even when given a diet that makes normal mice fat.[10]

In humans, high rates of insulin release from the pancreas due to genetic variants or other reasons cause weight gain.[11] People with type 1 diabetes who receive excess insulin predictably gain weight, whereas those treated inadequately with too little insulin lose weight, no matter how much they eat. Furthermore, drugs that stimulate insulin release from the pancreas are also associated with weight gain, and those that block its release with weight loss.[12]

If too much insulin drives fat cells to increase in size and number, what drives the pancreas to produce too much insulin? Carbohydrate, specifically sugar and the highly processed starches that quickly digest into sugar.[13] Basically, any of those packaged "low-fat" foods made primarily from refined grains, potato products, or concentrated sugar that crept into our diet as we single-mindedly focused on eating less fat.

Our Fat Cells Make Us Overeat

All this is just Endocrinology 101, well-established information every first-year medical student should know. But it leads to a stunning possibility. The usual way of thinking about the obesity epidemic has it backward. *Overeating hasn't made our fat cells grow; our fat cells have been programmed to grow, and that has made us overeat.*

Too much refined carbohydrate causes blood glucose to surge soon after a meal, which in turn makes the pancreas produce more insulin than would have ever been the case for humans in the past. High insulin levels trigger fat cells to hoard excessive amounts of glucose, fatty acids, and other calorie-rich substances that circulate in the blood. It's like those floor-to-ceiling turnstiles you might see at a ballpark or in the subway (see The One-Way Calorie Turnstile illustration below). People can pass freely in one direction, but horizontal crossbars prevent movement the other way. Insulin ushers calories into fat cells, but restricts their passage back out. Consequently, the body starts to run low on accessible fuel within a few hours, more quickly than normal. When that happens, the brain registers a problem and transmits an unmistakable call for help—in the form of rapidly rising hunger. Eating is a sure and fast way to increase the supply of calories in the blood, and processed carbohydrates act the fastest. The brain exploits this fact, making us crave starchy, sugary foods, more so than anything else. What would you rather have when your blood sugar is crashing: a bowl of fruit, a tall glass of full-fat milk, a large chicken breast, or a cinnamon sticky bun (each with the same number of calories)?

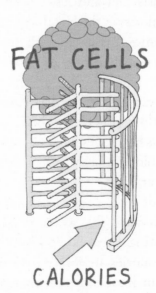

The One-Way Calorie Turnstile

As usually happens, we give in to temptation and have the sticky bun, or the myriad other formulations of processed carbohydrate so readily available today. But this solves the "energy crisis" only temporarily, sets up the next surge-crash cycle, and, over time, accelerates weight gain.

My Always Hungry Story

I've done all sorts of varieties of different things to lose weight. And I just always find myself, when challenged, in front of cake or cookies at an event, and I'll always just dive in, and then feel terrible afterward. The low-calorie diets never work, and after a while it just kind of tears you down mentally.

—*Eric D., 44, Catonsville, MD*
Weight loss: 21 pounds. Decrease in waist: 3 inches

The Brain's Emergency Alarm System

If we're on a low-calorie diet and resist the urge to eat more, the amount of accessible calories in the blood will continue to drift down, causing the brain to panic—understandably so, considering the catastrophic consequences of even a brief interruption in its fuel supply. Then, ancient parts of the brain that monitor metabolism activate the emergency alarm system: We become ravenously hungry, unable to concentrate on anything other than food, and increasingly weak. At the same time, stress hormones like epinephrine (adrenaline) and cortisol rush into the blood in an urgent attempt to unlock calorie stores in the fat and liver.

This combination of high stress hormones and low fuel levels resembles a state of starvation that wouldn't otherwise develop until after many hours of fasting. Eventually, either we succumb to hunger or some of the stored calories are forced back into the bloodstream. But if these cycles occur frequently, our metabolism suffers a slowdown, which can make weight loss nearly impossible. The usual "eat less, move more" approach misses the root cause of weight gain, produces side effects, and is destined to fail for most people. In this way, low-calorie diets may actually make matters worse.

Too Many Calories in the Body, But Too Few in the Right Place

This situation is similar to edema, a condition in which fluid leaks out of the blood vessels and accumulates elsewhere in the body (for example, in the legs), causing swelling. Despite having too much water in the body, people with edema may experience unquenchable thirst, because there's not enough water in the blood, where it's needed. Telling people with edema to drink less is no more effective than food restriction for weight loss, because it ignores the underlying cause. Insulin (and other influences, as we'll discuss later) has programmed fat cells into calorie-storage overdrive. People chronically overeat because they're trying to keep enough calories in the blood to feed the brain, compensating for those being siphoned off by overstimulated fat cells. But until the underlying problem is addressed, it's a never-ending battle, and those extra calories cause even more weight gain. The fundamental problem is one of distribution: not too many calories, but too few in the right place. Though we think of obesity as a condition of excess, it's actually a matter of starvation to the body!

This radically different way of thinking (illustrated in The Fat Cell Theory of Obesity on page 45), predicts that eating highly processed carbohydrate like that cinnamon bun or a bagel would cause an increase in the number of calories stored as fat, a decline in the number of calories available in the blood, hunger, and activation of brain regions involved in food cravings, all within a few hours. Over time, a diet based on those foods would slow down metabolism and have other major adverse effects on the body. And that's exactly what my colleagues and I have found in a twenty-year line of research.

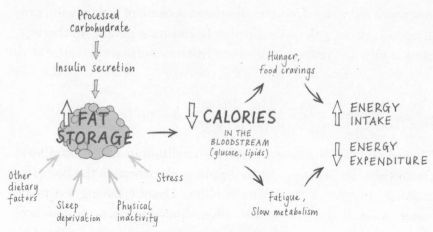

The Fat Cell Theory of Obesity

All Breakfasts Are Not Created Equal

In our first study, conducted in the mid-1990s and published in the journal *Pediatrics*,[14] we gave twelve adolescent boys three different breakfasts following separate overnight stays in the clinical research unit. Each breakfast had exactly the same number of calories, but varied in amount and type of carbohydrate. One breakfast was instant oatmeal, a highly processed carbohydrate. (Although instant oatmeal is technically "whole grain," the grain kernel has been pulverized into small particles and then cooked at high temperature.) The second breakfast, consisting of minimally processed carbohydrate, was steel-cut (also called Irish) oatmeal, in which the kernel structure is left mostly intact. Steel-cut oats take longer to cook and longer to digest than instant oats, producing a smaller rise in glucose and insulin. Both oatmeals had the same nutrients (about 65 percent carbohydrate, 20 percent fat). The third breakfast was a vegetable omelet with fruit. This meal had more protein and fat, less carbohydrate, and no grain products at all.

As expected, blood glucose and insulin levels initially rose to high, intermediate, and low levels following the instant oatmeal, steel-cut oatmeal, and omelet with fruit, in that order. But what goes up must come down. One hour after the instant oatmeal, blood glucose began to fall rapidly. By four hours, blood glucose was lower following the instant oatmeal (by about 10 milligrams per deciliter) than the other meals, even lower than after the overnight fast. This difference is large enough to provoke hunger and initiate eating.[15] Free fatty acids, the other major fuel in the bloodstream, were also lower following the instant oatmeal than the other meals at four hours, making for a metabolic double whammy.

Are these results mere scientific curiosities? Changes in the emergency stress hormones suggest not. Adrenaline surged at four hours after the instant oatmeal, but remained stable after the other meals, suggesting the brain had experienced *a true metabolic crisis*. Some of our participants looked frankly sweaty and shaky—signs of hypoglycemia—after the instant oatmeal.

We served the teens the same meals again at lunch, and then allowed them to eat as much or as little as they wanted throughout the afternoon from large platters of tasty foods—bread, bagels, cold cuts, cream cheese, regular cheese, spreads, cookies, and fruits. They ate substantially more on average after the instant oatmeal (about 1,400 calories) compared to the steel-cut oats (900 calories) or the omelet with fruit (750 calories). That's a 650-calorie difference following meals with the same number of calories, just in different forms!

Similar effects have been observed in more than a dozen studies by different research groups.[16] If only a small fraction of this 650-calorie difference happened for the general public meal after meal, day after day, it could account for much of the increase in body weight since the 1970s, as consumption of highly processed carbohydrate soared. Thus, meals with the same calories can produce dramatically different outcomes a few hours later, as depicted in the Hormones and Hunger after Eating Meals with and without Refined Carbohydrate figure on page 47.

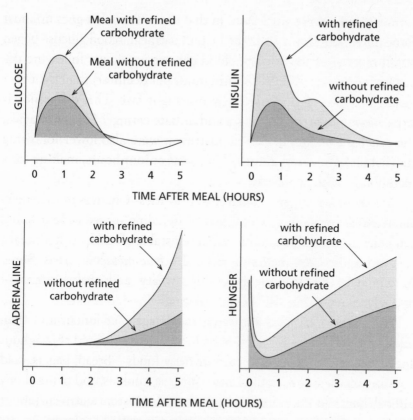

Hormones and Hunger after Eating Meals with and without
Refined Carbohydrate

Your Brain on Fast-Acting Carbs

What happens in the brain after eating too much refined carbohydrate, when accessible fuel levels in the blood crash? To answer this question, we gave twelve men with high BMI two milk shakes, one containing corn syrup (a highly processed and fast-acting carbohydrate) and the other with uncooked cornstarch (a slow-acting carbohydrate). Otherwise, the milk shakes had the same major nutrients (protein, fat, and carbohydrate) and similar sweetness, controlled by adding slightly different amounts of artificial sweetener. The milk shakes were given in random order, and neither the participants nor the study staff knew which came first.

The results were published in the *American Journal of Clinical Nutrition*.[17] Similar to our first study, blood glucose and insulin levels were higher after the fast-acting milk shake for the first hour or two. But by four hours after consuming the fast-acting shake, blood glucose fell to lower levels and reported hunger was greater, compared to the slow-acting shake. At that time, we conducted brain imaging scans, using a technique called functional magnetic resonance imaging (fMRI). The scans detected one brain region, called the nucleus accumbens, that lit up like a laser after the fast-acting shake. The effect was so strong and consistent, it occurred in every one of our participants, providing strong statistical confidence in the results. The nucleus accumbens is considered ground zero for reward, craving, and addiction—including alcohol, tobacco, and cocaine abuse. Activation of this brain region on a weight loss diet would erode willpower, making that sticky bun exceedingly hard to resist.

The concept of food addiction is controversial because, unlike substances of abuse, we need food to live. However, this study suggests that highly processed carbohydrates may hijack basic reward circuitry in the brain, not because they are inherently so tasty (both milk shakes had the same sweetness), but instead because of direct actions on metabolism. Hunger is hard enough to fight under any circumstances, but once the nucleus accumbens joins in, it's all over.

The Type of Calories You Eat Affects the Number You Burn

On the positive side, these short-term studies show that we're only one meal away from reversing this vicious cycle. However, they raise the question: Do the effects last longer than a single day? To examine this, we conducted a lengthy feeding study, providing twenty-one young adults all the foods they consumed for seven months. First, we reduced their weight 10 to 15 percent (about 25 pounds) by underfeeding. Next, we stabilized their weight at this new, lower level by increasing their food allowance. Then, we studied them for one month at a time on three diets, each with the same number of calories, but with different macronutrient breakdowns: high carbo-hydrate (60 percent), consistent with government recommendations; moderate carbohydrate (40 percent), similar to a Mediterranean diet; or low carbohydrate (10 percent), like the Atkins diet.

We found that the participants burned about 325 calories a day more on the low-carbohydrate compared to the high-carbohydrate diet. This difference is equivalent to about an hour of moderately vigor-ous physical activity, in effect without lifting a finger. They burned 150 calories more on the moderate-carbohydrate compared to the high-carbohydrate diet—equivalent to an hour of light physical activity.

The high-carbohydrate diet also had the worst effect on major heart disease risk factors, including insulin resistance, triglycerides, and HDL cholesterol. These results, published in *JAMA* in 2012,[18] indicate that all calories are not alike to the body. The *type* of calories going into the body affects the *number* of calories going out.

This study has two limitations. First, despite attempts to con-trol as many aspects of diet and lifestyle as possible, our participants didn't remain under direct observation at all times. We can't know with certainty how well they complied with the diet at home, when attending parties, or when traveling. Second, each diet lasted only one month. To understand the true effects of a diet over time, much longer interventions are needed, and that can be extremely costly and challenging to do properly with humans. For that reason, we also studied a species whose diet and environment can be precisely controlled for as long as we wish.

My Always Hungry Story

I took an active metabolic assessment at my gym. This test measures where your body is obtaining energy from, at increasing levels of activity. After warming up and getting into the test, my coach asked me if I had changed my diet recently. I said yes and told him about leaving sugar and simple carbs behind and eating lots of protein, vegetables, and full-fat. He was astonished at my results. He even called other trainers over to look at my readouts. The test breaks up the data into four training zones, and except for the highest effort, *all* of my energy (calorie burn) was coming from my fat cells—zero from carbs. He was totally impressed. Conclusion: With the right diet, our energy will be provided by our fat cells and the weight we are losing is actual fat! Totally awesome!!

—Dan B., 45, Lehi, UT
Weight loss: 15 pounds. Decrease in waist: 1 inch

Eating Fewer Calories, Yet Gaining More Fat

In a study published in *The Lancet*,[19] we examined two groups of rats from the same strain that were fed identical diets, differing only in carbohydrate type. One group ate the kind of starch found in beans, called amylose, a tough little molecule that digests slowly. The other group ate the kind of starch found in white potatoes, called amylopectin, a big fluffy molecule that digests quickly. We altered the total amount of food given to each animal, to keep the average weight in both groups the same throughout the eighteen-week study (which translates to about fifteen rat years).

Beginning at seven weeks, animals eating the fast-acting carbohydrate diet required less food compared to those eating the slow-acting carbohydrate diet to prevent excessive weight gain—*evidence that their metabolism was slowing down*. At the end of the study, we analyzed body composition by assessing how chemical tracers distributed in the animals' bodies. Even though both groups weighed exactly the same, the rats on the fast-acting carbohydrate diet had 70 percent more body fat (and a commensurate reduction of muscle tissue).

These findings completely defy the calorie-balance theory of obesity. According to standard advice, the best way to lose weight or avoid weight gain is to cut back on calories. And that's exactly what we did with the fast-acting carbohydrate group—in essence, we put them on a low-calorie diet. But despite having consumed *less* food, they had *more* fat. They also had significantly increased heart disease risk factors. Consistent with the Fat Cell Theory of Obesity figure (see page 45), the fast-acting carbohydrate increased insulin levels, causing calories to be stored as fat at the expense of the animals' lean tissues and overall health.

Rodents are, of course, not humans, and we ultimately need clinical trials of sufficient size, scope, and duration to provide definitive answers. Recently, though, data has begun to accumulate on how the composition of your diet can affect the composition of your body. Iris Shai of Ben-Gurion University in Israel, Meir Stampfer of Harvard, and their colleagues assigned a few hundred adults with large waist sizes to either low-fat or low-carbohydrate/Mediterranean diets, and carefully measured changes in body fat over eighteen months. Preliminary analyses suggest that the diets had profoundly different effects on fat content in the abdomen, heart, liver, pancreas, and other organs, above and beyond weight loss.* Along the same lines, researchers from Penn State had forty-eight adults consume cholesterol-lowering diets supplemented with about 250 calories from high-fat almonds or high-carbohydrate muffins for six weeks each. Belly fat decreased significantly while the participants consumed the almond-containing diet.[20]

Major observational studies like the Nurses' Health Study and Health Professionals Follow-Up Study also provide a consistent message about highly processed carbohydrate. Investigators from Harvard examined how changes in specific foods related to weight change during successive four-year periods ranging from 1986 to 2006. They reported the results in the *New England Journal of Medicine* in 2011.[21] Topping the list for weight gain were potato products and sugary beverages, with refined grains not far behind. In contrast, nuts, whole milk, and cheese either had no relationship with weight gain *or were associated with weight loss*. So it seems that those high-fat foods we've been avoiding for decades may be key to losing weight after all!

A Low-Quality Diet Keeps Calories Locked in the Fat Cells

Let's consider one more way to view the body's calorie-fuel management system, using a fuel tank as an analogy. Suppose a man had a cabin in the woods with an automated heating system fueled

---

* Unpublished results, with permission from Iris Shai.

by compressed natural gas, as depicted in the Natural Gas Heating System Analogy figure below. As the temperature inside drops, the thermostat sends an electronic message to the tank for more fuel, an outlet valve opens, and natural gas flows through pipes to a fireplace, generating heat. Once the cabin temperature rises to the desired setting, the thermostat sends another message to the fuel tank to close the valve.

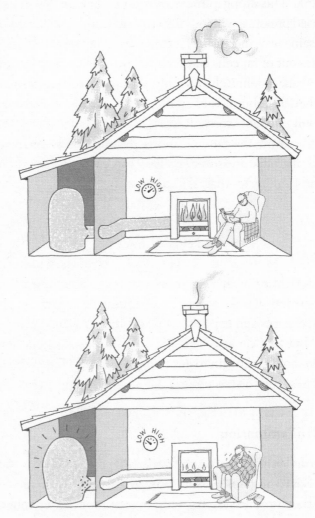

Natural Gas Heating System Analogy: Problems arise if the outlet valve becomes clogged and gas can't get out of the storage tank.

Now imagine what would happen if the man—in a misguided attempt to save money—filled the storage tank with low-quality fuel, and the outlet valve became clogged, partially restricting gas outflow. The fireplace wouldn't have enough fuel and the cabin would get chilly. Obviously, the sensible solution would be to clean the system and switch to higher-quality fuel. But instead, the tightfisted cabin owner decides to add more gas, increasing the pressure within the storage tank. This stopgap measure could work for a while, because the increased pressure will initially force additional fuel from the tank.

In the same way, increasing fat stores overcomes the difficulty of getting calories out of fat cells caused by a low-quality diet. But this strategy won't work indefinitely. As long as the fuel blockage remains—for the hypothetical cabin owner and for people with excess weight—the problem will only get worse. Residue will continue to clog the outlet valve (in the body, the fat cell calorie release mechanism), requiring ever-increasing tank pressures (body fat) to keep the cabin warm (our metabolism running)—that is, until the system reaches a critical state.

ANGRY FAT

Excessive weight gain can continue for quite some time with few serious consequences. Unlike other body organs, fat has a prodigious capacity to store calories and expand, while continuing to carry out its usual functions. But that capacity isn't limitless. Eventually, fat cells reach a critical threshold and begin to emit distress signals. Then, the immune system rushes in to the rescue, and that's when the trouble really starts.

Chronic Inflammation

Starvation and infection are among the two greatest threats to animals in nature. So it's perhaps not surprising that body fat, which stores calories, and the immune system, which fights invading microbes, would be closely linked. Fat tissue contains our most concentrated store of energy, a tremendous biological prize for invading bacteria, if they could get to it. Probably for this reason, infection-fighting white blood cells continuously circulate throughout fat tissue, in constant surveillance for foreign substances.[22] White blood cells and fat cells each produce a multitude of chemical messages that affect the other, helping to optimize metabolism, immunity to infection, and general health. However, this fine-tuned relationship becomes disrupted in obesity.

When fat cells reach a critical size—which can vary from person to person—many things go wrong. The cells' internal machinery may suffer under the strain of maintaining so much fat. Some cells may suffer oxygen deprivation, having outgrown their blood supply. Consequently, they become distressed and a few may actually die, releasing chemicals that signal tissue damage. Immediately upon receiving these danger signals, resident white blood cells call for reinforcements from immune cells elsewhere in the body and transform themselves into attack mode. This kind of rapid response could be lifesaving in the face of microbial invasion, but in this case, there is no infection to fight, and the response makes matters even worse.[23]

Normally, the immune system mobilizes only in response to foreign threat or injury, acting to destroy the invaders and clean up the damage. Once this work is done, the system quickly quiets down. However, if persistently activated, the immune system's powerful weaponry may become directed against the body, resulting in chronic inflammation. This harmful process occurs in an especially dramatic way with autoimmune diseases like Crohn's, rheumatoid arthritis, lupus, and multiple sclerosis.

In obesity, activation of the immune system by distressed fat cells leads to an escalating cycle of inflammation and injury, with potentially dire consequence (see the Insulin Resistance, Chronic Inflammation, and Systemic Disease figure on page 55). This situation is like that overpressurized gas storage tank: Sooner or later, the pipes will burst, releasing gas into the cabin and placing the cabin owner at immediate risk. Similarly, inflamed fat tissue spews a toxic brew of chemicals into the bloodstream, disseminating disease throughout the body. Chronic inflammation in the lining of the blood vessels causes narrowing of the arteries, called atherosclerosis, resulting in predisposition to a heart attack or stroke. In the liver, chronic inflammation can lead to hepatitis and cirrhosis; in muscle, to loss of lean body mass; in the lungs, to asthma; in the brain, to further metabolic disturbance and possibly neurodegenerative conditions like Alzheimer's (which some are now calling type 3 diabetes[24]).

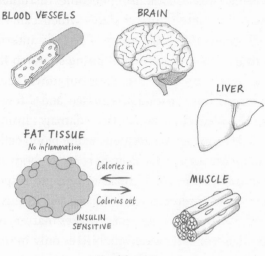

Healthy Fat

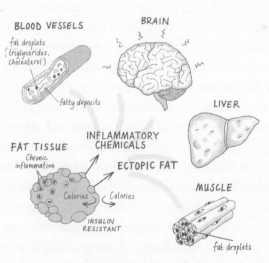

"Angry Fat"
Insulin Resistance, Chronic Inflammation, and Systemic Disease

Insulin Resistance, Type 2 Diabetes, and Other Health Issues

At this stage, after years of relentless increase, body weight may plateau, as chronic inflammation induces insulin resistance, disrupting the ability of fat cells to take up and store more calories. Insulin resistance is a complicated concept, but to understand the basic idea, think about insulin as a key that fits precisely into a lock (the insulin receptor) found on the surface of cells throughout the body. Normally, insulin easily unlocks this receptor, opening cellular doors that let in glucose. Insulin also stimulates cell processes related to growth, in part by altering the activity of many genes. With insulin resistance, the lock becomes rusty, causing insulin levels in the blood to increase in an attempt to force open the cell door. However, insulin resistance doesn't occur in a consistent way throughout the body, so that one organ may receive too little insulin stimulation (because the lock is especially rusty), whereas another may receive too much (because the lock remains relatively rust-free)—an imbalance that contributes to the medical consequences of obesity.

In any event, this weight plateau caused by insulin resistance isn't the blessing it might appear. Chronic inflammation also blocks the uptake and release of calories by fat cells, perpetuating hunger and overeating. But now, any excess calories consumed have no place to go, so they build up in abnormal locations, like liver and muscle. These abnormal fat deposits, called ectopic fat, worsen insulin resistance, setting the stage for development of diabetes.[25]

If the pancreas tires out and can't make enough insulin to compensate for insulin resistance, type 2 diabetes develops. When this happens, the body becomes unable to cope with carbohydrate, and blood sugar rises above the normal range (equal to or greater than 126 milligrams per deciliter fasting or 200 milligrams per deciliter two hours after consuming glucose). Chronic high blood sugar, together with other metabolic derangements in diabetes, puts organs in the body under additional stress, greatly increasing the risk for heart attack, kidney failure, blindness, limb amputation, and other problems.

Ironically, the standard treatment for diabetes since the 1970s has been a low-fat, high-carbohydrate diet—the same diet that contributed to the problem in the first place! We wouldn't give the milk sugar lactose to someone with lactose intolerance. What's the sense in giving so much carbohydrate to someone who, by definition, has carbohydrate intolerance?

My Always Hungry Story

When I started the program, I had high blood pressure, high triglycerides, and high CRP (a test for chronic inflammation). Just sixteen weeks later, these had all normalized. And my doctor said this was the first time in a number of years that she wasn't concerned about my diabetes because it was being so well controlled. It would be awesome if I could eventually get off the diabetes medications.
—*Ruth S., 65, Stillwater, MN*
Weight loss: 15 pounds. Decrease in waist: 2.5 inches

If chronic inflammation spreads to the hypothalamus, severe new problems arise.[26] The hypothalamus, an ancient part of the brain, is considered the master controller of metabolism. To locate it, visualize where two imaginary lines would intersect, one from between the eyes to the back of the head, and the other from the top of one ear to the other. The hypothalamus integrates signals from the body, such as the fat cell hormone leptin (discussed in chapter 2), and elsewhere in the brain, adjusting hunger and metabolic rate to prevent wild fluctuations in body weight. Damage to this brain region can cause an extreme form of obesity that resists almost every attempt at treatment.

In laboratory studies, normal mice develop hypothalamic inflammation soon after being placed on an obesity-inducing diet, producing brain cell injury in that region. In contrast, mice genetically engineered to block inflammation in the hypothalamus are protected against obesity.[27] Preliminary studies in people with obesity have identified brain injury similar to that seen in animals.[28] These findings suggest that, unless measures are taken to reverse hypothalamic inflammation, weight gain may become virtually irreversible.

Inevitably, cardiovascular complications mount, including high blood pressure, high triglycerides, low HDL (good) cholesterol, and fatty liver—components of what's called "metabolic syndrome." Modern drugs may control some of these conditions for a while, but heart attack and stroke loom, unless the underlying problems—high insulin and chronic inflammation—are addressed.

My Always Hungry Story

I was scared about the high-fat diet in Phase 1, especially because I have high cholesterol. We have been told to not eat a lot of fat. But by the end of the program, my lab tests improved so much that my doctor cut my cholesterol medication in half.

—Betty T., 76, Garland, TX
Weight loss: 17 pounds. Decrease in waist: 3 inches

After cardiovascular disease, cancer is the leading cause of death in the United States and, for many people, their greatest health fear. Here, too, an unhealthful diet may put us at risk. Insulin not only fertilizes the growth of fat cells, but also stimulates tissues throughout the body. In adults with obesity, cells throughout the body may be overstimulated by insulin and other growth-promoting substances (including hormones in the "insulin-like growth factor" family) for decades. Eating too much highly processed carbohydrate exacerbates this situation. Eventually, some cells may break free of the normal molecular control system that restrains growth, leading to cancer. Chronic inflammation may accelerate this malignant transformation, as has been described in cancers of the esophagus, stomach, colon, pancreas, lung, prostate, and breast. The American Society of Clinical Oncology recently concluded that obesity causes almost one hundred thousand cancers each year, increases risk for recurrence, and accounts for 15 to 20 percent of all cancer-related mortality.[29]

Calming Down Angry Fat

In large observational studies, body weight tracks closely with obesity-related chronic disease,[30] but this relationship is not perfect. Some people have the ability to store large amounts of fat in a healthy way, especially if it's on the hips, buttocks, and thighs (a pear-shaped body), without developing insulin resistance and chronic inflammation, at least for a while.[31] For others, including those with excess belly fat (an apple-shaped body), the transition from normal to inflamed fat tissue can occur at a relatively low body weight—a condition termed TOFI ("Thin Outside, Fat Inside").[32] For this reason, remaining lean does not, by itself, keep you safe from the ravages of insulin resistance and chronic inflammation. Indeed, millions of people in the United States with technically normal body weight are nevertheless at risk for all the complications discussed previously, based on a combination of genes and diet.

For fifty years, we've been told that a low-fat diet would protect us against chronic diseases. That notion inspired the Women's Health Initiative clinical trial which started in 1991 (whose disappointing results were discussed in chapter 2—see page 19) and also informed the design of the Look Ahead study, launched a decade later. The goal of Look Ahead was to reduce heart disease, a common complication of diabetes. The study, conducted in sixteen clinical centers in the United States, assigned about five thousand adults with type 2 diabetes to either a low-fat diet with intensive lifestyle modification or to usual care. The study, published in the *New England Journal of Medicine* in 2013,[33] was terminated prematurely for "futility." Analysis by independent statisticians found *no* reduction of heart disease among participants assigned to the intensive low-fat diet, and *no* prospect of ever seeing such a benefit emerge.

By coincidence, another study called PREDIMED was published in the same prestigious journal the very same year.[34] This study assigned about seven thousand five hundred Spanish adults with heart disease risk factors to one of three diets: Mediterranean with lots of olive oil, Mediterranean with lots of nuts, or a conventional low-fat diet. The interventions did not involve a calorie restriction or weight loss goal. PREDIMED was also terminated early, but in this case because effectiveness *exceeded* expectations. Both higher fat groups had such significant reductions in cardiovascular disease (about 30 percent) that continuation of the trial would have been unethical for the participants in the conventional group.

These two recent studies should seal the coffin on the standard low-fat diet. More broadly, they show that modest improvements in diet—specifically, more fat and less processed carbohydrates—can prevent obesity-related disease at any body weight. A high-quality diet seems to calm down "angry fat" even without weight loss. With weight loss, the health benefits could be huge.

CRAVINGS, BINGE EATING, AND "FOOD ADDICTION"

Most of us have lost control of eating at one time or another, only to regret it later. Who hasn't felt uncomfortably full after at least one Thanksgiving dinner? But why do so many people habitually succumb to food cravings and binge, despite intense feelings of guilt and an earnest desire to lose weight? In a way, everyone with excessive weight (that is, most adults in the United States) could be considered to have disordered eating, because by definition, they repeatedly overeat.

Disordered eating is commonly treated as a psychological problem of poor impulse control. For this reason, treatment typically involves behavioral therapy, with the goal to avoid triggering situations, reduce exposure to "danger foods," and develop alternative coping strategies. Yet this approach often fails, because it disregards the biological drivers of food cravings.

Consider Addison's disease, a form of severe adrenal gland failure that can strike adolescents and young adults. In this disease, the adrenal glands lose the ability to make aldosterone, a hormone that helps the kidneys hold on to sodium. Although Addison's can be effectively treated by hormone replacement therapy, the diagnosis is often initially missed, and the body can become dangerously deficient in sodium. If this happens, the brain responds in a logical way—increasing craving for salt, in an attempt to compensate for the ongoing urinary loss. Now picture a teenager with undiagnosed Addison's who begins to experience uncontrollable urges to eat chips, pretzels, and other salty foods. The parents, alarmed by this change in eating behavior, might consult a psychologist. The psychologist might suggest counseling to explore the emotional roots for these unusual cravings. But no amount of therapy will work, because the problem is biological in origin—too much salt loss in the urine.

Similarly, psychological approaches to binge eating will have limited effectiveness, if fat cells take in too many calories and leave too few for the rest of the body. It's impossible to know whether a behavioral problem like disordered eating has a psychological (or even psychiatric) origin, until potential biological contributors have been treated.

As we saw earlier in this chapter, the excessive insulin levels provoked by highly processed carbohydrates cause fat cells to suck up too many calories, leaving too few calories in the right places. When the bloodstream runs low on calories, the brain triggers an alarm system, leading to hunger, and cravings. We specifically crave highly processed carbohydrates—chips, cookies, crackers, candy, cake, and the like—for one simple reason: They make us feel better within a few minutes. The problem is, they also make us feel worse for hours afterward, setting up the next addictive cycle. In a sense, highly processed carbohydrates are akin to drugs of abuse, whose fast absorption rates increase addictiveness.[35] For example, unprocessed coca leaf (which takes a while to chew and digest) has a long record of safe use in South America for altitude sickness and other purposes. But when the active ingredient, cocaine, is refined and concentrated for rapid action, serious physical and psychological addiction results.

My Always Hungry Story

Well, today I had an old-fashioned doughnut. I used to love these. I ate it and when I was finished I realized I didn't enjoy it. It did not meet my expectations. I expected to enjoy every single bite...and nothing. I guess my body is changing. I ate it because I remember loving these—I wasn't hungry. I didn't crave it. It was just there. I plan to remind myself how much better real foods really are.

—Angelica G., 50, Sacramento, CA
Weight loss: 11.5 pounds. Decrease in waist: 3 inches

Let's do a thought experiment. Imagine you've just had an upsetting argument with your spouse. You can't reach your best friend to talk about it, and wind up in the kitchen, seeking comfort from food. Now suppose you could find only these four items, each with about 400 calories:

Bread—5 slices (highly processed carbohydrate)
Berries—6 cups (unprocessed carbohydrates)
Butter—½ stick, or about 12 teaspoons (fat)
Beef jerky—five 1-ounce portions (protein)

Which could you eat the quickest? Which would elicit the fewest cautionary feedback signals in your body (such as fullness, discomfort, or even nausea)? Which would leave you feeling hungry again the soonest? Which would most likely provoke a binge? You probably chose bread as the answer to each of these questions. It's much harder to binge on the other items, and if you did, you'd probably feel disinclined to do so again anytime soon.

Of course, some people suffer from serious eating disorders, like bulimia, that may require specialized psychiatric help. And even the highest-quality food can't fill emotional emptiness. Psychological counseling can play an important role in helping address life's challenges and promote positive behavior change. But highly processed carbohydrates set the stage for a binge, no matter what our psychological state is. Eliminate them and food-related behavioral problems may improve spontaneously. With most whole foods, your body will tell you in no uncertain terms when it's had enough.

My Always Hungry Story

It's actually possible to not have food cravings! I didn't think it was possible but when I am following this program, I am at ease and don't have anxiety about food or think about food obsessively. I now recognize that being full from carbohydrates is a different physical sensation, one that's not so comfortable—more like a beached whale. Before, I'd have that lousy full feeling but still be craving something else.
—*Pamela G., 56, Chantilly, VA*
Weight loss: 8 pounds. Decrease in waist: 3.5 inches

FOOD FOR THOUGHT

Optimal health depends upon careful calibration of opposing biological actions—contraction and relaxation of the heart, in breath and outbreath, wakefulness and sleep. If the heart repeatedly contracts too hard, or the breath is too deep, the body suffers. And so it is with nourishment. After a meal, calories flow into the body, replenishing energy stores. A few hours later, the tide turns, and calories flow in the other direction, out of storage sites. Normally, this back-and-forth choreography occurs smoothly, with gentle, health-promoting effects on the body. But our modern industrial diet has upset this natural rhythm (see the Hormones and Hunger after Eating Meals with and without Refined Carbohydrate figure on page 47), inundating the bloodstream with excess calories immediately after eating, then leaving us deficient soon thereafter. The body copes with each extreme as best it can, by increasing insulin levels during the calorie flood and increasing stress hormones during the drought. But these exaggerated swings in hormones and metabolism take a toll on the body. It stands to reason that they would also affect the brain.[36]

In a carefully controlled feeding study, researchers from the

University of Wales in the United Kingdom gave seventy-one female undergraduate students slow- or fast-digesting carbohydrate-based breakfasts and then tested their cognitive functioning. They found that memory, especially for hard words, was impaired throughout the morning after the fast-digesting breakfast. This effect was most pronounced several hours after the meal (a 33 percent deficit).[37] Similar results were obtained in Toronto among twenty-one patients with diabetes. Following a meal with fast-digesting carbohydrate, verbal memory performance, working memory, selective attention, and executive function were worse compared to a meal containing the same amount of carbohydrate in slow-digesting form.[38]

These cognitive deficits in children and young adults, if persistent, may lead to a diagnosis of attention-deficient disorder (ADD). Of course, there are many reasons why kids today may have difficulty concentrating, ranging from too much screen time to too little sleep. But these and other studies suggest that overconsumption of highly processed carbohydrates could be contributing to the problem.

Suppose you gave your twelve-year-old son a "whole-grain" bagel with fat-free cream cheese and a glass of 100% juice for breakfast, as was encouraged by the Food Guide Pyramid (see The Food Guide Pyramid of 1992 on page 4). Though these foods might sound healthy, they're highly processed, and contain little protein and fat to counterbalance the fast-digesting carbohydrate. By mid-morning, the calories in his blood would probably crash, and stress hormones would surge—hardly a biological recipe for calm concentration and

My Always Hungry Story

I suffer from depression, but it's not something I openly discuss because of the stigma. With this program, I have happiness in my life. I can't explain it, just as I cannot explain the depression. I feel that I am changing from the inside. This is going to be a life-changing program for me.

—*Joyce D., 70, Roswell, GA*
Weight loss: 8 pounds. Decrease in waist: 4.5 inches

learning. Curiously, the stimulant drugs used to treat ADD have broadly similar biological actions to the stress hormone adrenaline. Could it be that these drugs help counteract the swings in blood sugar that occur on the highly processed diets children consume today?

How has our general well-being fared, amid the assault on body and mind by our modern hyperprocessed diet? To get a sense of this, consider our general use of medicines and mood-altering substances—including some of the most heavily advertised products on TV. We take caffeine to wake up in the morning, alcohol to calm down in the evening, and tranquilizers to rest at night. We need ibuprofen for pains, antacids for indigestion, and pills for erectile dysfunction. Many rely upon drugs to manage fatigue, irritability, anxiety, inability to focus, depression, and other mental symptoms. Could the right diet—by controlling insulin levels and calming chronic inflammation—help end this chemical dependency? Much scientific evidence suggests so.

My Always Hungry Story

The number one benefit of this program is mood stabilization and ability to stop my antidepressant! I'm amazed at how the sugar cravings have gone away but what's more exciting is that I'm off the medication I've been taking since my second son was born seven years ago. I still have sad times but not to the same degree and not feeling out of control at night like I used to. I'm sure my weight will continue to drop but the real benefit is the overall wellness I feel.

—Karen L., 44, Savage, MN
Weight loss: 7 pounds. Decrease in waist: 2 inches

THE REASON WE'VE BEEN CONFUSED

Every year, the pharmaceutical industry sponsors many state-of-the-art clinical trials testing the effectiveness of new medicines, each with the potential to generate billions of dollars in annual sales. With so much profit at stake, drug companies make sure this research is done right. These "Phase 3" trials have huge budgets (sometimes exceeding $100 million); a large number of participants (typically many thousands); lengthy follow-up time (often many years); highly trained research staff; measures to ensure the protocol is correctly followed (such as giving participants the drug at no cost); and comprehensive quality-control procedures.

In striking contrast, nutrition research struggles by on a shoestring budget. Despite the massive cost savings that would result from improving our diet to prevent and treat obesity, no wealthy company stands to profit directly. Federal funding through the National Institutes of Health has dwindled, as costs for clinical research continue to escalate.[39] Consequently, most weight loss diet studies are drastically underfunded—rarely with more than a few hundred thousand dollars—and quality suffers. The vast majority of these studies have several dozen (or occasionally a few hundred) participants, short study duration (one year or less), staff with variable levels of expertise, limited resources to ensure behavior change, and inconsistent quality control. Typically, the interventions involve only instruction in what to eat, but no actual assistance with food purchasing or meal preparation. With such limited support, most participants in diet studies don't change their behavior very much, and the comparison groups (for example, people assigned to a low-fat versus a low-carbohydrate diet) don't wind up eating much differently from each other. Not surprisingly, these studies produce very little weight loss in any group.

Such research has sometimes been misinterpreted to mean that "all diets are alike," or "sticking to a diet, any diet, is the only thing that matters." But these conclusions are simply wrong. This sort of faulty reasoning wouldn't withstand scrutiny in other areas of clinical research. Should we abandon a promising new cancer drug, simply because participants in the experimental group didn't take most of the medicine?

Fortunately, a few diet studies have done it right. The DIRECT study, published in the *New England Journal of Medicine* in 2008,[40] compared a conventional diet (low-fat), a Mediterranean diet (medium-fat), and an Atkins-type diet (high-fat) among 322 participants with high BMI. The intervention was conducted at a work site in Israel, where—in addition to standard nutrition education—participants received their main meal of the day according to dietary assignment. In this way, the researchers could be assured that the three groups actually ate differently. Spouses were also instructed in the diets, to increase support at home. The study lasted two years, allowing enough time to see longer-term differences emerge.

Even though the dietary targets were not fully met, the findings of this remarkable study stand in stark contrast to the inconclusive outcomes of lower-quality research. Weight loss was greatest on the high-fat diet, intermediate on the medium-fat diet, and lowest on the low-fat diet—differences that were strongly significant from a statistical perspective. In addition, the higher fat diets produced more favorable changes in triglycerides, HDL-cholesterol and, among participants with diabetes, measures of blood sugar control. We need more carefully controlled research like this to end the reigning confusion about weight loss diets.

THE FALLACY OF THE "EMPTY CALORIE"

A fundamental problem with the calorie balance view of obesity is that it considers all calories alike, regardless of source, in some obviously awkward ways. According to this view, a pastry and a peach would affect the body in the same way, so long as we consume them in the same amounts—violating basic nutritional common sense. If this were true, why would we need dietitians at all, whose primary job is to advise which foods to eat and which to avoid? Some calories seem to be more equal than others! To get around this predicament, nutrition experts have come to rely on the notion of the empty calorie. Sure, having too many soft drinks may not be advisable, as this thinking goes, but not because of any negative effects of sugar itself. The only concern is that added sugar—which lacks fiber, vitamins, minerals, and other essential nutrients—will take the place of other foods that contain more of these nutrients. This argument was succinctly stated in an editorial in the prestigious *American Journal of Clinical Nutrition* in 2014:[41]

> As a card-carrying dietitian in good standing, I certainly am not going to tell people to eat more sugar. But we must be clear that added sugars provide 4 [calories per gram] just like any other digestible carbohydrate and are no more likely to cause weight gain than any other calorie source. The rationale to reduce intake of added sugars…is to reduce calories and thereby increase nutrient density.

But are we really to believe that a cup of Coke would be as healthy as a large apple (both with about 100 calories), if we drank it with a serving of Metamucil and a multivitamin pill?

Which isn't to say that nutrients don't also matter. Knowledge of nutrients helped conquer diseases of undernutrition, like pellagra (deficiency of a B vitamin), scurvy (deficiency of vitamin C), and rickets (deficiency of vitamin D). But a primary focus on nutrients has proven utterly ineffective in addressing the epidemics of chronic disease caused by overnutrition.[42] In fact, as discussed throughout this chapter, foods with similar nutrients can affect hormones and metabolism in profoundly different ways, determining whether we store or burn calories, build fat or muscle, feel hungry or satisfied, struggle with weight or maintain a healthy weight effortlessly, and suffer from or avoid chronic inflammation. In the next chapter, we'll see how these novel aspects of food can be used to create a powerful prescription for weight loss and disease prevention.

My Always Hungry Story

I have a friend who started a low-calorie diet program the same day that I started mine. She thinks it's "silly and restrictive" that there are some things that I just don't eat anymore. As we continued to describe our plans, I mentioned to her that I am eating full-fat dairy and putting cream in my coffee—a fact she found totally bizarre, that I would add things that "make you fat" and delete others that she considers healthy. As she went on and on about the poor psychology of deleting some foods entirely, I was starting to feel pretty ridiculous and defensive. But then she said, "See, my program is great because if I want to have Cheetos for breakfast, it tells me how many I can eat. I had Cheetos for breakfast this morning and that's fine." Yeah, I am *so* glad I don't have to wonder how many Cheetos I can have for breakfast anymore! I remember now how insane that felt.

—Holly C., 37, Raleigh, NC
Weight loss: 5 pounds. Decrease in waist: 2 inches

CHAPTER 4

The Solution

Forget calories.
Focus on quality.
Let your body do the rest.

In chapter 3, we saw why conventional diets rarely work. Excessive weight gain occurs when fat cells suck up and store too many calories, leaving too few for the rest of the body. Low-fat, low-calorie diets don't solve this basic problem, and can make matters worse. Faced with calorie deprivation, the body goes into starvation mode and fights back. Hunger and food cravings rise and metabolism slows—the perfect recipe for weight regain and disordered eating habits.

A more effective approach is to *reprogram your fat cells* to lose weight, by eating in a way that lowers insulin levels and reduces inflammation. When this happens, fat cells calm down and release their excess calorie stores. As the body begins to enjoy better access to fuel, metabolism runs better, hunger and cravings subside, and weight loss occurs naturally. It's diet without deprivation.

In this chapter, we'll take a deeper look into the components of this approach. But feel free to jump right to the Always Hungry Solution in part 2 if you've had enough science for now.

THE MAJOR NUTRIENTS—
CARBOHYDRATE, PROTEIN, AND FAT

Mini Quiz #1:

What is the minimum amount of carbohydrate required for long-term survival?

(Answer on page 73.)

What major nutrients does the body require to run effectively? The answer may be surprising. The body needs a few ounces of protein from the diet on a daily basis to repair tissues and to run the biochemical reactions that make up our metabolism. It needs a fraction of an ounce of fat (specifically, the essential *omega*-3 and *omega*-6 fatty acids) for cell membranes and cell-to-cell communication. Beyond these minimal amounts, our nutritional requirements can be satisfied with almost any combination of the major nutrients. The one nutrient we don't need at all is carbohydrate.

In the absence of carbohydrate from the diet, the body can produce all the fuel needed by the brain from protein and fat alone. We have enormous biological flexibility in which major nutrients to eat. That's why Inuits in the Arctic could survive on traditional diets consisting almost exclusively of sea and land animals. In contrast, many hunter-gatherers living at less extreme latitudes eat plant-based diets, with meat as a supplement.[1]

Today, we also have a virtually unlimited choice of foods, leading to a key question: What is the optimal proportion of carbohydrate, protein, and fat for weight control and chronic disease prevention? More than any other, this question distinguishes most popular weight loss diets, ranging from the very-high-carbohydrate Ornish diet to the ultra-low-carbohydrate ketogenic diet (see A Comparison of Popular Weight Loss Diets graph on page 72).

Phase 1 of the program is located to the right side of the figure,

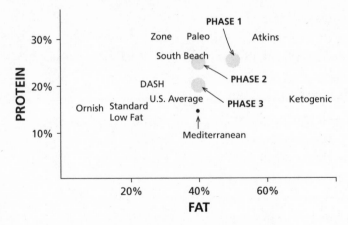

A Comparison of Popular Weight Loss Diets

near—but not as stringent as—the Atkins diet. Phase 2 resembles in nutrient composition the South Beach, Zone, and Paleo diets. Phase 3 moves closer to a typical Mediterranean diet. This final phase resides squarely in the middle of the figure, one indication that it is among the least restrictive of all options.

We cut total carbohydrate in half for the two weeks of Phase 1, from about 50 percent typically consumed in the United States to 25 percent of total calories (100 to 150 grams, based on energy requirements). Decreasing carbohydrate is the quickest and easiest way to lower insulin levels and jump-start weight loss. In Phases 2 and 3, total carbohydrate increases moderately, to about 40 percent of total calories. The type of carbohydrate also matters critically in all phases, which we'll consider in the next section.

Beyond basic biological requirements, protein plays an important role in weight control, in part by triggering release of the hormone glucagon.[2] Glucagon, also made in the pancreas, performs the opposite functions of insulin, by pulling fuels out of storage and helping to prevent the calorie crash a few hours after eating. In this way, glucagon and insulin have complementary effects on metabolism. Protein in the right amounts counterbalances carbohydrate.

But before digging in to that 20-ounce steak, keep in mind that the biological range for dietary protein is substantially smaller than for the other major nutrients. Intakes above 35 to 40 percent of total calories exceed the liver's capacity to process amino acids (the building blocks of protein), resulting in buildup of ammonia to toxic levels.[3] People naturally tend to avoid getting anywhere near that upper limit. On this program, you will consume 100 to 140 grams of protein a day, which works out to approximately 25 percent of daily calorie intake in Phases 1 and 2. Protein proportion then decreases to 20 percent in Phase 3, as body weight and calorie intake stabilize.

The remainder of calories comes from fat, with an emphasis on the types found in olive oil and nuts. As we saw in chapter 3, these fats are among the healthiest components of the diet. They slow digestion rate, help you feel full for hours after eating, and powerfully lower risk for heart disease. They also make for delicious recipes—no Spartan low-fat dressing, sauces, or spreads here! In Phase 1, fat comprises 50 percent of total calories, displacing all processed carbohydrate. This high amount will lower insulin secretion, help soothe fat cells, and get metabolism back on track. Fat proportion decreases to 40 percent by Phase 3, approximately equal to carbohydrate (based on individual tolerance), providing flexibility in food choices.

(Mini Quiz #1 Answer: 0)

LOW CARBOHYDRATE OR SLOW CARBOHYDRATE?

Mini Quiz #2:

Which of the following raises blood glucose and insulin the most after consumption, calorie for calorie?

1. white potato (baked)
2. ice cream
3. pure table sugar

(Answer on page 78.)

People with major metabolic problems, like severe insulin resistance or type 2 diabetes, may benefit from long-term carbohydrate restriction—to 25 percent of daily calories as in Phase 1 or sometimes even lower. Preliminary studies report that some individuals experience remarkable improvements in health by eliminating virtually all carbohydrates on a ketogenic diet.[4] Without carbohydrate, insulin secretion plummets and the body switches from the sugar glucose to ketones (chemicals derived directly from fat) as its main fuel. Some scientists consider ketones to be a sort of "superfuel" that might enhance mental performance, physical endurance, and general well-being, and possibly slow down the aging process.[5] However, ketogenic and other very-low-carbohydrate diets can be quite challenging to follow over the long term, and the possibility of adverse effects has not been ruled out. Usually, such severe restriction isn't necessary.

Just as calories differ according to how they affect the body, so too do carbohydrates. All carbohydrates break down into sugar, but the rate at which this occurs in the digestive tract varies tremendously from food to food. This difference forms the basis for the glycemic index (GI).[6]

The GI ranks carbohydrate-containing foods according to how they affect blood glucose, from 0 (no affect at all) to 100 (equal to glucose). Gram for gram, most starchy foods raise blood glucose to very high levels and therefore have high GI values. In fact, highly processed grain products—like white bread, white rice, and prepared breakfast cereals—and the modern white potato digest so quickly that their GI ratings are even greater than table sugar (sucrose). So for breakfast, you could have a bowl of cornflakes with no added sugar, or a bowl of sugar with no added cornflakes. They would taste different but, below the neck, act more or less the same. Minimally processed grains, nonstarchy vegetables, whole fruits, beans, nuts, and unsweetened dairy products have more gentle effects on blood glucose and, consequently, lower GI values.

A related concept is the glycemic load (GL), which accounts for the different carbohydrate content of foods as typically consumed (see the Glycemic Load of Carbohydrate-Containing Foods chart in

Appendix A, page 305).[7] Watermelon has a high GI, but relatively little carbohydrate in a standard serving, producing a moderate GL. In contrast, white potato has a high GI and lots of carbohydrate in a serving, producing a high GL. If this sounds a bit complicated, think of GI as describing how foods rank in a laboratory setting, whereas GL as applying more directly to a real-life setting. Research has shown that the GL reliably predicts, to within about 90 percent, how blood glucose will change after an actual meal—much better than simply counting carbohydrates as people with diabetes have been taught to do.

Hundreds of studies have examined the effects of GI and GL on body weight and numerous other health outcomes.[8] In the largest clinical trial of its kind ever done,[9] 773 adults from eight European countries who had achieved at least 8 percent weight loss on a standard diet were randomly assigned to diets varying in GI and protein. After six months, the group on the low-GI/high-protein diet (which would be lowest in GL) showed complete weight loss maintenance, with no weight regain at all—an impressive accomplishment for a diet study. Participants on the high-GI/low-protein diet (highest in GL) regained the most weight, and those on the other two combinations—low-GI/low-protein and high-GI/high-protein (both medium in GL)—regained an intermediate amount of weight. These data resemble a dose-response curve, common in drug studies but rarely seen in nutrition. The findings are clear: Each stepwise decrease in GL produced progressively better results.

Even controlling for body weight, high-GI and -GL diets are associated with chronic disease in observational studies. A major analysis, including all published data on the topic, found that people with high-GI diets had 20 percent increased risk for diabetes compared to those with low-GI diets.[10] It stands to reason that the excessive rise and fall of blood glucose on a high-GI diet would put stress on the insulin-producing cells of the pancreas. If those cells are already struggling because of insulin resistance, chronic inflammation, or genetic risk factors, a high-GI diet could be the last straw.

High-GI and -GL diets are also strongly associated with risk for heart disease. In one study of about 75,000 women, a high-GL diet increased risk for coronary heart disease twofold over ten years.[11] These results suggest that switching from a high- to a low-GL diet could cut heart disease risk in half—and that's exactly what's been seen in clinical trials of drugs like acarbose that act by slowing down digestion of carbohydrates in the gut.[12] (Though unlike a low-GL diet, these drugs have side effects.)

In addition, high-GI and -GL diets have been linked to cancer (breast, endometrial, colorectal), stroke, gallbladder disease, fatty liver, and depression in observational analyses, but more research is needed on these relationships.[13]

Despite strong evidence favoring a low-GI diet, small or short-term studies do show some inconsistencies in outcomes, as is virtually always the case in nutrition research. Researchers from Boston and Baltimore gave 163 adults four diets varying in carbohydrate and GI, keeping calorie intake constant throughout the study. They reported that the low-GI diets produced no improvements in insulin sensitivity, lipids, or blood pressure after 3.5 to 5 weeks.[14] However, as my colleagues and I recently argued, this study may simply not be long enough to see potentially important effects.[15] For example, 316 adults in the United Kingdom were randomly assigned to three groups and provided varying amount of whole grains for sixteen weeks. Even though the duration of this study was more than three times longer than the Boston and Baltimore study, there were no effects on any of twenty-two cardiovascular disease risk factors, including body weight, lipids, and blood pressure.[16] We wouldn't abandon the recommendation to substitute whole grains for refined grains based on short-term studies. In any event, other clinical studies of low-GI diets have reported significant improvements in insulin resistance, chronic inflammation, and serum lipids, especially when calorie intake and body weight were allowed to fluctuate naturally.[17]

Compared to severely restricting carbohydrate as with the Atkins diet, the effects of a low-GI diet are less dramatic at first. But many people can't remain on very-low-carbohydrate diets indefinitely. A low-GI diet may be more like the tortoise than the hare—it takes a bit longer, but gets you there in the end. Thus, switching from highly processed carbohydrates to low-GI alternatives can reduce body weight and lower risk for chronic disease without having to abandon a whole class of nutritious (and delicious) foods.

Another benefit of a minimally processed, low-GL diet may be fewer gastric bypass surgeries.[18] Because whole foods tend to digest slowly, some of their nutrients travel down the full length of the small intestines, simulating powerful hormones that rev up metabolism and help us feel full (a feedback mechanism called the "ileal brake"). Highly processed industrial foods—epitomized by modern fast foods—digest in the first segments of the intestines, too quickly to trigger this built-in weight-regulating mechanism. Not surprisingly, fast-food consumption is strongly linked to obesity and type 2 diabetes.[19] To deal with the consequences of too much highly processed foods (which comprise the majority of the American diet[20]), we're increasingly resorting to weight loss surgery. The most common procedure of this type (called roux-en-Y gastric bypass) reroutes the gastrointestinal tract, so that even rapidly digestible food reaches farther down in the intestines. As a result, people experience intense feelings of satiety regardless of what they eat. From this perspective, we seem to have a choice—bypass the gastrointestinal tract or bypass the highly processed diet.

Whole, natural, slow-digesting foods provide the foundation for all phases of the program. In Phase 1, you'll eliminate—for just two weeks—grain products, potatoes, and concentrated sugars (except for a small amount in very dark chocolate). Instead, carbohydrate will come from the lowest GL foods, including nonstarchy vegetables, non-tropical fruits, beans, and nuts. But rest assured that with three meals and two snacks a day of rich, satisfying foods, you won't feel hungry or deprived, and your cravings will quickly subside. You might be surprised how easily you can do without all the processed carbohydrates!

In Phase 2, you'll add back minimally processed grains, starchy vegetables (except white potato), tropical fruits like banana, and a touch of sugar. And in Phase 3, some of the more processed carbohydrates can be mindfully reintroduced, allowing for maximum flexibility based on individual tolerance. For people following a gluten-free diet, the Always Hungry Solution is easily adaptable, with whole-kernel alternatives to wheat and other gluten-containing grains.

(Mini Quiz #2 Answer: 1. white potato)

TYPES OF FAT

Mini Quiz #3:

Which is less healthy for your heart—white bread or butter?

(Answer on page 81.)

For much of the last half century, fat was considered the least healthy of the three major nutrients, and saturated fat the worst possible type of fat.[21] Saturated fats, such as those in butter and coconut, form a solid at room temperature. In contrast, monounsaturated fats (in olive oil and nuts) and polyunsaturated fats (in fatty fish, some nuts, and vegetable oils) are liquid at room temperature.

Saturated fat got a bad reputation in the 1960s with the observation that it raised LDL cholesterol, a risk factor for heart disease. Since then, national nutritional recommendations have consistently advised reducing saturated fat intake to very low levels. Largely for that reason, consumption of margarine made from partially hydrogenated vegetable oils (also known as *trans* fats) surged in the 1970s and 1980s. Solid at room temperature, trans fats became an attractive alternative to butter for health-conscious consumers. Unfortunately, these unnatural fats turned out to be far worse than saturated fat, becoming the closest thing to poison among additives in the food supply.[22] Until recent efforts to ban their use, trans fats caused tens of thousands of deaths from cardiovascular disease each year in the United States.[23]

Recently, the pendulum has swung in the other direction, with some popular diet books lauding the nutritional benefits of saturated fat. Despite its negative effects on LDL cholesterol, saturated fat also raises heart-protective HDL cholesterol, leaving their ratio relatively unchanged. In contrast, high-GI carbohydrates lower HDL cholesterol and raise triglycerides, combined effects that appear to be worse for cardiovascular disease than saturated fat.[24] Danish researchers confirmed this possibility in a study of about fifty thousand adults followed for twelve years. They found that exchanging saturated fat for high-GI carbohydrates was associated with a 33 percent increased risk for heart attack.[25] Exchanging saturated fat with low-GI carbohydrates decreased risk, but that trade-off doesn't typically occur. When people in Western countries eat less saturated fat, they tend to have more refined starch and sugar—not fruits, beans, or nuts.[26]

Indeed, two highly publicized reviews showed essentially no relationship between saturated fat consumption and cardiovascular disease in the general population.[27] However, these analyses inevitably set the bar quite low. The average diet in the United States and other Western countries is loaded with highly processed foods and predisposes the entire population to cardiovascular disease and diabetes. For a dietary component not to increase risk beyond this already high level isn't saying very much.

Many studies show that diets high in unsaturated fat rather than saturated fat reduce disease risk. In an analysis of randomized controlled trials involving about thirteen thousand participants, substitution of polyunsaturated fat for saturated fat decreased cardiovascular disease by 19 percent, with even larger effects seen in the longest interventions.[28] Monounsaturated fats may provide similar benefits.[29] Of particular concern, saturated fat may also cause chronic inflammation and insulin resistance, the underlying biological events linking obesity to chronic disease. After just one meal, saturated fat adversely affected markers of inflammation in the blood, blood vessel elasticity, and insulin action compared to unsaturated fat.[30] In animal studies, a diet high in saturated fat has been shown to activate powerful inflammatory pathways, cause inflammation of the hypothalamus (the key brain region regulating hunger and metabolism), increase insulin levels, and alter fat cell activity.[31]

Two recent studies provide further evidence that, like carbohydrate, all fat calories are not alike. In one trial, thirty-nine adults of normal weight were overfed 750 calories a day with muffins containing either saturated fat (from palm oil) or polyunsaturated fat (sunflower oil). After seven weeks, both groups had gained about 3 pounds, as expected, but total body fat and liver fat were significantly greater in the saturated fat group, whereas lean body tissue was greater in the polyunsaturated fat group.[32] In the other trial, thirty-four young adults received diets that were high in either saturated (palmitic) or monounsaturated (oleic) fat during two separate three-week periods. Otherwise, the diets were the same, and neither the participants nor the researchers knew which type of fat was given first. Remarkably, participants consuming the saturated fat diet had slower metabolic rate at rest, were spontaneously less physically active, and reported higher levels of anger and hostility.[33] It's not so surprising that the quality of the fat we eat can influence our metabolism, body composition, energy level, and even emotions when you consider the profound effects that chronic inflammation and insulin resistance have on the body and the brain.

Furthermore, not all saturated fats are alike. The saturated fats in dairy appear to be healthier than those in red meat.[34] Shorter chain saturated fatty acids, such as the kind found in coconut, are metabolized quickly and don't stick around long enough to cause much trouble. And to make matters even more complicated, the amount and type of carbohydrate in the diet influences how dietary fat affects blood lipids, with saturated fat and processed carbohydrate being an especially dangerous combination.[35] So without bread, butter may be relatively benign.

In the raging debate about saturated fats, the truth probably falls in the middle. They are neither public health enemy #1 nor a health food.

With the Always Hungry Solution, you'll eat lots of unsaturated fats, but also saturated fats in moderate amounts. Some foods high in saturated fat—like cultured dairy products, coconut, and chocolate—can make a delicious contribution to a high-quality diet, and there is no reason to avoid them. And a dash of heavy cream with fresh berries makes a much healthier dessert than the usual sugar-laden options. In addition, the Always Hungry Solution includes several servings of fish each week to provide long chain omega-3 fats. These polyunsaturated fats are the building blocks of critical anti-inflammatory cellular signals,[36] and we generally don't eat enough of them in the United States. A fish oil supplement may also be helpful, especially for those with chronic inflammation. Vegetarians can satisfy this nutritional requirement with flax oil or some types of nuts, but the omega-3 fat in plants is short chain and somewhat less efficient in the body.

(Mini Quiz #3 Answer: white bread)

ANIMAL OR VEGETABLE?

Mini Quiz #4:

Which has the most protein, ounce for ounce?
1. hard-boiled egg
2. chicken nuggets
3. hot dog
4. tempeh (a soybean product commonly consumed in some Asian countries)

(Answer on page 82.)

Some diet books consider meat toxic. Others extol it as an exceptionally high-quality food. Here, too, the truth is likely in the middle.

Since the dawn of our species, animal products have made a major contribution to human nutrition, with concentrated amounts of protein, fat, and other vital nutrients. But today's factory-farmed cows and chicken are different from those allowed to graze freely, which our grandparents would have eaten, and certainly from the wild animals our ancestors hunted.[37] Industrial animal production also raises major ethical and environmental issues. And there simply aren't enough wild animals for the world's 7 billion people.

For adults, nutritional needs can be satisfied with a vegetarian diet containing dairy and eggs, or a (carefully managed) vegan diet containing no animal products at all. Contrary to common belief, some plant products provide high amounts of protein, such as tempeh with 23 grams in 4 ounces—comparing favorably to similar-size portions of hard-boiled eggs (13 grams), chicken nuggets (14 grams), or hot dog (12 grams).

There's also some indication that replacing carbohydrate with plant rather than animal foods has special health benefits. Among approximately eighty thousand women in the Nurses' Health Study consuming lower-carbohydrate diets, high consumption of vegetable protein and fat was associated with a 30 percent lower risk for heart disease over twenty years, whereas high consumption of animal protein and fat appeared to provide no such protection.[38]

One explanation for this finding is that the relative amounts of amino acids in animal protein stimulate more insulin and less glucagon release than those in plant protein—a hormone combination that has detrimental effects on serum cholesterol and fat-cell metabolism.[39] Other possible downsides of a modern, animal-based diet include a less healthful profile of dietary fats, excessive iron absorption (especially for men), and chronic exposure to hormones, preservatives, and environmental pollutants.

Ultimately, we have a choice about how much meat, dairy, and eggs to eat. This decision involves more than health; it's also a matter of personal preference, culture, ethics, and the environment. From an individual health perspective, the scientific evidence provides no reason to banish animal products. However, an emphasis on plants seems sensible, for ourselves and our planet. For this reason, the Always Hungry Solution provides vegetarian options for all recipes and meal plans.

(Mini Quiz #4 Answer: 4. tempeh)

PROBIOTICS, PREBIOTICS, AND POLYPHENOLS

Mini Quiz #5:

True or False: The microbes in our intestinal tract outnumber the cells in our body.

(Answer on page 85.)

Humans have always had an intimate relationship with microbes, from constant exposures through food, water, dirt, animals, and one another. Our digestive tract contains a vast collection of bacteria, viruses, and other microorganisms, estimated to total over 100 trillion[40]—compared to about 35 trillion of our own cells in the body. Most of these microorganisms are benign or even beneficial. However, in Western societies, the biodiversity and richness of this gut microbiome may suffer for a variety of reasons: reduced exposure to microbes in our modern "hygienic" environment, our highly processed diet, and frequent antibiotic use.[41]

In addition to helping digest food, the microbiome plays an especially important role in maintaining the health and integrity of the gut lining—the critical barrier separating intestinal contents from our internal bodily environment. With a proper diet, beneficial bacteria produce fermentation by-products (such as short chain fatty acids) that nourish the colon, helping to reinforce the normally impermeable connections between adjacent cells. Beneficial bacteria also keep the immune cells in the intestinal tract functioning calmly through a complex series of interactions that are only now being identified. However, if the microbiome contains the wrong type or amount of bacteria, the intestinal lining may become damaged and leaky, allowing incompletely digested food and microbial breakdown products to be absorbed directly into the bloodstream. Long-term exposure to these toxic substances puts the immune system into overdrive, increasing the risk of diabetes and other obesity-related complications.[42] In addition, leaky gut has been linked to an astonishing number of other diseases, including asthma, arthritis, eczema, psoriasis, irritable bowel syndrome, chronic fatigue syndrome, depression, schizophrenia, multiple sclerosis, Alzheimer's, and more.[43]

What does this have to do with weight loss? The gut microbiomes of people with obesity and those without appear to differ in consistent ways.[44] When Danish researchers examined 192 adults of varying body weight, they were able to identify two distinct groups based on gut bacteria composition. Compared to individuals with high bacterial richness, those with low richness had more insulin resistance and chronic inflammation, and tended to gain more weight.[45]

In a study that would have seemed straight out of science fiction a few years ago, separate groups of mice raised in a germ-free environment were given fecal transplants from human twin pairs who differed in body weight (one lean, the other heavy). Astoundingly, mice that received transplants from the heavy twins became significantly fatter than mice receiving transplants from the lean twins. Furthermore, cohousing the animals together allowed bacteria from the lean mice to spread to the other group, protecting them from excessive weight gain.[46]

How do we maintain a healthy microbial garden in our gut? Clearly, the answer isn't to abandon handwashing and other hygienic practices. Instead, by analogy to an actual garden, we need to plant the right seeds, fertilize the soil, and carefully eliminate weeds. This is accomplished with probiotics, prebiotics, and polyphenols.

Probiotics are live beneficial bacteria (and sometimes yeast) present in certain foods and nutritional supplements. Prebiotics are the components of plants, typically grouped under the term "fiber," that can't be digested in the small intestines and instead provide food for beneficial bacteria in the colon. And polyphenols are plant-derived chemicals, abundant in colorful fruits and vegetables (especially berries), that can slow the growth of toxic microbes—allowing beneficial bacteria to flourish.[47] In addition, some polyphenols, like curcumin from the spice turmeric, can be absorbed from the intestinal tract and exert an anti-inflammatory effect throughout the body.[48] Whole plant foods and live fermented products provide these three microbiome-enhancing factors, helping to keep this internal ecology working for rather than against us.[49]

Whether you choose standard or vegetarian options, all phases of the Always Hungry Solution provide an abundance of whole plant foods that will cultivate a vibrant and well-behaved microbiome. Yogurt also appears frequently on the meal plan—make sure to choose products with live cultures. Try to include other dietary sources of probiotics as often as possible, such as authentic fermented pickles (not the versions made with vinegar), sauerkraut, kimchi, and kefir. You may also want to consider taking a high-quality probiotic supplement. In addition, the recipes use a liberal amount of spices, to provide both flavor and rich sources of polyphenols. And avoid emulsifiers (like carboxymethylcellulose, polysorbate-80, and lecithin) which may break down the intestine's protective mucus lining.[50]

(Mini Quiz #5 Answer: True)

SUGAR AND ARTIFICIAL SWEETENERS

Mini Quiz #6:

Is fructose toxic?

(Answer on page 88.)

In the 1990s, sugar was commonly considered harmless and sugary beverages were touted as "fat-free."[51] Today, some notable experts regard high consumption of fructose, a primary component of sugar, to be the main problem with the American diet, uniquely responsible for the twin epidemics of obesity and diabetes.[52] As with some other dietary debates addressed in this chapter, the truth is probably more nuanced.

Most sugars are composed of three basic building blocks— glucose, fructose, and galactose—singly or combined in various ways.

The common sweeteners, such as table sugar (sucrose), maple syrup, honey, and high-fructose corn syrup, contain approximately equal proportions of glucose and fructose. Since fructose tastes much sweeter than glucose or galactose, sugars without this component (such as lactose and maltose) have limited use.

With the obsessive focus on decreasing fat intake since the 1970s, consumption of fructose-containing sweeteners rose substantially, especially in the form of sugary beverages.[53] Might this trend have contributed to the obesity epidemic? Unlike glucose, which can be used by all cells in the body, fructose is metabolized almost exclusively in the liver. Too much at one time overwhelms the liver, with the excess being diverted into the production of new molecules of fat. Eventually, fatty liver and other metabolic problems may result.

Several studies have documented insulin resistance, higher triglycerides, higher blood pressure, and increased belly fat among research participants given diets with about 150 grams of fructose per day compared to diets with an equivalent amount of glucose.[54] However, these studies have been criticized for providing unrealistically large amounts of fructose, triple the average intake of about 50 grams.[55] Moreover, high consumption of fruit—the primary natural source of fructose—is associated with better, not worse outcomes in observational studies.[56] In possibly the only clinical trial of its kind, seventeen South African adults were instructed to follow diets consisting primarily of fruit for a minimum of twelve weeks, with small amounts of nuts to satisfy nutritional requirements. The participants consumed on average twenty servings a day or more, likely containing at least 200 grams fructose. At the end of the study, the investigators observed virtually no adverse effects. To the contrary, body weight and other heart disease risk factors tended to improve despite this massive dose of fructose.[57]

Similar to the concept of glycemic index, the main concern with fructose probably isn't total amount, but rather the rate of absorption into the body.[58] High-GI bread has an adverse impact on metabolism compared to low-GI beans, though both have about the same amount of carbohydrate in a serving. After we eat conventional sweeteners like high-fructose corn syrup, table sugar, or honey, fructose hits the liver rapidly. Eating more than a small amount of any of them can cause fructose to spill over into metabolic pathways leading to fat production. By contrast, fructose in whole fruit is absorbed slowly, because it's surrounded by fiber and sequestered within the cells of the fruit. For this reason, even large amounts of whole fruit generally won't overtax your liver. The situation is like alcohol, another compound metabolized primarily in the liver. The liver can usually handle one drink, but seven at one time would cause damage.

Fructose isn't inherently toxic, and whole fruit is among the healthiest foods we can eat. Nor is glucose benign when present either in sweeteners or rapidly released with digestion of high-GI foods. Simply replacing fructose-containing sweeteners with highly processed, glucose-based carbohydrate (either fructose-free sugar or starch) may miss the point, as suggested by two small clinical trials from the 1970s. In one study, nineteen men on an Antarctic expedition were given a standard diet with 400 calories a day from table sugar, or an experimental fructose-free diet using glucose from corn syrup. The investigators reported no difference in calorie intake and body weight, and no consistent differences in blood sugar levels after at least fourteen weeks on each diet.[59] In another study, nine adults were examined in a metabolic ward on a high-sugar diet (70 percent of carbohydrate as table sugar, an average of about 675 calories a day) or a sugar-free diet with additional wheat and potato starch. After four weeks on each diet, there were no differences in body weight, glucose tolerance, insulin levels, or serum lipids.[60] We certainly need more research on the topic, but as I see it, the similarities among all concentrated sugars and refined starch outweigh their metabolic differences.

How about artificial sweeteners, which contain no fructose or glucose at all? With saccharin instead of sugar, can we have our cake and eat it, too? Although artificial sweeteners—also including acesulfame, aspartame, neotame, and sucralose—have essentially no calories, they still affect the body.[61] These synthetic chemicals stimulate taste receptors for sweetness hundreds to thousands of times more powerfully than sugar, with possible detrimental effects on diet quality. People who regularly consume artificial sweeteners may find naturally sweet foods (like fruit) unappealing, and unsweet foods (like vegetables) intolerable. Artificial sweeteners may also cause insulin secretion, driving calories into fat cells and stimulating hunger.[62] In addition, fat cells have been reported to contain sweet taste receptors—similar to those on the tongue. Artificial sweeteners may promote fat cell growth by stimulating these receptors or in other ways.[63]

In the Always Hungry Solution, you'll avoid all added sugar in Phase 1 (except for a small amount in dark chocolate). In Phases 2 and 3, you can add back a moderate amount, based on individual tolerance. But it's best to satisfy desire for sweetness mostly the old-fashioned way—with fresh fruit. When using added sweetener, choose pure maple syrup or honey instead of table sugar when possible. These less-refined sweeteners contain nutrients and polyphenols that may partially counterbalance the sugar. They also have stronger flavor, so you can get by with less. None of the recipes and meal plans contains artificial sweeteners. After giving up the hypersweetened stuff, you may be surprised to discover just how sweet and flavorful fresh seasonal fruit can taste.

(Mini Quiz #6 Answer: No)

SALT

Mini Quiz #7:

True or False: Sodium consumption should be reduced as much as possible.

(Answer on page 90.)

Many processed foods have a tremendous amount of salt that, together with sugar, helps make cheap industrial food products taste good. A single serving of Jack in the Box Crispy Chicken Strips contains 1,580 milligrams of sodium—more than the government recommended total daily limit for everyone over age fifty.[64] High intake of salt can cause hypertension, increasing the risk for heart attack, stroke, and kidney disease. Since only a small portion of the sodium in our diet normally comes by way of the kitchen saltshaker, eliminating highly processed foods naturally lowers salt consumption. But when it comes to salt, is less always more?

The concentration of sodium in the blood is controlled to within a very narrow range. When intake rises, the kidneys excrete the excess. When intake falls below 3 to 4 grams a day, the body compensates by activating powerful hormones, called the renin-angiotensin system (RAS), which helps the kidneys hold on tightly to salt.[65] The problem is, receptors for RAS are present not only in the kidneys, but also in fat cells, muscle, the pancreas, the lining of the blood vessels, and elsewhere. Overactivity of this system has been shown to cause fat cell dysfunction, insulin resistance, and inflammation—the fundamental problems linking obesity to diabetes and heart disease. Blocking RAS, such as with the widely used ACE inhibitors, lowers risk for these two major killers out of proportion to the drugs' effects on blood pressure.[66]

Based on this reasoning, excessive restriction of salt could have adverse consequences, a possibility supported by several lines of research. The Cochrane Collaboration (an international organization that sponsors systematic reviews of scientific evidence) examined 167 randomized clinical trials from 1950 to 2011 comparing low-salt to high-salt diets. They found that among whites without hypertension, sodium reduction produced a decrease in systolic blood pressure of only 1 millimeter of mercury and no decrease in diastolic blood pressure. African Americans and people with hypertension experienced somewhat greater improvements in blood pressure, ranging from 2 to 6 millimeters of mercury. However, sodium reduction also increased RAS activity, adrenaline, cholesterol, and triglycerides, suggesting that it may worsen insulin resistance.[67]

In a recent study in the *New England Journal of Medicine* that followed about one hundred thousand people for an average of four years, the risk of major cardiovascular disease or death was lowest among those with sodium intakes ranging from 3 to 6 grams—well above currently recommended levels—compared to either lower or higher amounts.[68] These findings received a great deal of attention in the media, but must be interpreted cautiously. Individuals at risk for heart disease might be more likely to follow medical advice and reduce their salt consumption. So the increased risk in this observational study among those consuming a low-salt diet might reflect preexisting disease, rather than the effects of sodium itself.

The jury is still out regarding optimal levels of intake. But one thing seems clear: A fast-food, junk-food diet provides too much salt in addition to all the highly processed carbohydrate (an especially bad combination for heart health). For people with hypertension or other special risk factors, low sodium intake significantly lowers blood pressure—a major public health goal. But for everyone else, sodium reduction from average to very low levels appears to have negligible benefit for blood pressure and may cause metabolic problems. Potentially more effective ways to control blood pressure may be to lower intakes of added sugar[69] and other highly processed carbohydrates,[70] reduce stress, and increase physical activity—all components of the Always Hungry Solution.

The amount of sodium on the program diet will total less than 3 grams a day for most people (depending on how much salt you add to your meals), below average levels in the United States throughout the last half century.[71] But if you are following a low-sodium diet, the recipes and meal plans can be easily adapted to your needs.

(Mini Quiz #7 Answer: False)

FOOD ADDITIVES AND POLLUTANTS

Mini Quiz #8:

How many food additives are FDA approved?

(Answer on page 91.)

Ultraprocessed industrial foods lack a great many health-promoting qualities, such as high-quality fats, slow-digesting carbohydrates, essential vitamins and minerals, fiber, probiotics, and polyphenols. They do contain a staggering array of preservatives, colorants, flavorings, emulsifiers, and other artificial ingredients. In addition, pesticides, plastics, antibiotics, heavy metals, and other pollutants inadvertently find their way into our food and water supply. Some of these substances interfere with hormones in especially harmful ways for fat tissue.[72] Recently, two physicians from the University of Chicago made the provocative (and alarming) argument that our fat cells are "under assault" from the toxic chemicals in our environment.[73] As just one example, rats exposed to low-dose bisphenol A (BPA)—a chemical that was widely used in plastic food containers—around the time of birth gained excessive weight and showed extensive changes in the behavior of their fat cells.[74]

In truth, most artificial additives and pollutants in our food have never been thoroughly tested for long-term health effects.[75] And who knows how these chemicals interact in various combinations inside the body? By emphasizing whole, natural foods, the Always Hungry Solution reduces these exposures substantially. You can further reduce exposures by purchasing organic or pesticide-free produce when feasible and using a good-quality water filter at home.

(Mini Quiz #8 Answer: More than 3,000, not including substances "Generally Recognized as Safe"[76])

BONUS—Mini Quiz #9:

True or False: Sour Triple Berry Shock Fruit Gushers contain berries.

(Answer below.)

(Mini Quiz #9 Answer: False. The ingredients include pears from concentrate, sugar, dried corn syrup, corn syrup, modified cornstarch, fructose, grape juice from concentrate, partially hydrogenated cottonseed oil, citric acid, maltodextrin, cottonseed oil, carrageenan, glycerin, monoglycerides, sodium citrate, malic acid, potassium citrate, ascorbic acid, flavors, agar-agar, artificial colors, and xanthan gum.[77])

PERSONALIZED DIETING—PREPARING FOR PHASE 3

Mini Quiz #10:

> Which biological factor best predicts how individuals will respond to diets with varying amounts of carbohydrate?
> 1. Blood type
> 2. Eye color
> 3. Insulin secretion
>
> *(Answer on page 95.)*

On average, human DNA is 99.9 percent identical from one person to the next. So it's not surprising that the contours of a healthful diet—one that satisfies all nutritional requirements and keeps levels of insulin and inflammation low—don't differ among people very much. A diet based on whole, natural, slow-digesting foods lowers everyone's risk for chronic disease, regardless of body weight, age, sex, race, or country of origin.

But just as risks for many specific diseases vary between individuals, so too does tolerance for poor eating patterns. Some people have a resilient and adaptable metabolism, especially when young and physically active. Others seem to be exquisitely sensitive to processed carbohydrates, certain types of fat[78] (potentially explaining some of the controversies previously considered in this chapter), or wide variations in the relative proportions of major nutrients in the diet. My collaborators and I have explored this issue for more than a decade and found that insulin secretion plays a key role.

After eating carbohydrate, the pancreas secretes insulin to keep blood sugar from rising too high, but the amount and timing of insulin secretion varies substantially from person to person. To assess this difference in research, we give volunteers (or sometimes experimental animals) an oral glucose solution and then measure insulin in the blood thirty minutes later—the test is called the Insulin-30 level.

In a study published in the *American Journal of Clinical Nutrition*,[79] we followed 276 middle-aged adults in Quebec for six years, dividing them into categories based on diet. Overall, the participants gained about 6 pounds (quite typical for this age group), but with huge individual variation—ranging from a 20-pound weight loss to a 30-pound weight gain. For those consuming a high-carbohydrate/low-fat diet, Insulin-30 strongly predicted this variation. That is, people with low insulin secretion gained on average virtually no weight, whereas those with high insulin secretion gained on average more than 10 pounds. In contrast, Insulin-30 had no relationship to weight gain among those consuming a low-carbohydrate/high-fat diet. Furthermore, hypoglycemia several hours after consuming glucose was more severe in the high-carbohydrate/low-fat group, and predicted weight gain.

This study suggests that some people are especially sensitive to carbohydrate for biological reasons. A high-carbohydrate diet exacerbates their underlying tendency to secrete too much insulin, creating a vicious cycle of high insulin followed by low blood sugar that leads to excessive weight gain. But these individuals can reduce this risk by switching to a lower carbohydrate diet—or, as we'll see next, a low-GI diet.

In chapter 3, we considered an animal study published in *Lancet*[80] that found greater body fat among rats fed a high-GI diet compared to those fed a low-GI diet. Here, too, Insulin-30 strongly predicted how much weight and fat each animal in the high-GI group gained, accounting for about 85 percent of the total variation. (This is a remarkably high figure; for comparison, all known genes account for less than 10 percent of the variation in body weight among humans.) In the low-GI group, Insulin-30 was unrelated to weight gain (see the Insulin Secretion and Weight Gain figure on page 94).

My colleagues and I tested this hypothesis in a long-term clinical trial published in *JAMA*.[81] We measured insulin secretion in seventy-three young adults and then randomly assigned them to a low-GL or low-fat diet for eighteen months, providing the same amount of dietary counseling and other supports to both groups.

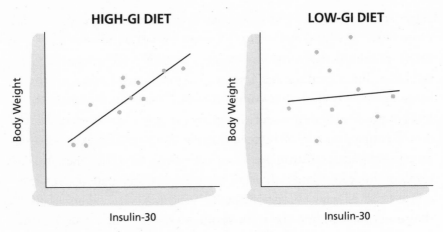

Insulin Secretion and Weight Gain Among Rats Fed High- or Low-GI Diets

Among individuals with low Insulin-30, weight loss did not differ significantly between the two diet groups. However, individuals with high Insulin-30 (above 57.5 microunits per milliliter) lost 10 pounds more on the low-GL diet compared to the low-fat diet. Moreover, those with high insulin secretion assigned to the low-fat diet tended to drop out of the study more than anyone else—an indication that this diet wasn't working for them.

The good news is that a person's susceptibility to diet may not be set in stone. After just one month on a low-carbohydrate diet, the cells in the pancreas that make insulin seemed to calm down, allowing individuals with high Insulin-30 to be able to tolerate more carbohydrate without a slowdown in metabolic rate (at least for a while).[82] In this way, Phases 1 and 2 of the Always Hungry Solution may reset metabolism, allowing previously sensitive people to have some processed carbohydrates in Phase 3 without adverse effects.

Undoubtedly, there are other biological differences among people that affect response to different diets (though the evidence for blood type is lacking). In addition, physical activity level plays a role. Research participants given five daily servings of sugary drinks showed increases in triglycerides, inflammation, and insulin when they were limited to walking no more than 4,500 steps per day. But these adverse changes did not occur when the participants walked more than 12,000 steps a day.[83] Eating lots of white rice may not cause metabolic problems for peasants in China doing regular manual labor. But as millions of Chinese migrate from farms to cities—bringing their high-carbohydrate diet and leaving behind the high level of physical activity—rates of diabetes have skyrocketed.[84]

Of course, on top of biological differences, we all have specific food preferences, cultural practices, time availability and constraints, levels of discipline, and individual health goals. For that reason, we've crafted the Always Hungry Solution with maximum flexibility, so that everyone can find the right balance between their body's needs and their personal preferences. Phases 1 and 2 are designed to retrain fat cells, boost metabolism, and help you find the optimal weight for your body. Phase 3 allows for personalization. Use the Daily Tracker and Monthly Progress Chart (see Appendix B) to follow your weight, hunger, cravings, energy level, and overall well-being. If these remain stable as you add back some processed carbohydrate, then feel free to enjoy the extra flexibility your metabolism allows (within reason). If not, cut back, or return to Phase 2 permanently. And remember, the fleeting moments of pleasure from eating poor-quality food pale in comparison to the enduring rewards of feeling good.

(Mini Quiz #10 Answer: 3. insulin secretion)

You've now reached the end of part 1, where we explored a radically different way to think about diet, body weight, and chronic disease prevention. In part 2, we put all this information together into the three-phase program to achieve permanent weight loss.

Part Two

THE ALWAYS HUNGRY SOLUTION

Welcome to the Program!

For the next few months—and perhaps the rest of your life—I invite you to forget about calories, focus on food quality, eat when hungry until fully satisfied, and follow a few simple lifestyle prescriptions.

In this way, you can conquer cravings, retrain your fat cells, and lose weight permanently.

My Always Hungry Story

I haven't been that hungry since we started this diet. I actually haven't been hungry at all.

—*Matthew F., 36, Roslindale, MA*
Weight loss: 31 pounds. Decrease in waist: 5.5 inches

CHAPTER 5

Prepare to Change Your Life

HOW THE PROGRAM WORKS

Standard low-fat diets aim to squeeze calories out of fat cells by restricting calorie intake. But after a few weeks of deprivation, hunger skyrockets and metabolism slows. The problem is, cutting calories does nothing to address the underlying cause of weight gain.

The Always Hungry Solution targets weight gain at its sources—fat cells stuck in calorie-storage overdrive. By decreasing insulin levels and calming chronic inflammation, we can reprogram fat cells to release excess calories. When this happens, hunger diminishes, cravings subside, metabolism speeds up, and you lose weight naturally.

We'll do this through three progressive phases:

- Phase 1—A two-week boot camp to conquer cravings and jump-start weight loss.

- Phase 2—A hunger-free plan to retrain your fat cells and reach your new, lower body weight set point. This can last anywhere from several weeks to six months or more, depending upon how much weight you have to lose.
- Phase 3—A customized diet for your body's unique needs so you can keep the weight off permanently.

In chapters 6 to 8, I'll provide step-by-step instructions, including recipes, meal plans, and tracking tools to help you follow the program easily. Each chapter also includes "Life Supports"—recommendations for good sleep habits, enjoyable physical activities, and stress reduction techniques that work with diet to support optimal weight loss and health.

Together with my team of nutrition and culinary experts, I developed the recipes and meal plans with three goals in mind:

1. To translate the latest scientific insights into a powerful prescription for weight loss *without hunger*, providing maximum benefits with minimum effort.
2. To be convenient and simple enough for anyone, with most meals taking 30 minutes or less to prepare.
3. To be delicious, satisfying, and adaptable for special diets—including vegetarian and gluten-free.

Many of the recipes resemble classic favorites, but each has been updated with modern flavors and calibrated for optimal results. If you've been counting calories, many previously forbidden foods—like whole eggs or heavy cream—will once again be welcome on your plate. You may be surprised how quickly some of your biggest craving triggers like sugar lose their appeal and new, more healthful foods become regular favorites. You may be shocked to realize how pervasive highly processed carbohydrates have become—and how much more satisfying it is to eat real, whole foods.

Popular weight loss plans often promise rapid, sensational weight loss, but require severe diets and arduous workouts. Sadly, the results of these restrictive regimens almost never last. Of course, the fastest way to lose weight is to simply stop eating. But I don't recommend it! In contrast, the Always Hungry Solution is designed to produce progressive, sustainable weight loss. After a few days on the program, you'll probably feel better, not worse, as your fat cells calm down and begin to share calories with the rest of the body. Energy level will improve, as will motivation—the opposite of what happens with time on many other diets.

Consider two ways to weigh about 50 pounds less in one year. Lose 4 pounds a week for 3 months by eating 1,200 fewer calories and working out every day, then struggle for the next 9 months to keep the weight off. Or lose 4 pounds a month for 12 months straight, eat whenever hungry, and feel great. Which would you prefer?

My Always Hungry Story

After eight weeks on the program, I have seen my weight decrease steadily and at a consistent level. Didn't see a "crazy" loss of 10 pounds one week that just comes back the following week with a vengeance. Very sustainable. The plan has recipes that I love and that I can turn to, to keep me on track (and happy!).
—*Esther K., 38, Flower Mound, TX*
Weight loss: 11 pounds. Decrease in waist: 3.5 inches

Most people in the pilot initially lost 1 to 2 pounds a week, a few lost even more, some a bit less. The rate of weight loss on the Always Hungry Solution will vary from person to person, based on individual metabolism, overall health, starting weight, age, physical activity level, and also how prepared you are to follow the plan. The program is designed to lower your body weight set point—the weight that the body fights to maintain—creating the right internal conditions to achieve and maintain optimal weight loss. Just follow the meal plan, eat when hungry until satisfied, and let your body (not a diet book author) determine the best rate of weight loss for you. Forcing weight down quickly with calorie restriction is nothing more than symptomatic treatment. It doesn't work for long, so why bother?

In any event, the change apparent on a scale provides only a rough measure of a diet's true effectiveness. A 50-pound weight loss entirely from fat tissue would affect appearance, fitness, and health much differently than the same weight loss, half coming from muscle. As you know from chapter 3, the Always Hungry Solution targets fat cells directly, producing more favorable changes in body composition (the ratio of lean muscle mass to fat tissue). In fact, some of our pilot participants reported decreasing waist size before major weight change, suggesting that they selectively lost fat and preserved lean muscle mass. Most important, participants consistently experienced benefits beyond weight loss, such as enhanced:

- energy level
- physical fitness
- mood
- emotional stability
- mental function

They also experienced improvements in a range of medical problems, including:

- diabetes
- heart disease risk factors
- gastroesophageal reflux and indigestion
- arthritis
- chronic fatigue
- depression

Of course weight loss is important for many people today—and it may have been one of the main reasons you picked up this book. This program will help you lose weight and keep it off permanently, but the ultimate goal of the Always Hungry Solution is radiant health and well-being.

Now, let's prepare for a successful start.

My Always Hungry Story

My body is moving so much better. I feel like I did when I was younger. My brain is clearer, too. "Arthritis"-type pain is gone. Amazing. The fact that I have lost weight eating so well is incredible to me. To bottom-line it: I went from an almost nonfunctional state to seemingly gaining back years of my health, and feeling back in the saddle of my life. Honestly.

—Nan T., 53, Birmingham, AL
Weight loss: 7.5 pounds. Decrease in waist: 1 inch

THE 7-DAY COUNTDOWN

Day -7: The Overview: Become familiar with the nutritional goals of the program.

Day -6: Take Your Health Snapshot—and Start Tracking: Collect your baseline health metrics, learn how to use the Daily Tracker and Monthly Progress Chart...and start tracking!

Day -5: Movement, Sleep, and Stress Relief Strategies: Discover how these three key lifestyle factors can accelerate weight loss and support long-term success.

Day -4: Your "Big Why" and "If-Then" Plans: Articulate your overarching goals and craft a plan for staying on track.

Day -3: Gather Your Cooking Tools and Clean Out Your Kitchen: Prepare your home and kitchen for a new way of eating.

Day -2: Go Shopping: Restock the fridge and cupboards with Always Hungry Solution–approved foods.

Day -1: Roast Nuts, Make Sauces, and Get Mentally Ready: Use your final Prep Phase day as a springboard to Phase 1.

My Always Hungry Story

I've had problems controlling my weight since puberty, though the worst has been in the last ten to fifteen years. My biggest issue has been managing (or failing to manage) cravings. The wonderful thing is the usual problems I have with dieting have not occurred with this plan. The biggest one for me is my depression and mood swings are gone. I'd tried antidepressants, but they made me feel sort of flat emotionally. This new way of eating has solved the problem, completely. Now I'm a normal person—I still get annoyed and sad sometimes, like anyone, but it doesn't rule my life the way it used to, and I'm growing in self-confidence. This is by far the most successful weight loss I've ever experienced, and the diet has been surprisingly easy for me. I expected to quit after a week or two, but I'm still doing it three months later. In fact, I think I can do this for life.

—Anne C., 48, Austin, TX
Weight loss: 18 pounds. Decrease in waist: 6 inches

PREPARE WITH A 7-DAY COUNTDOWN*

The most powerful changes in our lives often depend on preparation and motivation. To set yourself up for success, I suggest taking the week leading up to Phase 1 to get *really* ready—with your kitchen fully equipped and yourself mentally prepared for change. As we walk through the 7-day countdown, I'll explain the specifics of the diet, what foods are in and out, how you'll track your progress, and more. When Phase 1 begins, you'll have all the tools and information needed for a great start.

The timing of the Prep Phase will work best if you begin with Day -7 on a Monday. To make your Prep Phase period more manageable, consider designating a specific time each day for prep work. These brief daily assignments will help break down preparation into simple steps. Or, if you'd prefer to prepare at your own pace, no

---

* I recommend that you discuss participation in the program with your health care provider before getting started, especially if you have any medical problems. This would also be a good time to request baseline laboratory tests, if you plan to do them.

problem—the diet was designed for flexibility, and I encourage you to adapt this and any other component of the program to your individual preferences and needs. Simply read through all the Prep Phase tasks and schedule them at your own convenience. (Just try to divide them up over several days, so you don't get caught doing all the tasks at the last moment.)

To help stay organized, you also might want to pick up a sturdy folder or three-ring binder to keep the shopping lists, tracker sheets, and other program information in one place. (All these forms can be downloaded at www.alwayshungrybook.com.) As you move through the program, you'll gather lots of data about your hunger and cravings, energy level and mood, diet, and lifestyle activities, as well as weight and waist size. This information will allow you to monitor your progress, examine how your body responds to specific changes in diet, and fine-tune the program for your long-term individual needs.

My Always Hungry Story

I've experienced much less to no symptoms of gastroesophageal reflux. Blood work, glucose, cholesterol are the best in ten years. I used to need naps four to five days a week. Now I rarely take one. My former high energy level is returning. Obviously, future benefits will be better health, feeling better, better sex, getting more done, enjoying life more.

—Michael B., 65, New Market, MD
Weight loss: 10 pounds. Decrease in waist: 3 inches

Day -7: The Overview

For this first day of Prep Phase, let's step back and look at the broad strokes of the eating plan. You'll completely abandon the calorie-counting approach to weight loss. Instead, you'll focus on eating the right foods in the right combinations to reprogram fat cells so they release their excess calorie stores. The fastest way to do this is by replacing refined carbohydrates (the primary driver of insulin secretion) with fat, and achieving the right proportions of unprocessed carbohydrate and protein at meals and snacks. With the proper balance of nutrients, your body will feel well nourished rather than deprived, transition out of starvation mode, and begin to lose weight without struggle. *Just follow the meal plan, eat when hungry until satisfied—and then stop.*

One of the most dramatic results of this approach is that food cravings diminish or disappear, in some cases from day one.

Understanding Phase 1: Conquer Cravings

Phase 1 is essentially the opposite of a standard low-fat diet. During Phase 1, you'll eat a high proportion of fat (50 percent of your total calories), a lower amount of total carbohydrates (25 percent), and modestly more protein than you might be used to (25 percent), as shown in the figure below. During these two weeks, you'll eliminate all grain products, potatoes, and added sugar. But don't worry about feeling deprived. You'll fill up on rich sauces and spreads, nuts and nut butters, full-fat dairy, and other high-fat foods that calorie-restricted diets won't let you go near. As in all phases of the program, high-quality proteins play an important role, with vegetarian options available.

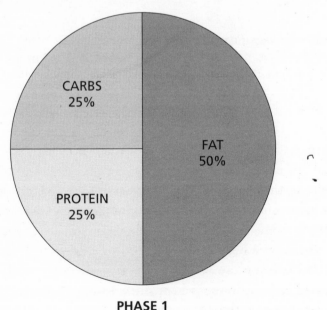

PHASE 1

What Phase 1 Will Look Like

My Always Hungry Story

Wow! It is so amazing to eat a meal and say, "I wonder if I had enough fat with that meal?" Love it!

—*Angelica G., 50, Sacramento, CA*
Weight loss: 11.5 pounds. Decrease in waist: 3 inches

Phase 1 is the most restrictive part of program, but it's not nearly as severe as very-low-carbohydrate and ketogenic diets, which aim to eliminate this major nutrient almost entirely. You'll still be able to enjoy whole, natural carbohydrates such as fruits, beans, and a full range of nonstarchy vegetables. This phase, just two weeks in length, is designed to jump-start weight loss, not as a permanent diet for everyone. Most people can tolerate more carbohydrate, and the next phases will allow for greater flexibility, variety, and adaptability to personal preferences. However, those with more extreme metabolic problems, like severe insulin resistance or prediabetes, may do best in Phase 1 on a longer-term basis.

Understanding Phase 2: Retrain Your Fat Cells

In Phase 2, you will slightly decrease fat (to 40 percent of your total calories) and increase carbohydrate intake (to 35 percent), by adding in some minimally processed whole-kernel grains (such as brown rice, steel-cut oats, barley, and quinoa) and starchy vegetables other than white potato. The sources and proportions of protein will remain the same (25 percent). Phase 2 is designed to retrain your fat cells so that your weight decreases progressively until stabilizing at its new, lower set point. This process can take a few weeks or months for some people, possibly many months for those who begin the program at a high weight. Phase 2 is intended to be your basic plan, to which you can always return as needed. If you're sensitive to processed carbohydrates (which you'll test in Phase 3), you may do best remaining on this phase indefinitely. As with all phases of the program, let your hunger be your guide.

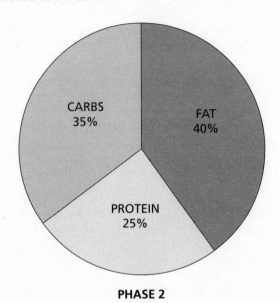

PHASE 2

What Phase 2 Will Look Like

Understanding Phase 3: Lose Weight Permanently

The ratio of carbs to protein to fats in Phase 3 is similar to the way many Americans ate in the 1950s and 1960s, before the low-fat craze hit—with 40 percent fat, 40 percent carbohydrate, and 20 percent protein. (Versions of the Mediterranean diet also have a similar nutrient ratio.) At this point in the Always Hungry Solution, you'll probably need more food than in prior phases because you're no longer burning off calories from stored body fat.

A major focus of Phase 3 is experimentation, to see how much diet flexibility your body can handle. Some people, after weight loss and improvements in metabolism, can tolerate a few servings of processed carbohydrate a day without triggering cravings or weight gain. For others, even a moderate amount of these foods will cause problems. The goal of this phase is to discover your body's unique needs and create a personalized blueprint to follow, rather than relying on an arbitrary nutrient prescription. The Daily Tracker and Monthly Progress Chart (described in more detail on page 121) become especially important in this phase.

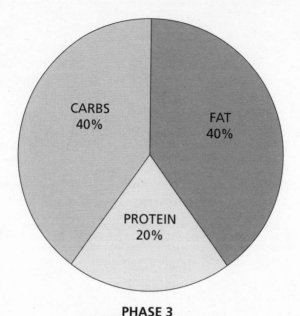

PHASE 3

What Phase 3 Will Look Like

My Always Hungry Story

My main obstacle to completing any weight loss program was a real difficulty managing hunger and cravings. I was ravenous most of the time but somehow never felt satiated.

From the first day, I noticed the food was amazingly good. I can't even tell you how great I felt after breakfast. I guess the nutrient ratios on that meal just hit a high note with my body. I have thoroughly broken my addiction to sugar, soda, and bread. It's rather remarkable. The psychological impact of feeling like I have dominion over my own cravings is huge. I just don't have a taste for that stuff any longer. That's not to say I won't ever have a piece of birthday cake or other refined carbs. But I don't crave them with a burning passion. It's more like, "Well, that might be nice. Think I'll have *one*." Before, it was, "How much of those can I eat without anyone noticing?" I am so pleased about this.

—Holly C., 37, Raleigh, NC
Weight loss: 5 pounds. Decrease in waist: 2 inches

Program Foods Phase-by-Phase

The diet in the Always Hungry Solution is rich, luscious, and satisfying, featuring many foods that are forbidden on conventional diets. You'll enjoy hearty favorites like Shepherd's Pie, Eggplant Parmesan, and Taco Salad, and treats like Chocolate-Drizzled Fruit (yes, we've included dessert most nights). And if you've never been a vegetable-lover, the meals on this plan may change your mind. You'll eat salads drenched with full-fat dressings, zucchini and other greens sautéed in garlic and olive oil, and a variety of vegetables layered into tasty casseroles. Here's a closer look at the foods you'll eat in each of the three phases, as well as foods to limit or avoid.

	PHASE 1: Conquer Cravings	PHASE 2: Retrain Your Fat Cells	PHASE 3: Lose Weight Permanently
GRAINS			
Includes (but not limited to): Amaranth Barley Buckwheat Corn Millet Oats Quinoa Rice Spelt Teff Wheat *Note:* Refer to the Guide to Cooking Whole Grains in Appendix C, page 317.	No	Yes, with limits Have up to 3 servings per day (no more than one per meal) of "intact" 100% whole-kernel grains. *Note:* "Intact" means the actual grain, or thickly cut grain—not flour or rolled grains. (For example, steel-cut oats are OK, but not Cheerios or rolled oats.) No bread, pasta, or couscous (even whole-grain products). No refined grains, such as white rice. A serving is about ½ cup cooked grain.	Yes, as tolerated Have up to 4 servings per day, primarily whole-kernel grains. May include up to 2 servings per day processed grains in this total as tolerated. *Note:* If eating processed grains, emphasize products made with whole grains (such as whole wheat bread). A modest amount of refined grain product (like white bread or white rice) may be OK, depending on your tolerance. A serving size is 1 slice of bread, or ½ cup cooked grain or pasta.

	PHASE 1: Conquer Cravings	PHASE 2: Retrain Your Fat Cells	PHASE 3: Lose Weight Permanently
STARCHY VEGETABLES			
Includes (but not limited to): Acorn squash Beets Buttercup squash Butternut squash Kabocha squash Peas Potatoes (white and sweet) Winter squash Yams	No	Yes, with limits Eat any starchy vegetable at meals in place of grains, *except white potato.* *Note:* A serving is ½ to 1 cup cooked vegetable.	Yes, as tolerated Eat any starchy vegetable at meals in place of grains. *Note:* Consider white potato equivalent to a processed grain, to be eaten sparingly.
LEGUMES			
Includes (but not limited to): Black beans Black-eyed peas Edamame (soybeans) Garbanzo beans (chickpeas) Kidney beans Lentils Lima beans Peanuts Pinto beans Red beans White beans (cannellini, great northern, etc.)	Yes *Note:* Legumes are the only sanctioned starchy foods in Phase 1. Legumes have a nice balance of carbs and protein; don't spike blood sugar; and are rich in fiber. Serving size is ½ to ¾ cup. Canned or dried beans are fine. Avoid products with added sugar, like Boston baked beans.	Yes	Yes
GREENS AND OTHER NONSTARCHY VEGETABLES			
Includes (but not limited to): Arugula Beet greens Bell peppers (green, red, yellow, orange) Broccoli	Yes *Note:* Nonstarchy vegetables are a mainstay of every lunch and dinner, and even show up in some breakfasts and snacks.	Yes	Yes

	PHASE 1: Conquer Cravings	**PHASE 2:** Retrain Your Fat Cells	**PHASE 3:** Lose Weight Permanently
GREENS AND OTHER NONSTARCHY VEGETABLES *(continued)*			
Broccoli rabe Brussels sprouts Cabbage Carrots Chard Collards Dandelion greens Fennel Hot peppers Kale Mushrooms Mustard greens Romaine and other lettuce Spinach Tomatoes *Note:* Refer to the Guide to Cooking Vegetables in Appendix C, page 313.	Vegetables help round out a meal when most starches are off the table (and provide an excellent vehicle for the luscious sauces and dressings included in the program).		
FRUITS			
Includes (but not limited to): **Non-tropical:** Apples Apricots Blackberries Blueberries Figs Grapefruit Grapes Oranges Peaches Pears Plums Raspberries Strawberries	Yes, with limits Have 2 or 3 non-tropical fruits daily. *Note:* "Fruit" means a whole fruit, such as an orange or apple, or a cup of cut-up fruit. Fruit, with its "just right" sweetness, helps wean taste buds off hypersweetened junk food.	Yes *Note:* Enjoy any fruit you like, but eat tropical and dried fruits sparingly. Serving size for dried fruit is 1 to 2 tablespoons. Continue to avoid fruit juice (it's highly concentrated in sugar).	Yes *Note:* Adjust and personalize your fruit intake.

	PHASE 1: Conquer Cravings	**PHASE 2:** Retrain Your Fat Cells	**PHASE 3:** Lose Weight Permanently
FRUITS *(continued)*			
Tropical: Banana Cantaloupe Dates Mango Papaya Pineapple Watermelon	Avoid the following in Phase 1: -Tropical fruits -Dried fruit (such as raisins) -Fruit juice		
HIGH-PROTEIN FOODS			
Includes (but not limited to): Beef Cheese Eggs and egg whites Fish Lamb Other game and meats Poultry Protein powder Shellfish Tempeh Tofu Vegetarian cold cuts Yogurt (Greek)	Yes Have a serving at every meal. *Note:* A protein serving is: -3 to 6 ounces of meat, poultry, fish, other seafood, tofu, tempeh, or vegan cold cuts -3 eggs -1 cup (3 ounces) grated cheese -1 cup Greek yogurt -5 tablespoons protein powder (see serving size on package) Greek yogurt contains about twice the protein as the regular varieties. Legumes can make a substantial contribution to the protein of a meal, especially for vegetarians.	Yes Have a serving at every meal.	Yes Have a serving at every meal.

	PHASE 1: Conquer Cravings	**PHASE 2:** Retrain Your Fat Cells	**PHASE 3:** Lose Weight Permanently
FATS AND HIGH-FAT FOODS			
Includes (but not limited to): Avocado Avocado oil Butter Coconut oil Flax oil Heavy cream Mayonnaise (no added sugar) Nuts and nut butters Olive oil Peanuts and peanut butter (no added sugar) Safflower oil (high oleic) Seeds and seed butters Sesame oil (plain or toasted) Sour cream	Yes Have at every meal. *Note:* If the high-protein source in your meal is high in fat (such as poultry with skin, fatty meat, cheese, tofu, or tempeh) then add: -2 to 3 teaspoons oil, butter, or mayo -1 to 2 tablespoons nuts -¼ avocado Double these amounts if the protein source is *not* high-fat (skinless poultry, lean meat, seafood, vegan cold cuts, or protein powder).	Yes Have at every meal, about 25% less than in Phase 1.	Yes Have at every meal, about 25% less than in Phase 1.
DAIRY AND NONDAIRY MILKS			
Includes (but not limited to): Almond milk Coconut milk Kefir, full-fat Milk, whole Soy milk Yogurt, full-fat	Yes *Note:* A serving is typically 1 cup. Natural yogurt and kefir have live probiotic cultures—"good" bacteria that play a critical role in health and well-being. Choose these over plain milk as often as possible. Choose only unsweetened products (with no added sugar or artificial sweetener).	Yes	Yes

	PHASE 1: Conquer Cravings	PHASE 2: Retrain Your Fat Cells	PHASE 3: Lose Weight Permanently
HIGH-CARB SWEETS AND SNACK FOODS			
Includes (but not limited to): Baked goods (cookies, cake, pie, etc.) Candy Chips French fries Fruit juice Ice cream Other sweets Sorbet Sweetened beverages (soft drinks, iced tea, sports and energy drinks, etc.)	No *Note:* Dark chocolate (minimum 70% cocoa content) is relatively low in sugar and permitted in all phases (up to 1 ounce daily).	No	Yes, based on individual tolerance *Note:* Limit total servings of processed carbohydrates (anything with refined grains or concentrated sugars) to 2 a day. Avoid highly sweetened beverages (containing sugar or artificial sweetener).
SUGAR			
Includes (but not limited to): Agave syrup Barley malt Brown sugar Cane juice Cane sugar Corn syrup Date sugar Dextran Dextrose Florida crystals Fructose Fruit juice concentrate Glucose Grape sugar High-fructose corn syrup	No (except for the small amount of sugar in dark chocolate, 70% minimum cocoa content)	Yes, with limits Up to 3 teaspoons (12 g) of added sugar daily, preferable in the form of honey or maple syrup. *Note:* 1 teaspoon of maple syrup, honey, or other sweetener contains about 4 g of sugar. Limit sugar in beverages to 1 g per ounce or less (e.g., a maximum of 2 teaspoons in a cup of coffee or tea).	Yes, as tolerated Up to 6 teaspoons (24 g) of added sugar daily, preferable in the form of honey or maple syrup. *Note:* Continue to limit sugar in beverages to 1 g per ounce.

	PHASE 1: Conquer Cravings	PHASE 2: Retrain Your Fat Cells	PHASE 3: Lose Weight Permanently
SUGAR *(continued)*			
Honey Hydrolyzed starch Maltodextrin Maltose Maple syrup Molasses Rice syrup Sucanat Sucrose Sugar Turbinado			
CAFFEINATED BEVERAGES			
Includes (but not limited to): Coffee (drip, French press, espresso) Tea (black, green, oolong)	Yes, with limits Up to 2 to 3 servings per day. *Note:* Caffeine causes insulin resistance, but coffee and tea have health-promoting plant substances called polyphenols. Ideally, drink green tea (or coffee, if necessary to avoid headache). Avoid sweeteners. Feel free to add cream or whole milk. OK to have decaf coffee in unlimited amounts.	Yes, with limits Up to 2 to 3 servings per day. *Note:* You may add 1 to 2 teaspoons sugar (4 or 8 grams), if desired (as part of 12 gram daily sugar maximum).	Yes, as tolerated *Note:* You may add 1 to 2 teaspoons sugar, if desired (as part of 24 gram daily sugar maximum).

	PHASE 1: Conquer Cravings	PHASE 2: Retrain Your Fat Cells	PHASE 3: Lose Weight Permanently
DIET DRINKS AND ARTIFICIAL SWEETENERS			
Includes (but not limited to): Aspartame (Equal) Diet drinks Diet sodas Saccharin (Sweet'N Low) Stevia (Truvia) Sucralose (Splenda)	Avoid *Note:* Although they have no calories, artificial sweeteners can prevent the taste buds from appreciating the natural sweetness present in whole foods like fruit. In addition, research suggests that these additives can have negative effects on metabolism. Stevia is a natural, sugar-free sweetener. Avoid stevia-containing products (for example, Truvia) in Phase 1.	Avoid *Note:* Occasional, small amounts of stevia are OK.	Avoid *Note:* Small amounts of stevia are OK.
ALCOHOL			
Includes (but not limited to): Beer Gin Rum Vodka Whiskey Wine	No (it's just 2 weeks!)	Yes, with limits 1 to 2 drinks a day (ideally limit alcohol to weekends or special occasions). *Note:* A drink is: -5 ounces dry wine -12 ounces beer -1½ fl ounces liquor If this amount interferes with your progress, cut back or avoid altogether.	Yes, as tolerated 1 to 2 drinks a day *Note:* If you drink, take note of how it affects your weight, sleep patterns, energy, and mood. Limit your intake to an amount that doesn't interfere with your well-being.

My Always Hungry Story

What is great is this plan realizes not everyone's body works the same! I was a bit worried about my preferences not to eat gluten, soy, and beans (I wasn't feeling great with them every day). But I am now feeling more energetic! Feels like I should have *gained* weight with all the food I was eating!

—Lisa K., 43, Albertville, MN
Weight loss: 8 pounds. Decrease in waist: 2 inches

Now that you have a general understanding of the meal plan guidelines, you can begin to visualize how your diet will change on the program. But before you head out to stock up, we have a few more things to accomplish. Next, let's gather your baseline personal data.

Day -6: Take Your Health Snapshot—and Start Tracking

Today, you'll begin tracking key personal health data. Capturing this information now will give you a definitive starting point and help you follow your progress through the program. Many of the pilot participants found consistent data collection to be both motivating and instructive.

Gather Your Pre-Program Data

Weigh yourself. Weigh yourself first thing in the morning, after you've used the bathroom but before eating or drinking anything. Wear only light clothing. This first measurement represents your starting weight, even though you won't begin the diet until next week. Record this number in your Monthly Progress Chart (see page 121).

Once you've obtained this measurement, please stow your scale out of sight for a while. I recommend you weigh yourself just once a week throughout the program.

Body weight naturally varies by up to several pounds daily, based on hydration state and other factors. For this reason, changes from one day to the next have very little significance. More important, as we touch upon above, weight is only a rough measure—especially at first—of a diet's true effectiveness. A critical aspect of the Always Hungry Solution is to gain a better understanding of your body's internal weight-regulating signals. Unfortunately, many of us have lost track of these signals and no longer respond to our body's needs—for healthful foods, adequate sleep, stress relief, and regular physical activity. Conventional diets actually make this mind-body disconnect worse, by specifically requiring us to ignore hunger (a primal biological signal) and focus instead on external numbers, like calories in our food and changes on the scale.

In contrast, young children are naturally in tune with their internal body signals. In one study, children of different ages were given varying amounts of macaroni and cheese and allowed to eat as much or little as they liked. The younger children ate the same amount regardless of portion size, but the older children ate more as portion size increased.[1] Perhaps exposure to the modern environment of supersized, superprocessed foods eventually overrides our innate abilities to recognize how much is enough.

Eliminating highly processed foods will automatically help heal this mind-body disconnect. But for some, it may take a while to relearn how to recognize the body's signals of hunger and fullness. Ignoring the scale for a while, rather than your hunger, will also help. Trust that once you've given your body what it wants, it will give you what you want.

My Always Hungry Story

I now have the strongest connection between my mind and my body than I think I've ever had in my life. I used to live from the head up with no understanding of how to nurture myself. Being disconnected from my body meant I could eat crap (mostly refined carbs), drink too much alcohol, and not exercise, all with a subconscious end goal of burying any feelings of unease in a fog of overindulgence. Now I really want to know how managing my sleep, anxiety levels, movement, and food consumption affects my overall well-being—I'm checking in with myself all the time. I also have a new confidence that I can trust my body to tell me what it needs to be healthy. It's not about denial or following rules, it's about a partnership...paying attention to how I feel when I eat certain things/amounts. And paying attention to when I've eaten enough or need a snack. Knowing that feeling "out of control" (cravings, crabby, tired) is my body telling me that I need to tweak something (sleep, foods, meditation, movement) and that stress can't be "fixed" by eating junk. And how absolutely amazing that I now know what feeling at peace feels like!

—Nancy F., 64, Eden Prairie, MN
Weight loss: 14.5 pounds. Decrease in waist: 7 inches

Take your waist measurement. Though weight usually gets most of the attention, waist circumference is actually more important, because it specifically measures how much fat we carry in the highest-risk location, around the midsection. Consider two hypothetical people on a diet who each decreased their waist size by 4 inches. One lost a total of 20 pounds and the other lost only 10 pounds. All things being equal, which one would have benefited the most? Although both individuals experienced a similar decrease in fat mass (based on change in waist circumference), the one who lost less weight would have preserved more muscle—a definite advantage for appearance, health, and likelihood of successful weight loss maintenance. Waist circumference predicts long-term risk for heart disease, diabetes, and other weight-related complications better than weight itself.

Wrap a fabric measuring tape around your waist, in line with your belly button and just above your hips. Obtain your measurement to the nearest half inch. Repeat this measurement on a monthly basis and record the results in the Monthly Progress Chart.

Take your height (optional). Your height will enable you to determine BMI, if you wish to do so. (See www.alwayshungrybook.com for a BMI calculator.) You probably already know how tall you are. But bodies can shift and settle over the years. If it's been a while since you measured yourself, ask a friend to help or stand next to a wall and use a pencil to mark your height, then use a yardstick or tape measure to obtain your measurement to the nearest half inch.

Get blood tests (optional). Consider obtaining these tests prior to beginning Phase 1. Your health care provider may have some from a prior laboratory test that you can use as a baseline. These tests provide a snapshot of your metabolic health, and changes in them will indicate how your body responds to the program, from the inside.

- Fasting lipid profile—including HDL cholesterol, LDL cholesterol, triglycerides (cardiovascular disease risk factors)
- Fasting glucose, fasting insulin, and HgA1c (diabetes risk factors including insulin resistance)
- C-reactive protein, high sensitivity (CRP, a measure of inflammation)

Have your blood pressure taken (optional). Since blood pressure is usually measured at medical visits, chances are your health care provider has this information on record.

The Tracking Tools

The Daily Tracker and Monthly Progress Chart are important components of the program that will help you tune in to crucial body signals, monitor progress, determine how you respond to changes in diet and lifestyle, and individualize Phase 3 based on your unique biological needs. In addition, regular use of these tools can be very motivating. (Copy the trackers in Appendix B, page 309, or download electronic copies at www.alwayshungrybook.com.) As their names imply, you'll need one copy per day of the Daily Tracker and one copy per month of the Monthly Progress Chart. Begin using these tools today, and if you're working with hard copies, keep them in your program folder or binder.

The Daily Tracker asks questions about your overall experience of hunger, cravings, satiety, energy level, and well-being throughout the day on a scale of 0 (worst) to 4 (best). Record your ratings for each of these symptoms, and add them up to determine your Total Score (ranging from 0 to 20). Next, indicate the number of processed carbohydrates you ate on that day. Once you begin the program, you'll also note whether or not you engaged in the lifestyle supports related to stress reduction, physical activity, and sleep, but skip this section during the Prep Phase. Finally, plot your Total Score on the Monthly Progress Chart, using an ink color corresponding to the amount of processed carbohydrates you ate that day (green for 0, yellow for 1 to 2, and red for 3 or more). This way, you will be able to see how your symptoms, body weight, and waist circumference change throughout the program, and how variations in your diet might influence your results.

My Always Hungry Story

The Tracker made me more aware of hunger and satiety. If I would feel excessively hungry, I'd ask myself, "What did I do differently? What is causing this?"

—Renee B., 49, West Roxbury, MA
Weight loss: 12.5 pounds. Decrease in waist: 5.5 inches

Day -5: Movement, Sleep, and Stress Relief Strategies

Diet has a dominant effect on fat cells, but other behaviors also play an important role. Too little sleep or physical activity, or too much stress, can raise insulin levels, promote chronic inflammation, keep fat cells in calorie storage overdrive and counteract the benefits of a good diet. In our modern, fast-paced social environment, many of us have difficulty getting enough sleep, physical movement, and relief from stress. For this reason, all three phases of the program devote attention to these three key "life supports." Small changes in any of these areas can produce important synergies: Reducing stress improves sleep quality; feeling well rested encourages physical activity; and all enhance motivation to eat well. As with diet, our strategy emphasizes enjoyment, not deprivation.

Joyful Movement and the "**Passeggiata.**" If weight loss were simply a question of calories in and calories out, you could spend 20 grueling minutes on a treadmill, but a handful of raisins (just ½ cup) would negate all your hard work. Thankfully, in addition to burning a modest number of calories, physical activity also improves insulin resistance, setting the stage for weight loss. You needn't work out for hours for these effects. A study involving older adults at risk for diabetes found that three 15-minute walks after meals improved their ability to regulate blood sugar for the following 24 hours. These three short walks were at least as effective as one long 45-minute walk taken during the day.[2] The habit of taking multiple walks during the day also gets you up and away from your desk or couch, and may lower stress levels.

Italians have a name for this type of walk: the *passeggiata*. You won't see anyone wearing a pedometer or spandex during an Italian *passeggiata*—these walks are purely for pleasure, to get outside and see the neighbors, to reconnect as a family after a long day, and to enjoy the last bit of sunlight. The movement and light that you take in during your *passeggiata* before nightfall can also recalibrate your body clock. The *passeggiata* is a moment of joyful movement that helps support healthy digestion and insulin action, while simultaneously relieving stress and helping you sleep better.

No matter how fit you are, the *passeggiata* can reintroduce you to movement as a pleasurable, easy, stress-relieving activity—not a chore to be sweated out and endured. Start in Phase 1 by adding one short walk a day, right after dinner. If you already have a fitness habit, fantastic—your fat cells have a head start. But try not to overdo it during Phase 1, as your body adapts to a new way of eating. Add the *passeggiata* but reduce your current workout intensity by one-third for now.

In Phase 2, you'll continue the *passeggiata* and add (or continue with) 30 minutes of enjoyable, moderate to vigorous physical activity, three to four days each week, depending on your fitness level and health care provider's advice. Some people, due to many years of poor diet and sedentary lifestyle, have low muscle mass, a condition called sarcopenia. For these people, physical activity is especially important, not primarily to burn calories, but rather to increase muscle mass and improve insulin sensitivity. In Phase 3, you'll add (or transition to) an activity that you do purely for enjoyment and can continue for the long term.

Regardless of your fitness level, the low-glycemic load food combinations will help fuel your physical activities by improving access to stored fat—the body's most efficient energy source.[3]

Safeguarding Your Sleep. Over 30 percent of adults in this country get less than six hours of sleep per night[4] though most bodies function optimally with at least seven or eight hours. We're so eager to pack more tasks into our days that we keep lights, televisions, computers, and phones on until the last second before bed—and then wonder why we have such a tough time falling or staying asleep. We pay for those lost minutes of sleep with our health. The exposure to bright light suppresses the release of melatonin (which is *supposed* to help us fall asleep), and the resulting sleep deprivation dysregulates the normal release of stress hormones (which are *supposed* to help us stay awake).[5] After a sleepless night, we may become irritable and snap at colleagues or loved ones, creating even more stress. With sleep deprivation, the reward system in our brains reacts differently in response to the sight of junk food, and we tend to eat more calories, primarily from high–glycemic load foods, than during times of healthy sleep.[6] (We also tend to eat them at the worst time of day for our fat cells: at night.)

Fat cells are among the biggest victims of sleep deprivation. A University of Chicago study found that sleep deprivation for just four nights (4.5 hours per night) decreased insulin sensitivity of fat cells substantially.[7] Another study suggests that unhealthy changes in insulin sensitivity and metabolism can develop after just one night of restricted sleep.[8] Over the long term, sleep deprivation increases risk for obesity, type 2 diabetes, and heart disease.[9]

Today you will do the Bedroom Cleanout—six simple steps that will help create optimal conditions for nourishing sleep. Weaning ourselves from bad sleep habits may take some time, but the results can be life-changing. Safeguard your bedroom as a sanctuary reserved solely for The Three Rs: Rest, Reading, or Romance.

1. *Turn down the thermostat:* A cool room promotes deeper sleep, and preliminary research suggests it might also help improve metabolism by stimulating fat-burning brown adipose tissue.[10]

2. *Turn off the television:* Watching TV late at night—especially the shocking or violent content in some TV dramas or the news—can wreak havoc on the nervous system and stimulate the release of stress hormones at the very moment you need to be calming down for rest. On the Always Hungry Solution, you'll focus on improving the quality of your food, but also consider what your brain is ingesting: Is it high quality? Does it nourish you? After eight p.m. is not the right time to be updated on the latest news you'll no doubt hear about the following day.

3. *Turn off the phones and computer, too:* Catching up on work or Facebook on your laptop or phone is no different than watching TV—in fact, it might be worse. We tend to hold our laptops or phones very close to our face in bed, increasing our exposure to sleep-disrupting blue light. In the two to three hours before sleep, you can use a computer app such as f.lux (justgetflux.com) that automatically dims and filters this light to lessen the effect. But a blanket ban would be even better—no screens in the bedroom! Those e-mails—work related or personal—will wait until morning.

4. *Keep lights low:* For the same reason, turn off overhead lights and use low-wattage incandescent bulbs in bedside lamps. If streetlights or the morning sun are a problem, consider blackout curtains or curtain liners (like those used in hotels). For an easy alternative, wear an eye mask.

5. *Block out the noise:* Remove all sources of noise from the area around your room to create a quiet, calm environment. If this is not entirely possibly—for example, if your bedroom faces a busy street

or you have noisy neighbors—try using a white noise sleep machine or app, running a fan on a low setting, or wearing earplugs.

6. *Create a pre-sleep ritual:* We are creatures of habit, and pre-bed routines have a powerful impact on sleep quality. Designate a regular bedtime that will let you get a minimum of seven to eight hours of rest (or longer, for those who need it) and adjust your evening activities to accommodate it. Pick a few soothing activities, and do them in the same sequence every night. Instead of an after-dinner coffee, take your *passeggiata* with family, friends, or the dog. Turn off most lights as early as possible, signaling to the brain that you're "shutting down" for the night. Do some stretches. Take a steamy shower or—a personal favorite of mine—a hot mineral bath (dissolve 2 cups Epsom salts in the tub, add a few drops of lavender oil, and soak for 10 to 15 minutes). Do your 5-minute stress-reduction relaxation. Listen to a recording of relaxing nature sounds—ocean waves, water flowing in a creek, wind blowing through the trees. Cuddle with your partner. Do whatever works for you, just try to do the same activities every night. You'll help your brain and body downshift into drowsy autopilot and be all the more ready for sleep when you finally flick off the bedside lamp.

We all can slip back into old habits—every night will not be perfect. Do your best and remember the many benefits of a good night's sleep. There's a reason many notable Hollywood celebrities consider sleep their number-one beauty regimen. Don't pollute your nightly fountain of youth! Sleep is sacred, and your bedroom is your sanctuary. Protect it.

My Always Hungry Story

I fall asleep easier and don't wake up so often during the night. After lunch, I used to get what I call the "Sleepies," where I would feel overwhelmingly tired and often find myself napping at my desk. I haven't had that since starting the diet.

—*Donna A., 51, Selah, WA*
Weight loss: 22 pounds. Decrease in waist: 5 inches

Creating Your Own Stress Relief Habit. Sporadic moments of positive stress can be energizing and motivating, like developing skills in a challenging sport or making a big presentation at work when fully prepared. But too much stress for too long can upset the body's precisely calibrated hormonal balance and program fat cells for weight gain. Cortisol, the ultimate stress hormone, erodes bone and muscle and builds up belly fat. We can help neutralize these dangerous effects by taking a few moments each day to consciously de-stress.

Starting today, I'd like you to adopt a regular relaxation practice that feels right for you, whether it's progressive muscle relaxation, yoga, tai chi, deep breathing exercises, meditation, prayer, journaling, or something else. A recent study found that a single session of guided relaxation reduced the expression of genes linked to insulin resistance and inflammation, even among people who had never done it before (though the effect was strongest among those who practiced regularly).[11] Other studies have found that these stress-reducing practices may lower blood pressure, alleviate pain, lessen insomnia, and relieve anxiety and depression as effectively as antidepressants.

To begin to experience these benefits, we'll start with just 5 minutes a day. You may already have a stress-relieving practice that works for you. If that's the case, please feel free to continue. Either way, I recommend in Phase 1 that everyone include a 5-minute stress-reduction practice at night before bed. In Phase 2, you'll add a second session earlier in the day, whenever is most convenient (and most needed) in your life. Once you have a steady practice going, you can expand both of these sessions, with an ultimate goal of reaching 30 minutes per day in Phase 3. But please note: The daily practice, not the number of minutes, is the most important factor here. It's better to practice 5 minutes every day than 35 minutes once a week.

With these few small daily practices, we can help shift our body into weight loss mode, as we embrace enjoyment in many aspects of our lives.

My Always Hungry Story

I have noticed a clearing in my head. The fog has lifted. It sort of feels like my insides have relaxed. I had no idea this could happen and it's amazing. I see a therapist and, because I am not in any type of crisis, I often only see her about once a month. She didn't know I was starting the pilot program and the first time I saw her, about three weeks in, she just looked at me and said, "What's up with you? You seem beautifully calm."

—Ann R., 61, Windsor Heights, IA
Weight loss: 6 pounds. Decrease in waist: n/a

Day -4: Your "Big Why" and "If-Then" Plans

Your "Big Why"

As you have probably come to appreciate, the Always Hungry Solution rejects the deprivation model of weight control and aims to produce changes in the body that will help you feel less hunger, have more energy, and experience a greater sense of well-being. With reduced carbohydrate cravings, it's just easier to say no to unhealthful temptations. In addition, the meal plan is delicious.

But even with tangible benefits, change can still be challenging. It may take time to modify long-standing lifestyle patterns and avoid old familiar habits that don't serve us. When you define a clear and compelling reason for making changes—your "Big Why"—you create a touchstone for support during moments of temptation, or when feeling off track.

Your Big Why should center on the most important issues in your life—lifelong goals, relationships with loved ones, your highest aspirations for the future. Maybe it's geared around adventure, such as getting into shape for a backpacking trip with your spouse, children, or grandchildren. Perhaps your goal will have a bit more urgency if, for example, you've been told you have prediabetes and want to avoid getting the full-blown disease.

It's easy to place excessive value on immediate rewards (that molten chocolate cake) while discounting long-term goals (losing weight). Our busy, stressful lives can make wise decision-making that much more difficult. If you connect with your Big Why during moments of temptation, you'll be more likely to stick to your plan. Here are a few ways to help you do that.

My Always Hungry Story

Creating my Big Why was challenging at first. In the past it has been too easy to just let the "whys" succumb to my food addiction. I am still struggling with old habits, and I find it still easy to binge on fast food and sweets (especially cookies and ice cream), but the power they held over me is diminishing more and more every day. I still have a long way to go, but I can see me doing it—and that's exciting.

—*Dan B., 45, Lehi, UT*
Weight loss: 15 pounds. Decrease in waist: 1 inch

Put it in writing. Turn your Big Why into a contract with yourself: "I will run a 10K by May of next year" or "I will lower my heart disease risk factors by my next medical appointment." And then imagine the moment that you've achieved your goal: "I see myself crossing the finish line with a big smile on my face" or "I see my health care provider's look of happy surprise." Then sign it! The act of putting your signature on this document increases your personal investment and your chances of following through.

Create a Big Why amulet. Just like the old-fashioned string tied around your finger as a reminder, visual cues can help remind you of your goal in the moment. You can designate a bracelet or watch, or create a simple armband or pin that symbolizes your Big Why. If you don't like physical adornments, pick a photo or image that best represents your Big Why, then frame it and place it in a conspicuous location—on your desk, bathroom sink, or bedside table. Whenever your amulet grabs your attention, take a few seconds to reconnect with your Big Why, to keep it in the front of your mind.

Think "as-if." During your 5-minute stress reductions, experiment with expanding your visualization. Sink all the way into the sensory experience of achieving your Big Why—what does it sound like, smell like, feel like to have achieved your goal? Where are you? Who is with you? What are you thinking in that moment? This type of mental rehearsal is akin to what actors, musicians, and athletes do to prepare for performances and games, and can help make your Big Why more immediate and real.

"If-Then" Plans

When trying to make positive changes in lifestyle, the things that most often trip people up are unanticipated stressors and challenges: "I would be doing just fine if X hadn't happened." There's no doubt that change is much easier with no obstacles in your way. But, alas, life is rarely like that. Chances are, you will encounter some obstacles as you follow the program—so the question to ask yourself is, "What am I going to do about it?"

Behavioral psychologists have found that if-then planning—also termed "anticipating obstacles and problem solving"—is one of the best ways to create strong and lasting habits, because it helps you create automatic responses to challenges you might face. When encountering those challenges, you don't have to wonder, "What should I do now?" and simply default to old habits. You've already created a solution and a plan, so you'll be more likely to follow through on that plan.

The key is to develop an if-then plan for every tricky scenario you expect to encounter, then *practice, practice, practice* until it becomes second nature. Some of this practice can be mental—just envisioning yourself reaching for the vegetables and (rich, full-fat) dip instead of the chips can help prepare you for the real thing.

If you keep a journal, write a list of all the new habits you would like to adopt for support on the Always Hungry Solution. For each one, answer the following three questions. Here's an example involving a person who used to eat out most nights but now would like to cook dinner every night:

1. *Which new habit do you want to establish?*

    I want to cook dinner at least five nights a week.

2. *When, where, and how will you do it?*

    Monday through Friday, at six p.m.

    In my kitchen

    By knowing in advance what I'm going to cook

3. *What could hinder you from doing it (could be a barrier) and how can you overcome it?*

    I might get busy at the end of the day and think, "It's too late to cook," so I'll just pick up takeout on the way home.

    Solution: I can stop at the precut veggies section in the grocery store and get fresh food that will be easier to cook than my planned dinner.

    Then form if-then plan for cooking dinner:

    If it's Monday through Friday at six p.m., then I will cook dinner.

    If I get delayed at work, then I will stop by the grocery store to pick up precut veggies, so the meal will be easier and faster to prepare. Or I will keep precut veggies in my fridge for quick access anytime I need them.

Now, roll this solution over in your mind—is it feasible? Is it practical? Are you likely to do it? If so, you have your if-then plan for that barrier. If not, take some time to figure out a solution that seems as easy as the takeout option, but helps you fulfill your weight loss goals.

Once you have a number of if-then plans, you may want to write them out on 3 by 5-inch index cards and carry them with you to review every day. That mental practice will help ensure that when the situation arises, you'll snap right into your planned response.

You're getting closer to the start of Phase 1.* Now we'll move into the room most important for your success: the kitchen.

My Always Hungry Story

My if-then plans have helped tremendously! I have been able to plan ahead of known challenging situations like an all-day meeting with lunch being served. Also, bringing healthy snacks along helps in those situations where I am away from my normal patterned eating regimen. With two children, we never have enough time to cook, so these prepped meals are a huge benefit to us. I hope to set a pattern in our house of eating well.

—Eric D., 44, Catonsville, MD
Weight loss: 21 pounds. Decrease in waist: 3.5 inches

Day -3: Gather Your Cooking Tools and Clean Out Your Kitchen

With a bit of prep cooking over the weekend, many weeknight dishes can be ready in less than 20 minutes. Throughout the program, I'll explain how to make every dish, step-by-step, and show you techniques that transfer from recipe to recipe. You'll be able to prepare these meals starting from the very first day.

If you're already a regular cook or you have a fully equipped kitchen, feel free to skip ahead. But if you tend not to cook for yourself, please take the time to read this section. The Always Hungry Solution is about getting back in touch with your food—literally. Cooking is a powerful way to reconnect with food, control the quality of your diet, and save on the costs of eat-out/takeout at the same time.

With the basic tools in the list below, you will be able to make all the recipes on the meal plan. Note the ones you have, and then try to obtain the others before you begin Phase 1. These tools make for an excellent investment that will provide returns for years to come.

---

* To break up the big first shopping trip later in the week (see page 138) into two, consider purchasing nonperishable items on Day -4 or Day -3—especially if you're shopping for a big family.

KITCHEN ESSENTIALS

Tools/Utensils
2 large cutting boards (14 x 8-inches or larger; one for fish, poultry, and meat, the other for fruits and vegetables)
1 sharp paring knife and 1 large sharp knife (for cutting vegetables and meats; sharp knives save time and effort)
1 whisk (not necessary if you have an immersion blender with a whisk attachment)
1 large salad bowl
2 or 3 medium bowls (about 8-inch diameter)
12 pint-size (2-cup) wide-mouth glass mason jars such as Ball canning jars (Use to make sauces—the immersion blender fits right into them!— and to store sauces and roasted nuts.)
3 or more glass or clear plastic containers with lids (for storing cut vegetables, fruits, or leftovers)
1 set of measuring cups for measuring dry ingredients
1 set of measuring spoons
1 or 2 clear glass or plastic measuring cups (2-, 4-, or 8-cup size) for measuring liquid ingredients
1 can opener
1 garlic press (optional)
1 mesh skimmer (for scooping blanched vegetables from hot water)
1 salad spinner (optional, but very useful to prevent watery pools of dressing!)
Machines
1 blender (optional if you have an immersion blender)
1 immersion blender (with whisk and optional food processor attachments)
1 food processor or immersion blender food processor attachment (optional, makes chopping large quantities of vegetables easier)
For the Stove
1 large skillet or saucepan with lid (12-inch stainless steel)
1 heavy-bottomed skillet (optional; 12-inch cast-iron skillet with glass or stainless steel lid; or coated cast-iron skillet with lid, like Le Creuset)
1 large pot with lid (7-to 8-quart, preferably a Dutch oven)

For the Stove (continued)
1 small to medium pot with lid
1 steamer basket (to fit into saucepan or larger pot)
1 baking pan (9 x 12 inches, metal or glass) or 6 ramekins (4- to 5-inch diameter)
1 baking pan (8 inches square, metal or glass)
1 loaf pan (4 x 8 inches) or 6 ramekins (about 3 inches diameter)
1 large cookie sheet (about 10 x 14 inches, no sides or very short sides)

My Always Hungry Story

A set of 1- and 2-cup Pyrex glass containers with lids makes it very easy to grab something healthy when it is already prepared and measured out into a container. Additionally, I notice that my children are more likely to eat something in the fridge when they can see what it is—apparently, it takes too much effort to open an opaque or semi-transparent box!

—Monica M., 45, Great Falls, VA
Weight loss: 11 pounds. Decrease in waist: 2 inches

Kitchen Cleanout

Nothing says "starting over" like a kitchen purged of unhealthy foods and restocked with nutritious ingredients. Let's clean out your kitchen so you'll have space for all the delicious and nutritious foods to come starting next week. The list below tells you which foods to throw away and which to keep. (For specific foods required on the Phase 1 and 2 meal plans, please consult the shopping lists online at www.alwayshungrybook.com.)

If you feel guilt about wasting any items in your kitchen, just remember: The cost of getting rid of those unhealthy foods is nothing compared to the value of your health. You'll head out for your first shopping trip tomorrow.

THE KITCHEN CLEANOUT

	TOSS	SAVE FOR PHASE 2	KEEP (OR STOCK—SEE SHOPPING LISTS FOR DETAILS)
Freezer	**Fruit/Vegetables** • Frozen fruit with added sugar • Frozen vegetables with seasoning that contains sugar (e.g., glazed carrots) • Orange juice, lemonade, or other fruit juice concentrates **Baked Products** • Bread, rolls, piecrust shells, or similar items **Entrées/Meals** • Frozen entrées or meals containing grains (such as rice or pasta), or added sugar • Frozen pizza **Sweets** • Ice cream, sorbet, and other frozen sweets • Cakes, cookies, cookie dough or other desserts	**Fruit/ Vegetables** • Frozen tropical fruit, such as mango, papaya, or pineapple • Frozen corn or vegetable mixtures containing corn • Frozen peas or other starchy vegetables	**Fruit/Vegetables** • Frozen vegetables such as broccoli, spinach, carrots • Frozen lima beans, edamame, or other beans • Unsweetened frozen nontropical fruit (such as blueberries, blackberries, peaches, strawberries, and raspberries) **Seafood/Meat/Poultry/ Vegetarian Protein** • Frozen shrimp, fish, or other seafood (without sauces containing sugar) • Beef, lamb, poultry, or other meats • Veggie burgers made from soy, other beans, or vegetables but without processed grains, white potato, or added sweeteners
Fridge	**Baked Products** • Bread, tortillas, canned biscuit dough **Beverages** • Juice of any kind • Sugar-sweetened beverages of any kind (containing either sugar or artificial sweetener), such as regular or "diet" soft drinks, sweetened iced tea, fruit punch, vitamin waters, and sports drinks	**Sweeteners** • Maple syrup (100% pure only)	**Beverages** • Mineral water • Sparkling water (flavored is fine, as long as there's no sugar or artificial sweetener) • Unsweetened iced tea **Dairy/Soy Milk** • Whole milk • Whole plain, unsweetened yogurt (Greek or regular)

	TOSS	SAVE FOR PHASE 2	KEEP (OR STOCK—SEE SHOPPING LISTS FOR DETAILS)
Fridge *(continued)*	**Dairy** • Nonfat and lowfat milk (plain, chocolate, or other flavors) • Nonfat or lowfat plain or flavored yogurt **Fruits** • Jam and jelly with added sugar (save 100% fruit products for Phase 2) • Tropical fruit (banana, mango, papaya, pineapple, melon) **Meats** • Hot dogs and sausages (meat or vegan) that contain processed grains, white potato, or sugar among the ingredients **Sauces/Condiments** • Sweet pickles, relish • Sauces and spreads with added sugar (for example, many types of ketchup and mayonnaise) **Sweets** • Canned, sweetened whipped cream or other sweetened "nondairy" topping or flavored coffee creamer • Chocolate syrup and fudge sauce • Applesauce (sweetened) • Pudding, Jell-O, or other sweets		• Unsweetened soy milk, almond milk, or coconut milk (but not rice milk) • Cheese, regular—all types (not low-fat) • Butter • Sour cream, cream cheese (not low-fat) • Heavy cream **Eggs** • Eggs • Liquid egg whites in a carton (optional) **Fruit/Vegetables** • All non-tropical fruit (such as apples, berries, oranges, lemons, pears) • All vegetables except white potato **Meats/Vegetarian Proteins** • Deli cold cuts or vegetarian cold cuts • Tofu, tempeh, or other vegetarian proteins **Sauces/Condiments** • Sauces and spreads—no added sugar, such as soy sauce and mustard • Hummus • Olives, capers • Herbs and spices (basil, oregano, etc.) • Vinegar (distilled white, apple cider, white or red wine, unseasoned rice)

	TOSS	SAVE FOR PHASE 2	KEEP (OR STOCK—SEE SHOPPING LISTS FOR DETAILS)
Cupboards/ Countertop	**Beverages/Beverage Mixes** • Regular or diet beverages as listed under "Fridge," Kool-Aid mix, cocoa mix (with added sugar or artificial sweetener) **Canned/Jarred Goods** • Canned baked beans or other canned beans with added sugar • Fruit canned in syrup • Spaghetti sauce or plain tomato sauce with added sugar **Cereal** • Cold or hot cereal made with flour (refined or whole grain) • Rolled oats and muesli (or save for Phase 3) **Vegetables** • White potato **Grains, Flour, Mixes** • White rice (or save for Phase 3) • Pasta or couscous, white and whole grain (or save for Phase 3) • Flour, white and whole grain (or save for Phase 3) • Instant potato mix • Cornmeal, corn grits, popcorn kernels (or save for Phase 3)	**Canned Goods** • Canned corn (no sugar added) **Cereal** • Hot cereal such as steel-cut oats, mixed whole kernel **Fruit/ Vegetable** • Dried fruit • Sweet potatoes, yams **Sweeteners** • Honey • Maple syrup (100%)	**Beverages** • Tea (black, green, herbal) or coffee • Unsweetened cocoa • Beverages as listed under "Fridge" **Canned/Jarred Goods** • Canned beans (such as black beans, kidney beans, or other plain beans with no added sugar) • Canned salmon, tuna, smoked oysters, or other seafood • Spaghetti sauce (tomato based, with no sugar or other sweetener) • Salsa (with no sugar or other sweetener) **Nuts and Seeds** • All nuts (almonds, peanuts, walnuts, etc.) • All seeds (chia, flax, pumpkin, sesame, sunflower, etc.) • Nut and seed butters, such as almond or peanut butter (no sugar added) **Oil** • Avocado oil • Olive oil • Safflower oil (high oleic) • Sesame oil (plain or toasted) **Sweets** • Dark chocolate (minimum 70% cocoa content)

	TOSS	SAVE FOR PHASE 2	KEEP (OR STOCK—SEE SHOPPING LISTS FOR DETAILS)
Cupboards/ Countertop *(continued)*	**Bread/crackers** • Bread and other baked goods listed under "Freezer" • Crackers, rice cakes, bread crumbs, or croutons • Pita chips, corn chips, potato chips, or other chips • Granola bars, popcorn, pretzels, and processed fruit snacks **Sweets** • Candy (except for dark chocolate—at least 70% cocoa content) • Jell-O or pudding mix • Cookies or other sweet baked products • Brownie, cake, cookie, muffin, or other mixes		

My Always Hungry Story

My eye doc uses a tool to measure carotenoids in the bloodstream, since this is a key preventative for eye issues. My last score was above average—but now I am scoring at the top of their scale. All those photograph-worthy meals are paying off! The eye doc said that the eyes are made of the same stuff as the brain so not only will my eyes be stronger, my brain is benefiting, too.

—*Luisa G., 51, Menomonie, WI*
Weight loss: 6 pounds. Decrease in waist: 2.5 inches

Day -2: Go Shopping

Now the fun part begins: stocking the fridge and cupboards with healthy and delicious items for Phase 1. Today, you'll stock up on staples, obtain ingredients for a week of sauces and nuts (which you'll prepare tomorrow), and shop for three days of food (Monday through Wednesday).

Print a copy of the Prep Phase, Nonperishables Shopping List and of the Phase 1, Days 1–3 Shopping List at www.alwayshungrybook .com. If you've done the shopping for nonperishables on Day -4, you'll only need the second list. (If you've been out of the kitchen for a while and are feeling a little overwhelmed, have a look at the shortcuts on page 157 and the Simplified Meal Plan online at www.alwayshungrybook.com. The Simplified Meal Plan is great for one person and can also be scaled up for a family of any size.) Take the lists into your kitchen and check off any items you already have.

Scan through the Phase 1 Meal Plan on page 159 to see if there are any meals you absolutely won't eat because of allergies or sensitivities, and delete those ingredients from the shopping lists. But I encourage you to be adventurous. Some of the meals might initially seem a bit outside your comfort zone. Just for these two weeks, give them a try—you may be surprised. Sticking closely to the plan will not only introduce you to some exciting new flavors, but also ensure the best results. (Be prepared: If you haven't already purchased your nonperishables, this will be your largest shopping expedition of the program, since you'll be stocking up on items to be used for weeks to come.)

Then, go shopping! Enjoy the process of putting away your groceries and getting everything ready for the program. And check the Resources page at www.alwayshungrybook.com for recommendations on specific products.

Day -1: Food Prep for Phase 1, Week 1

The last day of the Prep Phase, before you begin Phase 1, is your first day of cooking. Today, you'll spend a couple of hours preparing sauces and roasted nuts—two fundamental (and tasty) components of the program—to be ready for your week. With regular food prep on the weekends, you'll be able to assemble a delicious weeknight dinner in 30 minutes or less, your breakfast or lunch in 15 minutes or less, and snacks in just a few moments. Familiarize yourself with the Phase 1 Meal Plan (see page 159) and recipes (chapter 9). See if there is anything else you can do to give yourself a head start on the week.

Weekly Prep Worksheet for Phase 1, Week 1

Premade sauces, dressings, and spreads make creating a full Always Hungry Solution meal quick and easy. For example, you could roast a fish fillet, serve it with Creamy Dill Sauce (page 270), and toss a salad with Mustard Vinaigrette (page 264). These sauces keep well in the refrigerator for 1 to 2 weeks—with the exception of the Creamy Lime-Cilantro Dressing (page 271), which is best used within 3 to 5 days.

My Always Hungry Story

I noticed that several of the sauces had similar ingredients, so I made an assembly line. I taped the recipes on the kitchen cabinet and placed an appropriately sized Ball jar under each. I started with one ingredient that was common to each recipe—like vinegar—and went down the line and put the correct amount in each jar. Then I went on to the next common ingredient, salt or lemon or whatever. Last, I did all the ingredients that were different. When each jar had all its proper ingredients, I took my immersion blender and went right down the line mixing each (just rinsing the blender in between). It worked great!

—*Pat M., 66, Maple Grove, MN*
Weight loss: 4 pounds. Decrease in waist: 0.5 inch

Nuts and seeds are also a mainstay of the Always Hungry Solution. Roasting them adds depth of flavor and a slightly caramelized taste. Fortunately, the process of roasting is really simple and takes just a few minutes. Read the instructions for roasting nuts and seeds in Appendix C. These keep well when stored in airtight jars or containers. Replace the candy jar on your desk or in your office with a jar of roasted nuts! Keep them in strategic snacking spots around the house, and stash a sturdy container in your bag or car to grab on the go.

My Always Hungry Story

What kind of amazes me is twofold. First, that after how many years of, "Oh, I can't eat all those nuts. Think of the fat!" I've actually given myself permission to eat them. And, second, that a handful of nuts when I'm feeling like I need a snack really takes care of it.

—*Pam M., 55, Confluence, PA*
Weight loss: 13 pounds. Decrease in waist: 2 inches

Throughout the program, choose a convenient day every week or two for food prep and use the Weekly Prep Worksheet as your guide. For the next three weeks, just follow the completed worksheets that correspond to the meal plans provided in Phase 1 (two full weeks) and Phase 2 (one full week). After that, you'll be prepared to fill out blank worksheets (online at www.alwayshungrybook.com), according to the meal plans you design. The Weekly Prep Worksheet for Phase 1, Week 1 is on page 142. You'll have a bit of extra work this week, but rest assured that prep day will become easier in future weeks, with sauces and roasted nuts on hand from previous weeks.

My Always Hungry Story

I had this stigma that changing our diet was this difficult task that would take hours a day. To make it work during the week, a lot of it does need to be done on Sunday afternoon. You can make a big dish and then integrate it into multiple meals during the week. I don't think my girlfriend was very excited by it at first. But once she saw we actually saved money, she was happy with that.

—*Benjamin P., 26, Natick, MA*
Weight loss: 14 pounds. Decrease in waist: 2 inches

WEEKLY PREP WORKSHEET

Prep Day for Phase 1, Week 1 Meal Plan

Since this is the first meal plan prep, you'll have a little extra work to do this week. Prep will become easier in future weeks, with previously made sauces and nuts available. **Note:** This worksheet is designed for the menu plan that serves two people. Make one of each recipe listed unless otherwise noted, or scale up or down according to your needs.

Sauces

- Lemon Tahini Sauce (page 269)
- Blue Cheese Dressing (page 263)
- Creamy Dill Sauce (page 270)
- Stir-Fry Sauce (page 260)
- Creamy Lime-Cilantro Dressing (page 271)

For the following items, use this week and save leftovers for week 2:

- Basic Mayonnaise (page 259)—Make a double batch or add store-bought mayonnaise with no added sugar to your shopping list.
- Lemon Olive Oil Dressing (page 269)
- Ginger-Soy Vinaigrette (page 267)
- Chocolate Sauce (page 289)
- Ranchero Sauce (page 272)—Use 1 cup this week; freeze 2½ cups for week 2 and ½ cup for Phase 2.

Snacks/Roasted Nuts & Seeds

- Hummus (page 290), or add premade hummus to your shopping list
- Roast 2 tablespoons walnuts (page 319—Guide to Roasting Nuts and Seeds) for Day 2 Chicken Salad with Grapes and Walnuts and ¼ cup peanuts for Day 6 Chicken Stir-Fry Lettuce Wrap—or add roasted nuts to shopping list in place of raw nuts

For the following items, use this week and save leftovers for week 2:

- Spicy Pumpkin Seeds (page 292)—or add roasted pumpkin seeds to your shopping list in place of raw seeds
- Trail Mix (page 291)—or add roasted nuts to shopping list in place of raw nuts

Ingredients to Prep (Proteins, Grains, Soups, etc., to Use Throughout the Week)

- If choosing vegetarian variations for any of the recipes: 1 pound Pan-Fried Tempeh or Tofu Strips (page 243) or Crumbled Tempeh (page 244)

Note: Phase 1 meal plan begins on page 159

A FINAL THOUGHT ABOUT HUNGER
BEFORE YOU START

As they prepared to begin Phase 1, some pilot participants expressed a bit of anxiety: *What do I do if I get hungry on this plan? I shouldn't really eat as much as I want, should I? How can I possibly lose weight?*

But consider this: Ultimately, the main reason people overeat is hunger. Ironically, conventional weight loss plans only make this problem worse by restricting the amount of food you eat, one way or another. Sure, you might lose 20 pounds in two months on a low-calorie diet—which can be exciting at first—but then the real work begins. The internal signals you ignored for a while only get louder as your body resists calorie deprivation with increasing ferocity. Gnawing hunger and plummeting energy level take an increasingly heavy toll. You can try to white knuckle through it, but for how long? Sooner or later, willpower weakens, motivation erodes, and the weight comes rushing back.

The Always Hungry Solution turns this approach on its head by encouraging you to eat until fully satisfied and snack whenever hungry. With a carefully calibrated meal plan—together with key lifestyle supports—fat cells can be coaxed to open up and release their stored calories. On this program, calories stay in the bloodstream and nourish the rest of the body longer, leading to long-lasting satiety. You will eventually eat less—and probably burn off more calories, too—but this way, with your body's active cooperation. It's similar to the way body temperature decreases after treating the underlying cause of a fever.

Use your Daily Tracker to help you tune in to your body. Start a meal when you're hungry (but not ravenous) and stop eating when you're satisfied—but not over-full. Put reasonable portions on your plate, eat at a leisurely pace, and check in with your body regularly during the meal. If you're still hungry, have more food. And if you get full before you clean your plate, stop eating.

Because this is expressly not a calorie-controlled diet, the serving sizes in the meal plans and recipes are just suggestions, designed for someone of typical size and activity level. Your requirements may differ, and your body will tell you if you need more or less. You don't need to deny yourself—you just need to pay attention. In fact, the longer you stay on this program, the *easier* it gets.

Part of that ease comes from learning to incorporate the program into your lifestyle. But the rest comes from an increasing sense of well-being, as hunger and cravings diminish, energy level increases, and weight declines naturally—signs that the program is working from the inside out.

My Always Hungry Story

From Prep Phase: Eating 50 percent fat sounds a little scary! I've been in the "fat is bad" environment so long. This will take a trusting shift in thinking.

From Week 1 (Phase 1): I'm noticing my body is content—no cravings or hunger to be white-knuckled through. Diets with 5-pound loss in the first week leave me feeling like I'm hanging on by my fingernails. This feels *so* different.

From Week 2 (Phase 1): Even without the scale budging this week, I feel trimmer and more content. I have cheekbones again!? Feels like I'm renegotiating with my body right now.

From Week 6 (Phase 2): I admit, I was skeptical at the start—would this be another failed diet? My energy was low, bad moods most of the time, no interest in sex, lots of aches and pains. I cringed when I looked in the mirror or squeezed into clothes. Fast-forward six weeks, and I feel like a new person. I sigh in utter pleasure during meals. I'm interested in sex again! Hot flashes have disappeared, sleep is better. My clothes fit better, and I have more options in my closet.

From Week 10 (Phase 2): I can calmly notice what's going on with my mind and body, key in to my hunger, and know that a moderate amount of nourishing food meets that need. I know what feeling good feels like (mentally and physically). Interestingly, it has less to do with the scale than I expected it to.

From Week 16 (Phase 3): I feel emotionally and physically renewed—it's amazing to me how far I've come learning to work *with* instead of against my body and biology. I've got more to lose, but I feel hopeful and in control…something I've only had glimmers of in the past.

—*Nancy F., 64, Eden Prairie, MN*
Weight loss: 14.5 pounds. Decrease in waist: 7 inches

YOU ARE READY

You've officially finished the Prep Phase. Tomorrow you begin Phase 1. Be sure to get a good night's rest in your sleep sanctuary this evening, so you can enjoy Day 1 to the fullest.

CHAPTER 6

Phase 1—Conquer Cravings

Having completed the Prep Phase, you're ready to discover your personal Always Hungry Solution! In each of the next three chapters, I'll outline the specific Life Supports (related to stress reduction, sleep, and movement), Diet Tools, and Meal Plans that will allow you to integrate the program into your life, in a way that works for you. In this chapter, we'll focus on Phase 1.

For the next fourteen days, you'll completely eliminate all grain products, potatoes, and added sugar (except the small amount present in very dark chocolate). To avoid any sense of deprivation, you'll replace these high–glycemic load calories with fat from olive oil, nuts, avocado, full-fat dairy products, and other sources. But this isn't a very-low-carbohydrate-type diet—you get to have slow-digesting carbohydrate in the form of nonstarchy vegetables, legumes, and fruits. Fat will total

50 percent of your calories, protein 25 percent, and carbohydrate 25 percent (see What Phase 1 Will Look Like, page 106).

My Always Hungry Story

I started to think, "Is there protein in this? Is there fat in this?" To think of fat not as a bad thing, which is quite honestly how I was raised and many people were raised—"cut down on the fat!"—but actually looking at it as a positive and thinking about how it was going to affect me for the rest of the day. And the effect was pretty profound.

—*Eric F., 42, Needham, MA*
Weight loss: 17 pounds. Decrease in waist: 3 inches

On the Standard American Diet, most people will have developed some degree of insulin resistance and chronic inflammation. The ratio of carbs to fat to protein in Phase 1 was designed to reverse these twin metabolic troublemakers rapidly. As in all phases of the program, you'll eat whenever hungry, as much as you need to feel satisfied (but not over-full), allowing the body to transition out of starvation mode. During these first two weeks, your body will probably experience major shifts in metabolism. Drink lots of water, take it easy, and follow the lifestyle supports related to sleep, stress reduction, and gentle movement as your body adjusts.

My Always Hungry Story

The first week of Phase 1, I had these crazy headaches, my body's way of detoxing all those things I shouldn't have been putting in. Then three weeks into the program, I definitely noticed a surge in energy. I work about twelve hours a day, and I have a three-hour commute. But after work, I needed to go to the gym to get out all this energy. I also noticed that while my amount of sleep didn't change, the quality of the sleep improved. I felt rested in the morning. Those nights when I have extra sugar or a bunch of carbs, the quality of sleep isn't there. Do you want to sacrifice that? I know I don't.

—*Amanda N., 28, Pepperell, MA*
Weight loss: 8 pounds. Decrease in waist: 5 inches

PHASE 1 LIFE SUPPORTS

Before we explore the diet in more detail, let's take a moment to review the three key Phase 1 supports for optimal weight loss.

Movement

With the start of Phase 1, you'll begin the *passeggiata*—your short walk after dinner (see page 123). These walks are intended to be a pleasurable time to commune outdoors with your neighborhood, your loved ones, your dog, or yourself—not "exercise." Rather than burn off many calories, the purpose of the *passeggiata* is to aid digestion, dampen the post-meal surge in insulin (acting synergistically with the diet), and stimulate metabolism. In addition, the *passeggiata* can be the first component of your pre-bed ritual. For those with a preexisting fitness program, reduce intensity by one-third for now—the Phase 1 diet will put your fat cells through their paces!—but don't omit the *passeggiata*.

My Always Hungry Story

For my *passeggiata*, I would just walk around the hospital where I work for five or ten minutes. Beyond whatever digestive health it was providing, the walk was relaxing and used up some of the added energy from eating this way. And while burning off some energy, it also kept me going, almost like a cup of coffee.

—*Benjamin P., 26, Natick, MA*
Weight loss: 14 pounds. Decrease in waist: 2 inches

Sleep

During the Prep Phase, you completed the Bedroom Cleanout, so your sleep sanctuary is ready for the Three Rs only: Rest, Reading, and Romance. As you develop your pre-sleep ritual (see page 126), remember to respect your designated bedtime—the cornerstone of good sleep habits. A good night's sleep reduces insulin resistance, helps keep stress hormone levels on an even keel, and makes it easier to adopt other positive changes in your life.

Stress Relief

As part of your pre-sleep ritual (see page 126), make time for your 5-minute stress reduction practice, whether it's meditation, prayer, yoga, journaling, or a breathing exercise. Consider doing some progressive muscle relaxation before you fall asleep. Play an audio recording of a meditation, visualization, guided relaxation, or pleasant sounds from nature.

My Always Hungry Story

Because I'm not constantly fighting cravings, I feel more free and less stressed. This happened overnight, within the first week of the diet. At first, I really couldn't name it or even identify it, but I knew there was something different going on inside.

—*Donna A., 51, Selah, WA*
Weight loss: 22 pounds. Decrease in waist: 5 inches

Other Supports

Your Big Why: Find a few moments to visualize or journal about your Big Why to connect with your long-term goals on a daily basis and maintain motivation.

Road Test Your If-Then Plans: Rather than wait to see whether your if-then plan will succeed in a moment of crisis, do a dry run. Pretend your "If" situation happened and implement your "Then." Did it work? If not, how can you shift your strategy to be successful when you really need it?

Use Your Tracker Every Day. To help remain connected with your body's hunger and satiety signals, be sure to complete your Daily Tracker regularly. Either copy page 310 or download the form from www.alwayshungrybook.com. The Daily Tracker will allow you to record your body's responses to the program—your level of hunger, cravings, satisfaction, energy, and sense of well-being—and related data. Plot your Total Score from the Daily Tracker each day and record your weight and waist circumference each month on the Monthly Progress Chart. Then watch how the trends change as you progress through the program phases. Do your results correlate with intake of processed carbohydrate? Or with attention to sleep, physical activity, and stress reduction? This information will help you tailor the program for your unique needs, especially in Phase 3.

My Always Hungry Story

If-then planning has helped immensely. The small practice of if-then planning has trained my brain to see options and helped me move from the rigid all-or-nothing thinking to feeling like I have tons of choices. It gives me a feeling of being capable and empowered.

—*Kim S., 47, South Jordan, UT*
Weight loss: 25 pounds. Decrease in waist: 3.5 inches

PHASE 1 TOOLS

A Guide to Portion Size

During Phase 1, pilot participants reported big declines in hunger, sometimes from as early as Day 1. As fat cells calm down and begin to release their excess calorie stores back into the body, your brain will register (perhaps for the first time in years) that it has enough fuel to run your metabolism in optimal mode. Since your body will be burning more fat, your need for external calories will decrease. You'll fill up with less food and stay full longer. However, these changes don't occur with everyone at the same time or in the same way. And as we considered in chapter 5, calorie requirements will differ between people based on size, age, physical activity level, and other biological factors.

The Always Hungry Solution rejects the one-size-fits-all calorie prescriptions common to conventional weight loss plans. The recipes and meal plans offer portion size suggestions for a typical person. But only you can determine the right amount of food to satisfy your needs and allow for a rate of weight loss that's right for your body. Start with an amount of food that seems appropriate for you, eat mindfully, and let your body signals guide you. As you begin a meal, pay attention to the way the food feels in your body. Is your hunger receding? Are your bites slowing down? Is your belly becoming pleasantly full? If you feel satisfied before finishing your meal, stop eating and don't worry about wasting food for now. (At your next meal, try taking a smaller portion to see if that satisfies you.) Still hungry after cleaning your plate? Then help yourself to more of everything in the meal (main dish *and* sides) to keep the nutrient ratios in balance. And if you get hungry between meals, feel free to reach for an extra snack.

Building a Phase 1 Meal

Phase 1 features a carefully calibrated Meal Plan (page 159) covering every meal and snack during these fourteen days—a boot camp for your fat cells (but not for you!). However, this plan is designed to be flexible. Feel free to adapt it for your specific needs, but do your best to follow recommended food combinations and reach the target nutrient ratio. This section and the following two (Lettuce Wrap and Vegetarian Substitutions) will show you how to create your own Phase 1–compatible meals, if you prefer to do so for any reason.

All Phase 1 meals follow this general formula:

START WITH A HIGH-QUALITY PROTEIN...	BULK UP THE PROTEIN IF NEEDED...	POUR ON THE FAT...	THEN ADD A CARBOHYDRATE
Higher protein/higher fat: -fatty meat or fish, poultry with skin (4 to 6 ounces) *Higher protein/lower fat:* -lean meat or fish, poultry without skin (4 to 6 ounces) -cold cuts (4 to 6 ounces) -protein powder (about 1 ounce) *Lower protein/higher fat:* -tempeh, tofu (4 to 6 ounces) -eggs (3) -cheese (3 ounces)	*For lower-protein items, add another source of protein:* -Greek yogurt (½ cup) -beans (½ cup) -cheese (1 to 2 ounces) -nuts or nut butter (2 to 3 tablespoons)	*For lower-fat items, add a larger portion of fat:* -dressings and sauces (2 to 4 tablespoons) -oils (1 to 2 tablespoons) -heavy cream or canned coconut milk (3 to 4 tablespoons) -nuts or nut butter (2 to 3 tablespoons) -½ avocado *For higher-fat items, add a smaller portion of fat:* -dressings and sauces (1 to 2 tablespoons) -oils (1 to 3 teaspoons) -heavy cream or canned coconut milk (1 to 3 tablespoons) -nuts or nut butter (1 to 2 tablespoons) -¼ avocado	*If your meal doesn't already have a carbohydrate, add one serving of the following:* -beans (½ cup) -bean or vegetable soup (1 cup) -fruit (non-tropical) (1 cup) **Note:** Include as many extra nonstarchy vegetables as you like (e.g., salad or cooked vegetables).

My Always Hungry Story

As I was eating my steak and blue cheese salad, which I ate over a luxurious twenty minutes, savoring every bite, I mused on the frozen meals I scarfed down in three minutes while on other diet programs. It feels really good to be eating quality foods and resetting my dietary programming. I feel like I've gone to a spa this week!

—*Nancy F., 64, Eden Prairie, MN*
Weight loss: 14 pounds. Decrease in waist: 7 inches

Lettuce Wrap

A secret to being efficient in the kitchen is knowing how to use leftovers creatively, altering them in ways that feel new and fresh. Lettuce wraps with sauces are an easy way to give your leftovers a makeover. Any leftover fish, chicken, or other protein can be your base for a wrap. Add a few vegetables and a sauce, and you have a fresh, quick, easy meal.

Choose one item from each of the categories below, and make a lettuce wrap.

WRAP	BASE INGREDIENT	ADDED VEGETABLE	DIPPING SAUCE
Large lettuce leaf like romaine, butter, Bibb, or red/green leaf Flavorful lettuce leaves like radicchio or endive	Leftover protein, such as rotisserie chicken, Herb-Roasted Chicken Thighs (page 241), broiled or baked fish, Salmon Salad (page 254), Pan-Fried Tempeh or Tofu Strips (page 243) Leftover casserole, either cold or stored separately and reheated prior to wrapping Can of salmon or sardines (skin on and bones in, for maximum omega-3 and calcium) Smoked salmon	Leftover blanched, steamed, or sautéed vegetables (only good for one day, so make fresh the previous dinner or at breakfast and pack for your lunch) Slices of tomato, avocado, shredded carrots, and/or other raw veggies	Any of your favorite sauces from the recipe list or that you make on your own Store-bought guacamole or sour cream Pairing suggestions: Creamy Dill (page 270) with most fish Creamy Lime-Cilantro (page 271) with Mexican Shredded Chicken (page 241) Blue Cheese (page 263) with beef Ginger-Soy Vinaigrette (page 267) with fish, chicken or tofu Lemon Tahini (page 269) with Mediterranean fillings

Vegetarian Substitutions

The meal plans emphasize an abundance of whole foods from a variety of plant sources but also include animal products. Because some people have chosen to minimize or eliminate animal foods from their diets for various reasons—such as health, taste preferences, allergies, or concerns about animal welfare and the environment—all recipes include vegetarian options. This chart guides substitution of all animal products used on the meal plan for vegan alternatives:

INSTEAD OF...	SUBSTITUTE...
Fatty meat, chicken, fish, or eggs	-Tofu -Tempeh
Lean meats	-Vegetarian deli cold cuts -Seitan* -Vegetarian protein powder
Cheese	-Nuts or nut butter (especially peanut) -Soy cheese
Yogurt	-Coconut yogurt, plain, unsweetened plus ½ serving vegetarian protein powder -Soy yogurt, plain, unsweetened
Heavy cream	-Coconut milk, canned
Sour cream	-Avocado -Guacamole -Dressing or sauce of choice

* Wheat gluten—avoid if sensitive to gluten-containing products

My Always Hungry Story

I have not been a fan of tofu, but the tofu and black bean hash is *wonderful*! I never expected this recipe to taste so good. This recipe is definitely a keeper.

—Angelica G., 50, Sacramento, CA
Weight loss: 11.5 pounds. Decrease in waist: 3 inches

Tips for Phase 1 Success

Here are a few additional pointers to keep you on track as you begin Phase 1.

Stick as close to the plan as possible. For the next fourteen days, do your best to follow the meal plan closely. This plan is designed to deliver a specific combination of protein, fat, and natural carbohydrates for fast changes in metabolism. If you need to make adjustments for personal reasons, refer to the guidelines on page 151 for Building a Phase 1 Meal. If you're unable to prepare your own foods, choose from the Restaurant and Grab-and-Go Recommendations in chapter 7 (page 186).

Portion sizes are truly up to you. The portions in the meal plan are designed for a typical person, but your needs may be greater or smaller. Eat until you are satisfied but not unpleasantly over-full. If you find that you need more or less, take larger or smaller portions. Add or omit a snack. As long as you eat the types of foods in the ratios prescribed, your body will do the rest.

Swap with similar items whenever possible. If you don't like a certain ingredient in the recipe, simply swap like for like: Trade broccoli for cauliflower, raspberries for strawberries, fish for chicken, and so on, as long as the foods are closely related in content of the major nutrients. Refer to Program Foods Phase-by-Phase (page 110) for guidelines.

Seasonings are a matter of personal preference. We have included a range of herbs and spices in the meal plan. By adding flavor to food, herbs and spices help displace sugar from the diet. In addition, they contain polyphenols that reduce inflammation. Get creative and find the ones you like. Store them in a convenient location (for example, a specially dedicated drawer or rack) for easy access.

Limit yourself to Phase 1 sweets only. If you tend to get cravings for sweets, you may find they're satisfied with the desserts accompanying most dinners on the meal plan. Pilot participants consistently reported reductions in desire for highly sweetened foods from very early into the program. However, if you need a little extra treat, have up to an ounce of dark chocolate—minimum 70% cocoa content—once a day. (And please don't be reluctant to eat the desserts on the plan. They're built into the nutritional ratios for each day, and will actually help you attain the best results.)

My Always Hungry Story

I used to think, "Oh, I'm tired—let me eat something sweet." But that just gives you a little bit of boost and then you crash again. By shying away from carbs and the sugar crashes, I'm maintaining an even level of that energy through the whole day.

—*Renee B., 49, West Roxbury, MA*
Weight loss: 13 pounds. Decrease in waist: 6 inches

Enjoy coffee or tea. You may have two or three cups of caffeinated coffee or tea a day. Add cream or whole milk if you wish (no need for the skim or low-fat versions), but steer clear of sugar and other sweeteners.

No alcohol—for now. Just for these two weeks, abstain from alcoholic beverages. You will have the option to reintroduce moderate amounts in Phase 2.

Supplements. Consider taking three supplements throughout the program:

- Vitamin D_3: With so many hours spent indoors and the increased use of sunscreens, many people do not get enough sun exposure to maintain adequate vitamin D levels. In addition to its importance for bone health, vitamin D may play a role in the prevention of cancer, autoimmune diseases, diabetes, heart disease and psychiatric problems.[1] (Note: D_3 has greater biological activity than D_2, and vegan versions are now available.)
- Fish oil: Fish oil is an excellent source of long chain omega-3 fatty acids (see page 81). Choose a product that has been concentrated, purified, and tested for contaminants. For vegetarians, flax oil and certain nuts provide short chain omega-3 fatty acids (which can be converted to the active, long chain form in the body).

- Probiotics: Take these supplements, which are available in capsules, for gut health, to supplement dietary sources like yogurt (see page 83).

If you're pressed for time, check out the Simplified Meal Plan. The Simplified Meal Plan (online at www.alwayshungrybook.com) offers a streamlined version of the Phase 1 Meal Plan (page 159), with a bit less variety, greater use of leftovers, and just-the-basics prep work. This version works well for one person. And if you have a busy family, multiply the Simplified Meal Plan instructions by the number of mouths to feed.

Use leftovers often, but always add something fresh. Several casseroles and one-pot dishes can be frozen in individual portions as backup meals. Add freshly prepared vegetables (cooked or raw) to reheated leftovers.

Use time-saving shortcuts. These "convenience" foods—all ingredients in recipes on this plan—will get you in and out of the kitchen more quickly. Buy Green Bags (www.evertfresh.com) for storage, to help your produce stay fresh in the refrigerator.

- Chopped vegetables found in the produce section, such as cauliflower, broccoli, celery (check for freshness)
- Washed, precut greens—spinach, kale, mixed greens, salad greens
- Shredded cabbage and carrots
- Frozen vegetables and fruits
- Rotisserie chicken
- Baked, seasoned, packaged tofu
- Canned, unsweetened legumes/beans, such as black beans, chickpeas, kidney beans (drained and rinsed well)
- Shredded cheese (full-fat, without additives)

Also use sauce as a time-saver. Make sauces or parts of recipes ahead of time so that meal preparation on busy days will be less time consuming. (Sauces could be a big part of your if-then planning: "If

I'm too tired, late, or uninspired, then I will use the sauces in the fridge to make a quick dinner.")

Get a sharp knife, keep it sharp, and learn how to use it. Not having a proper knife can cause a major slowdown while prepping and cooking. Knife work takes a bit of practice, but learning to use a sharp knife will save you precious time in the kitchen.

Don't forget your prep time. Try to block out a few hours every weekend to do shopping and meal prep for the coming week—those few hours will make the program much easier to follow.

Shopping Lists and Preparation for the Meal Plan

The shopping lists are designed for two trips to the market each week for perishables (you stocked up on the nonperishables during the Prep Phase). We suggest that you do one of these two trips on the weekend for the foods you'll eat Monday through Wednesday (supplies to make three days of meals plus sauces and nuts for the week); and the other one on Wednesday for foods you'll eat Thursday through Sunday (supplies for four days of meals). If you prefer to shop just once a week, combine the two perishable food lists, and freeze items intended for later in the week as appropriate. Sunday is prep day to make sauces and roast nuts for the entire week. Refer to the Weekly Prep Worksheets for Phase 1 (Week 1 in chapter 5, page 142, and Week 2 on page 166). And get ready for the next phase with the Weekly Prep Worksheet for Phase 2, Week 1 (on page 175).

Before each shopping trip, take a look at the Menus At-A-Glance Charts (online at www.alwayshungrybook.com) to see what's on the menu. If you have allergies or food sensitivities, make a note of any items that may present issues for you. Refer to the Program Foods Phase-by-Phase chart (page 110) to find alternatives. Then refer to the corresponding Shopping List online, and copy it or download the file from www.alwayshungrybook.com.

My Always Hungry Story

I grew up eating shepherd's pie with a *huge* layer of potato. I didn't think I could be fooled by this cauliflower-bean combo, but I was! It was delicious! These recipes continue to surprise me!
—*Amanda B., 35, Roslindale, MA*
Weight loss: 8 pounds. Decrease in waist: 2.5 inches

PHASE 1 MEAL PLAN AND PREP WORKSHEETS

The Meal Plan is designed for two people, and described per serving, but can be easily scaled up for families of any size. And if you're cooking just for yourself, either reduce recipes accordingly or refer to the Simplified Meal Plan online at www.alwayshungry book.com. (The Weekly Prep Worksheet for Week 1 is on page 142.)

My Always Hungry Story

On Day 1: Gosh, the food was good. I am really full though and am most likely going to skip dessert. Did I just say "skip dessert"? Wow!
—*Pam M., 55, Confluence, PA*
Weight loss: 13 pounds. Decrease in waist: 2 inches

MONDAY (DAY 1)

Breakfast

Huevos Rancheros

Fry 2 eggs plus 1 egg white in 1 teaspoon olive oil. Top with ½ cup *Ranchero Sauce* (page 272), 2 tablespoons shredded cheddar cheese. Serve with 1 cup raspberries and ½ cup plain whole-milk Greek yogurt.

Protein: 25%	Fat: 53%	Carbohydrate: 22%	Calories: 534*

Prep: Assemble and pack today's snacks.

Assemble today's lunch—Mozzarella, Tomato, and Chickpea Salad.

Snack

¼ cup *Trail Mix* (page 291)

Lunch

Mozzarella, Tomato, and Chickpea Salad

1 medium tomato, chopped; ½ cup cooked garbanzo beans (chickpeas), drained and rinsed; 3 ounces fresh mozzarella, sliced; 1 cup chopped romaine or other lettuce; 2 tablespoons *Lemon Tahini Sauce* (page 269); salt and ground black pepper; 2 ounces canned sardines (optional)

Without Sardines

Protein: 21%	Fat: 55%	Carbohydrate: 24%	Calories: 446*

With Sardines

Protein: 27%	Fat: 54%	Carbohydrate: 19%	Calories: 564*

Snack

Cold-Cut Lettuce Boats (page 294) with *Creamy Dill Sauce* (page 270)

Dinner

Soup, Herb-Roasted Chicken, and Vegetables

About 1½ cups *Creamy Cauliflower Soup*** (page 280—prepared without heavy cream); *Herb-Roasted Chicken Thighs*** (page 241); 1 cup broccoli and ½ small carrot, blanched (page 313—Guide to Cooking Vegetables), topped with 1 tablespoon *Lemon Olive Oil Dressing* (page 269)

Dessert

1 cup fruit with ½ ounce square chocolate (at least 70% cocoa content)

Protein: 24%	Fat: 52%	Carbohydrate: 24%	Calories: 661*

Prep: Assemble tomorrow's lunch—*Chicken Salad with Grapes and Walnuts* (page 252) using reserved portion of *Herb-Roasted Chicken Thighs* without the skin; store lettuce separately and add tomorrow before serving.

Store reserved portion of *Creamy Cauliflower Soup* for tomorrow's dinner.

---

* Calorie content provided for descriptive purposes only—not as a measure to limit food intake.

** To serve two people, make a full recipe and store reserved portions to be used in subsequent meals as directed in prep notes.

*** To serve two people, make ½ recipe.

TUESDAY (DAY 2)			

Breakfast

Phase 1 Power Shake
Phase 1 Power Shake (page 220)

Protein: 22%	Fat: 54%	Carbohydrate: 24%	Calories: 500*

Prep: Assemble and pack today's snacks.

Snack

Smoked Salmon and Dill Cream Cheese on Cucumber Rounds (page 295)

Lunch

Chicken Salad with Grapes and Walnuts
Chicken Salad with Grapes and Walnuts (page 252) (using chicken from previous night's dinner)

Protein: 23%	Fat: 53%	Carbohydrate: 24%	Calories 572*

Snack

About ⅓ cup *Basic Hummus* (page 290) with veggie sticks

Dinner

Soup, Steak and Onions, Vegetables
About 1½ cups *Creamy Cauliflower Soup* (from previous night's dinner) garnished with 1 tablespoon heavy cream; cook a 9-ounce tenderloin steak (follow cooking instructions from *Steak Salad*, page 253), or cook 8 ounces *Pan-Fried Tempeh Strips* (page 243)—use 5 ounces steak or 4 ounces tempeh for tonight's dinner and 4 ounces steak or tempeh for tomorrow's lunch; sauté ½ small onion in the pan juices on medium-high heat until caramelized; 1 cup blanched kale or other green vegetable (page 313—Guide to Cooking Vegetables) topped with 1 tablespoon *Lemon Tahini Sauce* (page 269)

Dessert

1 cup raspberries with 2 tablespoons heavy cream

Protein: 25%	Fat: 51%	Carbohydrate: 24%	Calories: 602*

Prep: Assemble tomorrow's lunch—*Steak Salad with Blue Cheese Dressing* (page 253) using reserved portion of steak or tempeh; store lettuce separately and add tomorrow before serving; pack a tangerine.

---

   * Calorie content provided for descriptive purposes only—not as a measure to limit food intake.
  ** To serve two people, make a full recipe and store reserved portions to be used in subsequent meals as directed in prep notes.
 *** To serve two people, make ½ recipe.

WEDNESDAY (DAY 3)

Breakfast

Black Bean Tofu Hash

*Black Bean Tofu Hash*** (page 222) topped with 2 tablespoons cheddar cheese, 1 to 2 tablespoons sour cream, ½ avocado, sliced, or 5 tablespoons guacamole

| Protein: 23% | Fat: 55% | Carbohydrate: 22% | Calories: 455* |

Prep: Assemble and pack today's snacks.

Store reserved portion of *Black Bean Tofu Hash* for tomorrow's lunch.

Snack

Cold-Cut Lettuce Boats (page 294) with *Lemon Tahini Sauce* (page 269)

Lunch

Steak Salad with Blue Cheese

Steak Salad with Blue Cheese Dressing (page 253) (using steak from previous night's dinner). Serve with a tangerine.

| Protein: 27% | Fat: 47% | Carbohydrate: 26% | Calories: 565* |

Snack

¼ cup *Trail Mix* (page 291)

Dinner

Broiled Fish and Sautéed Kale

*Broiled Fish with Garlic and Lemon**** (page 232) Remove fish and lemons from pan and sauté 1 cup kale in the pan juices. Top fish or kale with 2 tablespoons *Creamy Dill Sauce* (page 270). Serve with 1 cup salad greens with 1 tablespoon dressing of your choice.

Dessert

Poached Seasonal Fruit (page 288) with 1 to 1½ tablespoons *Chocolate Sauce* (page 289).**

| Protein: 25% | Fat: 50% | Carbohydrate: 25% | Calories: 594* |

Prep: Assemble tomorrow's lunch—Taco Salad (see Day 4 lunch), using reserved portion of *Black Bean Tofu Hash*; store lettuce separately and add tomorrow before serving.

Store reserved portion of *Chocolate Sauce* for Day 7 dinner.

---

* Calorie content provided for descriptive purposes only—not as a measure to limit food intake.

** To serve two people, make a full recipe and store reserved portions to be used in subsequent meals as directed in prep notes.

*** To serve two people, make ½ recipe.

THURSDAY (DAY 4)

Breakfast

Spinach Omelet

Heat 2 teaspoons olive oil in a skillet. Whisk 2 eggs with 1 egg white. Add 1 cup baby spinach leaves, salt, and pepper. Pour into a pan. Top with 3 tablespoons shredded cheddar cheese. Fold over and cook until done. Serve with 1 cup fresh fruit and ½ cup plain whole-milk Greek yogurt.

Protein: 25%	Fat: 54%	Carbohydrate: 22%	Calories: 524*

Prep: Assemble and pack today's snacks.

Snack

Small apple with 2 tablespoons peanut butter

Lunch

Taco Salad

1½ cups *Black Bean Tofu Hash* (page 222) (from previous day's breakfast), 1 cup chopped romaine or other lettuce, 1 small tomato, diced, 2 tablespoons salsa, 2 tablespoons cheddar cheese. Top with 3 tablespoons *Creamy Lime-Cilantro Dressing* (page 271).

Protein: 23%	Fat: 52%	Carbohydrate: 25%	Calories: 502*

Snack

¼ cup *Spicy Pumpkin Seeds* (page 292)

Dinner

Eggplant Parmesan and Salad

*Eggplant Parmesan*** (page 247). Serve with salad greens with 1 cup sliced cucumber, ½ cup shredded carrot, ½ sliced red pepper, and 1 tablespoon dressing of your choice.

Dessert

1 cup raspberries

Additional Cooking Prep: Make *Coconut Cashew Clusters**** (page 284); follow directions for 4 clusters and set aside for tomorrow night's dessert

Protein: 20%	Fat: 56%	Carbohydrate: 24%	Calories: 698*

Prep: Pack tomorrow's lunch—*Eggplant Parmesan* and 1 cup of raspberries.

---

* Calorie content provided for descriptive purposes only—not as a measure to limit food intake.
** To serve two people, make a full recipe and store reserved portions to be used in subsequent meals as directed in prep notes.
*** To serve two people, make ½ recipe.

FRIDAY (DAY 5)

Breakfast

Smoked Salmon and Dill Sauce

3 ounces smoked salmon, 1 ounce cheddar cheese, 1 medium tomato, sliced, and 1 small cucumber, sliced. Top with 3 to 4 tablespoons *Creamy Dill Sauce* (page 270). Serve with 1 cup fresh blueberries or fruit of your choice.

| Protein: 23% | Fat: 55% | Carbohydrate: 22% | Calories: 530* |

Prep: Assemble and pack today's snacks.

Snack

Cold-Cut Lettuce Boats (page 294) with sauce of your choice

Lunch

Eggplant Parmesan and Fruit

Eggplant Parmesan (page 247) (from previous night's dinner); 1 cup raspberries

| Protein: 24% | Fat: 54% | Carbohydrate: 22% | Calories: 549* |

Snack

About ⅓ cup *Basic Hummus* (page 290) with veggie sticks

Dinner

Chicken Stir-Fry

*Chicken or Tofu Stir-Fry*** (page 230). If using tofu, serve with ½ cup edamame appetizer.
Dessert
Coconut Cashew Clusters (made last night)

| Protein: 29% | Fat: 49% | Carbohydrate: 22% | 597 calories* |

Prep: Pack tomorrow's lunch—Lettuce Wrap (see Day 6 Lunch) using reserved portion of *Chicken Stir-Fry*; store lettuce, carrots, peanuts and *Ginger-Soy Vinaigrette* (page 267) separately and assemble before eating; pack a tangerine.

---

* Calorie content provided for descriptive purposes only—not as a measure to limit food intake.
** To serve two people, make a full recipe and store reserved portions to be used in subsequent meals as directed in prep notes.
*** To serve two people, make ½ recipe.

SATURDAY (DAY 6)

Breakfast

Grain-Free Waffles and Turkey Bacon

*Grain-Free Waffles or Pancakes with Fruit Sauce*** (page 223) and 3 tablespoons *Whipped Cream (page 230)* or 1 tablespoon almond butter; 1 slice turkey bacon

Protein: 26%	Fat: 51%	Carbohydrate: 23%	Calories: 441*

Prep: Assemble and pack today's snacks. Make a full recipe of *Cheesy Pinto Bean Dip* and keep the reserved portions for week 2.

Store reserved portion of *Grain-Free Waffles with Fruit Sauce* and *Whipped Cream* for Day 8 Breakfast.

Snack

About ⅓ cup *Cheesy Pinto Bean Dip* (page 290)

Lunch

Chicken Stir-Fry Lettuce Wrap

Divide a lunch-size portion of *Chicken Stir-Fry* (from previous night's dinner) with ½ cup shredded carrots and 2 tablespoons peanuts evenly among 3 or 4 large lettuce leaves (if using tofu, serve with edamame instead of carrots and peanuts), leaving plenty of room to fold and wrap each leaf around the filling. Place 2 tablespoons *Ginger-Soy Vinaigrette* (page 267) into a shallow container. Dip the wraps in the sauce. Serve with a tangerine.

Protein: 24%	Fat: 51%	Carbohydrate: 25%	Calories: 552*

Snack

Cucumber Boats with Turkey and Feta (page 294)

Dinner

Shepherd's Pie

*Shepherd's Pie with Cauliflower Topping*** (page 238); 1 cup snap peas or snow peas, blanched (page 313—Guide to Cooking Vegetables), with 1 tablespoon *Creamy Dill Sauce* (page 270)

Dessert

1 ounce square dark chocolate

Protein: 22%	Fat: 48%	Carbohydrate: 30%	Calories: 648*

Prep: Pack tomorrow's lunch—*Shepherd's Pie* and snap peas with 1 tablespoon dressing of your choice.

Pack and freeze reserved portions of *Shepherd's Pie* for future meals.

---

* Calorie content provided for descriptive purposes only—not as a measure to limit food intake.

** To serve two people, make a full recipe and store reserved portions to be used in subsequent meals as directed in prep notes.

*** To serve two people, make ½ recipe.

WEEKLY PREP WORKSHEET

Prep Day for Phase 1, Week 2 Meal Plan
Note: Worksheet is designed for the menu plan that serves two people. Make one of each
recipe listed unless otherwise noted, or scale up or down according to your needs.

Sauces
- Coconut Curry Sauce (page 266)
- Chipotle Mayonnaise (page 268)
- Tartar Sauce (page 261)
- Mustard Vinaigrette (page 264)
- Thai Peanut Sauce (page 262)

For the following items, use leftovers from week 1:
- Ginger-Soy Vinaigrette (page 267)
- Ranchero Sauce (page 272—thaw 2½ cups)
- Chocolate Sauce (page 289)
- Lemon Olive Oil Dressing (page 269)
- Basic Mayonnaise (page 259)—use to make Tartar Sauce (listed above)

Snacks/Roasted Nuts & Seeds
- Herb-Roasted Chickpeas (page 293)
- Roast ¼ cup pecans (page 319—Guide to Roasting Nuts and Seeds) or other
  nuts for Day 10 Dessert and ½ cup peanuts for Day 12 Thai Peanut Tempeh
  (page 258)—or add roasted nuts to shopping list in place of raw nuts

For the following items, use leftovers from week 1:
- Spicy Pumpkin Seeds (page 292)—or add roasted pumpkin seeds to
  shopping list in place of raw seeds
- Trail Mix (page 291)—or add roasted nuts to shopping list in place of raw nuts

Ingredients to Prep (Proteins, Grains, Soups, etc. to use throughout the week)
- Crumbled Tempeh (page 244) for Friday Dinner
- Salmon Salad (page 254) for Tuesday Lunch

If choosing vegetarian variations for any of the recipes—Additional Pan-Fried Tempeh or Tofu Strips (page 243) or Crumbled Tempeh (page 244)

SUNDAY (DAY 7)

Breakfast

Frittata with Fruit and Yogurt

*Dr. Ludwig's Favorite Frittata*** (page 225); 1 cup fruit, ⅔ cup plain whole-milk Greek yogurt

Protein: 25%	Fat: 47%	Carbohydrate: 28%	Calories: 468*

Prep: Assemble and pack today's snacks.
Store reserved portion *Dr. Ludwig's Favorite Frittata* for Day 9 Breakfast.

Snack

¼ cup *Trail Mix* (page 291)

Lunch

Shepherd's Pie and Salad

Shepherd's Pie with Cauliflower Topping (page 238) (leftover from previous night's dinner);
1 cup snap peas or snow peas, blanched, with 1 tablespoon dressing of your choice.

Protein: 26%	Fat: 47%	Carbohydrate: 27%	Calories: 518*

Snack

Small apple with 1 ounce cheese

Dinner

Coconut Curry Shrimp

*Coconut Curry Shrimp or Tofu*** (page 248)

Dessert

½ cup strawberries with 1 to 2 tablespoons *Chocolate Sauce* (page 289) (from Day 3 Dessert)

Protein: 23%	Fat: 52%	Carbohydrate: 25%	Calories: 567*

Prep: Pack tomorrow's lunch—Lettuce Wrap (see Day 8 Lunch) using reserved portion of
Coconut Curry Shrimp; store lettuce separately; pack an orange and optional dressing or lime
wedges.

---

 * Calorie content provided for descriptive purposes only—not as a measure to limit food intake.
 ** To serve two people, make a full recipe and store reserved portions to be used in subsequent meals as
    directed in prep notes.
*** To serve two people, make ½ recipe.

MONDAY (DAY 8)

Breakfast

Grain-Free Waffles and Turkey Bacon

Grain-Free Waffles or Pancakes with Fruit Sauce (from Day 6 Breakfast) and 3 tablespoons *Whipped Cream* (page 230) or 1 tablespoon almond butter (from Day 6 Breakfast); 1 slice turkey bacon

Protein: 26%	Fat: 51%	Carbohydrate: 23%	Calories: 440*

Prep: Assemble and pack today's snacks.

Snack

About ⅓ cup *Herb-Roasted Chickpeas* (page 293)

Lunch

Coconut Curry Shrimp Lettuce Wrap

Divide reserved portion of *Coconut Curry Shrimp or Tofu* (page 248) (from previous night's dinner) evenly among 3 or 4 large lettuce leaves, leaving plenty of room to fold and wrap each leaf around the filling. Serve with an orange.

Optional: Add a squeeze of lime or place 1 to 2 tablespoons *Ginger-Soy Vinaigrette* (page 267) in a shallow container. Dip the wraps in the sauce.

Protein: 26%	Fat: 46%	Carbohydrate: 28%	Calories: 480*

Snack

1 ounce dark chocolate

Dinner

Chipotle Mayonnaise Baked Fish and Kale

*Chipotle Mayonnaise Baked Fish*** (page 250). Steam 1 cup kale and 1 small carrot (about ½ cup shredded). Top with 1 tablespoon *Lemon Olive Oil Dressing* (page 269).

Dessert

1 cup blueberries with 2 tablespoons canned coconut milk

Protein: 23%	Fat: 54%	Carbohydrate: 23%	Calories: 591*

Prep: Pack tomorrow's lunch—Lettuce Wrap (see Day 9 Lunch) using *Salmon or Tofu Salad**** (page 254) (from Sunday's prep); store lettuce separately; pack with an apple.

---

   * Calorie content provided for descriptive purposes only—not as a measure to limit food intake.
  ** To serve two people, make a full recipe and store reserved portions to be used in subsequent meals as directed in prep notes.
*** To serve two people, make ½ recipe.

TUESDAY (DAY 9)

Breakfast

Frittata with Fruit and Yogurt

Dr. Ludwig's Favorite Frittata (from Day 7 Breakfast); 1 cup fruit, ²/₃ cup plain whole-milk Greek yogurt

Protein: 25%	Fat: 47%	Carbohydrate: 28%	Calories: 468*

Prep: Assemble and pack today's snacks.

Snack

¼ cup *Spicy Pumpkin Seeds* (page 292)

Lunch

Lettuce Wrap Salmon Salad

Divide *Salmon or Tofu Salad* (page 254) (from Sunday's prep) evenly among 3 or 4 large lettuce leaves, leaving plenty of room to fold and wrap each leaf around the filling. Serve with an apple.

Protein: 22%	Fat: 55%	Carbohydrate: 23%	Calories: 515*

Snack

About ⅓ cup *Cheesy Pinto Bean Dip* (page 290)

Dinner

Mediterranean Chicken

*Mediterranean Chicken or Tofu*** (page 245). Serve with 1 small tomato, sliced, with ½ small cucumber, sliced, and a few leaves of fresh basil topped with 1 tablespoon *Mustard Vinaigrette* (page 264).

Dessert

½ cup berries

Protein: 26%	Fat: 47%	Carbohydrate: 27%	Calories: 656*

Prep: Pack tomorrow's lunch—*Mediterranean Chicken or Tofu* and ½ ounce dark chocolate.

---

   * Calorie content provided for descriptive purposes only—not as a measure to limit food intake.
  ** To serve two people, make a full recipe and store reserved portions to be used in subsequent meals as directed in prep notes.
*** To serve two people, make ½ recipe.

WEDNESDAY (DAY 10)

Breakfast

Phase 1 Power Shake

Phase 1 Power Shake (page 220)

Protein: 22%	Fat: 54%	Carbohydrate: 24%	Calories: 500*

Prep: Assemble and pack today's snacks.

Snack

¼ cup *Trail Mix* (page 291)

Lunch

Mediterranean Chicken

Mediterranean Chicken or Tofu (page 245) (from previous night's dinner). Serve with ½ ounce dark chocolate.

Protein: 30%	Fat: 46%	Carbohydrate: 24%	Calories: 580*

Snack

Small apple with 2 tablespoons peanut butter

Dinner

Soup, Cabbage Casserole, and Vegetables

About 1½ cups *Carrot-Ginger Soup*** (page 282) garnished with 2 tablespoons coconut milk; *Cabbage Casserole*** (page 236); 1 cup kale, lightly blanched (page 313—Guide to Cooking Vegetables), or other green vegetable of your choice, topped with 1 tablespoon dressing of your choice

Dessert

2 tablespoons roasted pecans (from Sunday's prep)

Protein: 23%	Fat: 49%	Carbohydrate: 28%	Calories: 640*

Prep: Pack tomorrow's lunch—*Cabbage Casserole*; salad greens with 1 to 2 tablespoons *Mustard Vinaigrette* on the side.

Store reserved portion of *Carrot-Ginger Soup* with 2 tablespoons coconut milk for tomorrow's dinner.

---

* Calorie content provided for descriptive purposes only—not as a measure to limit food intake.

** To serve two people, make a full recipe and store reserved portions to be used in subsequent meals as directed in prep notes.

*** To serve two people, make ½ recipe.

THURSDAY (DAY 11)

Breakfast

Black Bean Tofu Hash

*Black Bean Tofu Hash*** (page 222) topped with 2 tablespoons shredded cheddar cheese, 1 to 2 tablespoons sour cream, ½ avocado, sliced, or 5 tablespoons guacamole.

Protein: 23%	Fat: 55%	Carbohydrate: 22%	Calories: 455*

Prep: Assemble and pack today's snacks.

Snack

Cucumber Boat with Turkey and Feta (page 294)

Lunch

Cabbage Casserole and Vegetables

Cabbage Casserole (page 236) (from previous night's dinner); 2 cups mixed greens with 1 to 2 tablespoons *Mustard Vinaigrette* (page 264).

Protein: 26%	Fat: 52%	Carbohydrate: 22%	Calories: 523*

Snack

About ⅓ cup *Herb-Roasted Chickpeas* (page 293)

Dinner

Soup, Broiled Salmon, and Garlic Herb Zucchini Rounds

About 1½ cups *Carrot-Ginger Soup* (page 282) (from previous night's dinner) garnished with 2 tablespoons coconut milk. Broil 10 ounces salmon per person—use *Broiled Fish with Lemon and Garlic*** (page 232—follow *Salmon Variation*) use half for dinner and half for tomorrow's lunch. Serve with *Garlic Herb Zucchini Rounds* (page 277).

Dessert

½ cup fruit with ½ ounce square dark chocolate

Protein: 26%	Fat: 51%	Carbohydrate: 23%	Calories: 598*

Prep: Assemble tomorrow's lunch—Salmon, Arugula, and Orange Salad (see Day 12 Lunch), using reserved 5 ounces salmon; pack arugula separately.

---

* Calorie content provided for descriptive purposes only—not as a measure to limit food intake.
** To serve two people, make a full recipe and store reserved portions to be used in subsequent meals as directed in prep notes.
*** To serve two people, make ½ recipe.

FRIDAY (DAY 12)

Breakfast

Huevos Rancheros

Fry 2 eggs plus 1 egg white in 1 teaspoon olive oil. Top with ½ cup *Ranchero Sauce* (page 272), 2 tablespoons shredded cheddar cheese. Serve with 1 cup raspberries and ½ cup plain whole-milk Greek yogurt.

| Protein: 25% | Fat: 53% | Carbohydrate: 22% | Calories: 534* |

Prep: Assemble and pack today's snacks.

Snack

1 ounce chocolate

Lunch

Salmon, Arugula, and Orange Salad

Combine 5 ounces salmon (from previous night's dinner), 1½ to 2 cups arugula or lettuce, 1 orange, sectioned and chopped, and ¼ avocado, diced. Toss with 2 tablespoons *Ginger-Soy Vinaigrette* (page 267)

| Protein: 26% | Fat: 52% | Carbohydrate: 22% | Calories: 474* |

Snack

½ cup shelled *Edamame*** (page 296)

Dinner

Thai Peanut Tempeh

*Thai Peanut Tempeh*** (page 258). Serve with ½ small cucumber, sliced, with a dash of salt and a squeeze of lemon.

Dessert

1 cup spiced chai with 1 to 2 tablespoons soy milk or whole milk

| Protein: 22% | Fat: 53% | Carbohydrate: 25% | Calories: 680* |

Prep: Pack tomorrow's lunch—Lettuce Wrap (see Day 13 Lunch) using *Thai Peanut Tempeh* garnished with 1 tablespoon peanuts; store lettuce, lime wedges, and sprouts separately.

---

   * Calorie content provided for descriptive purposes only—not as a measure to limit food intake.
  ** To serve two people, make a full recipe and store reserved portions to be used in subsequent meals as directed in prep notes.
*** To serve two people, make ½ recipe.

SATURDAY (DAY 13)

Breakfast

Grain-Free Waffles and Turkey Bacon

*Grain-Free Waffles or Pancakes with Fruit Sauce*** (page 223) and 3 tablespoons *Whipped Cream* (page 230) or 1 tablespoon almond butter; 1 slice turkey bacon

Additional Cooking Prep: Make an extra slice of turkey bacon for Phase 2, Day 1 Lunch.

Protein: 26%   Fat: 51%   Carbohydrate: 23%   Calories: 441*

Prep: Assemble and pack today's snacks.

Store reserved portion of *Grain-Free Waffles or Pancakes and Fruit Sauce* in the freezer for Phase 2, Day 6.

Snack

Cold-Cut Lettuce Boats (page 294) with sauce of your choice

Lunch

Thai Peanut Tempeh Lettuce Wrap

Divide a portion of *Thai Peanut Tempeh* (page 258) (from previous night's dinner) evenly among 3 or 4 large lettuce leaves, leaving plenty of room to fold and wrap each leaf around the filling. Top with sprouts, peanuts, and a squeeze of lime.

Protein: 24%   Fat: 48%   Carbohydrate: 28%   Calories: 562*

Snack

Small apple with 1 ounce cheese

Dinner

Soup, Ranchero Chicken, and Broccoli

1½ to 2 cups *Creamy Cauliflower Soup**** (page 280—prepared without cream); *Ranchero Chicken*** (page 257); 1 cup blanched broccoli topped with 2 tablespoons dressing of your choice

Dessert

1 ounce square dark chocolate

Protein: 27%   Fat: 49%   Carbohydrate: 24%   Calories: 612*

Prep: Assemble tomorrow's lunch—5-Layer Ranchero Chicken Bake, using reserved portion of *Ranchero Chicken*; pack avocado and sour cream toppings on the side.

---

* Calorie content provided for descriptive purposes only—not as a measure to limit food intake.

** To serve two people, make a full recipe and store reserved portions to be used in subsequent meals as directed in prep notes.

*** To serve two people, make ½ recipe.

SUNDAY (DAY 14)

Breakfast

Phase 1 Power Shake

Phase 1 Power Shake (page 220)

Protein: 22%	Fat: 54%	Carbohydrate: 24%	Calories: 500*

Prep: Assemble and pack today's snacks.

Snack

Small apple with 2 tablespoons peanut butter

Lunch

5-Layer Ranchero Chicken Bake

Layer 1 cup packed spinach leaves, 4 to 5 ounces *Ranchero Chicken* (page 257) (from previous night's dinner), ½ cup black beans, and 1 tablespoon cheddar cheese. Bake at 350°F until the cheese melts and spinach wilts. Top with ½ avocado, sliced, or ¼ cup guacamole and 1 tablespoon sour cream.

Protein: 32%	Fat: 44%	Carbohydrate: 24%	Calories: 554*

Snack

Snack of your choice

Dinner

Lamb Shanks

*Melt-in-Your-Mouth Lamb Shanks*** (page 233); *Sautéed Greens with Garlic* (page 274); 1 cup crudités (for example: ⅓ cup each celery, tomato, carrot) with optional sauce of your choice

Additional Cooking Prep:

Boil an egg for tomorrow's lunch.

While the lamb is cooking, make the *Roasted Sweet Potatoes* (page 279), using the baked whole potato variation, for tomorrow's dinner.

Dessert

1 cup berries

Protein: 29%	Fat: 49%	Carbohydrate: 22%	Calories: 613*

Prep: Assemble tomorrow's lunch—*Cobb Salad* (page 255), using reserved portion of turkey bacon (from yesterday's breakfast prep); pack dressing on the side.

Store reserved portion of *Melt-in-Your-Mouth Lamb Shanks* and *Whole Roasted Sweet Potatoes* for tomorrow's dinner.

---

* Calorie content provided for descriptive purposes only—not as a measure to limit food intake.

** To serve two people, make a full recipe and store reserved portions to be used in subsequent meals as directed in prep notes.

*** To serve two people, make ½ recipe.

WEEKLY PREP WORKSHEET

Prep Day for Phase 2, Week 1 Meal Plan

Note: Worksheet is designed for the menu plan that serves two people. Make one of each recipe listed, or scale up or down according to your needs.

Sauces
- Ginger-Soy Vinaigrette (page 267)
- Lemon Olive Oil Dressing (page 269)
- Honey Balsamic Marinade (page 273)—make half a recipe
- Stir-Fry Sauce (page 260)
- Creamy Lime-Cilantro Dressing (page 271)

For the following items, use leftovers from Week 2:
- Mustard Vinaigrette (page 264)
- Ranchero Sauce (page 272—thaw ½ cup)
- Chipotle Mayonnaise (page 268)

Snacks/Roasted Nuts & Seeds
- Roast ⅓ cup pecans (see Appendix C, page 319) for Thursday's Quinoa Salad with Pecans and Cranberries (page 277), ½ cup peanuts for Monday Breakfast and Sunday Lunch, and ¼ cup nuts of your choice for Wednesday Breakfast—or add roasted nuts to shopping list in place of raw nuts

- Prep Choice of Snacks:

_____

_____

_____

Ingredients to Prep (Proteins, Grains, Soups, etc., to use throughout the week)
- Crumbled Tempeh (page 244) for Day 2 Marinara Primavera (page 234)
- If choosing vegetarian variations for any of the recipes—Additional Pan-Fried Tempeh or Tofu Strips (page 243) or Crumbled Tempeh (page 244)

Note: Phase 2 meal plan begins on page 190

My Always Hungry Story

Phase 1 taught me two important, logical things: First, avoid sugar-added foods. Eat foods that have only natural sweetness. Once sugar is added, my body feels achy, so simple avoidance is the solution. Second, avoid wheat and gluten products. I am not gluten intolerant, but avoiding these products makes me feel naturally better. My wife has type 1 diabetes and, since we started this program, she has needed less insulin (she has a computerized pump).

—Paul G., 66, Aurora, IL
Weight loss: 27.5 pounds. Decrease in waist: 4.5 inches

CHAPTER 7

Phase 2—Retrain Your Fat Cells

Congratulations, you've finished Phase 1, the most challenging part of the program!

If you are like the majority of our pilot program participants, you've lost between 1 and 5 pounds so far, but the amount doesn't matter much right now. With calorie-restricted diets, weight loss occurs relatively easily for only a few weeks (and much of that is from body water or lean tissue, rather than fat). Then the real work starts, as you struggle to keep the weight off. In contrast, the Always Hungry Solution becomes progressively easier with time. If in the last two weeks you've experienced decreased hunger, fewer cravings, longer-lasting satiety after eating, or improved energy (and ideally, a combination of them), you can have confidence that the program is working from the inside out.

When people are deprived of calories in research studies, they of course lose weight. But when the study ends, weight usually pops right back up. After a period of force-feeding, the opposite happens— weight naturally drops back to where it started. These observations have led researchers to think in terms of a "body weight set point" that differs among people based on genes (see page 4). However, set points aren't set in stone. Our genes haven't much changed in the last few decades, as obesity rates have skyrocketed. And many of us gain weight continuously from teenage through late middle age. Clearly, factors in the environment must combine with genes to determine the set point for each individual, at each point in time.

The program is designed to lower body weight set point by targeting insulin resistance and chronic inflammation—through food *quality*, sleep, stress, and activity level.* With this approach, your weight may decrease more slowly at first than with conventional diets, but you'll be working with, not against, your body. You won't have to struggle with rapidly rising hunger and fading motivation.

My Always Hungry Story

Honestly, I almost cannot verbalize what I am feeling. Just ecstatic that I am eating so well, feeling *so* much better, and, to my amazement, *I've lost weight*? I hadn't ever been able to get my weight to budge!

—Nan T., 53, Birmingham, AL
Weight loss: 7.5 pounds. Decrease in waist: 1 inch

Phase 2 may range from a month or two, to six months or more, based on your starting weight and other individual factors. In time, you'll find that you need more food to control hunger and feel satisfied after eating. Your rate of weight loss will slow down. These are signs that your body has burned much of its excess fat

---

* If you're already at an optimal body weight and chose to follow this program for health benefits, your set point won't change.

stores and now must rely on the food you eat for an increasing proportion of your calorie requirements. Your weight may continue to drift down for a bit longer, and other health benefits will continue to accrue, but visible changes will become more subtle. From this point forward, the goal is sustainability—to make a healthful diet and lifestyle easy, enjoyable, and natural…for the rest of your life. Whatever the optimal weight for your body might be, the Always Hungry Solution will help you get there (Phases 1 and 2) and stay there (Phase 3).

Phase 2 meals share the same basic components as those in Phase 1, but allow you to choose from a wider range of foods for greater flexibility and sustainability. As shown in the figure on page 108, you will slightly decrease fat (to 40 percent of your calories) and increase carb intake (to 35 percent). The percentage of protein will remain the same (25 percent). You can now add moderate portions of intact whole grains, starchy vegetables (except white potatoes), and tropical fruits and melons. And you can opt to have a touch of natural sweetener (such as honey or maple syrup) in desserts or coffee/tea.

PHASE 2 LIFE SUPPORTS

Now that you've been living the Always Hungry Solution for a couple of weeks, you're probably starting to feel the benefits of your new movement, sleep, and stress-relief strategies. Perhaps you have more energy and look forward to your daily *passeggiata*. You're hopefully feeling more rested and less stressed. In Phase 2, we'll continue to build on the practices in Phase 1 to accelerate weight loss.

Movement

As you know from chapter 5, the Always Hungry Solution emphasizes enjoyable physical activities to tune up your metabolism, rather than burn a lot of calories. In Phase 2, you'll continue the *passeggiata*—your daily walk after dinner—and in addition include 30 to 40 minutes of enjoyable, moderate to vigorous physical activity three or four days a week (depending on your physical fitness and doctor's advice). You can add another walk at a more vigorous clip, go for a gentle jog or hike in nature, take a Zumba or yoga class, work in the garden, play tennis—whatever you enjoy. Aim to engage in an activity that makes you breathe a bit faster, so that you can still carry on a conversation but would find it difficult to sing. Consider which activities will be the most rewarding and absorbing. Do you find yourself losing track of time dancing, playing a sport, or taking a swim?

My Always Hungry Story

I own a Fitbit and wear it daily. Since starting this program, I've had so much energy, and have been so busy cooking, I raised my average steps by about 3,000 or 4,000 steps a day!

—*Leasa E., 43, Jacksonville, FL*
Weight loss: 5.5 pounds. Decrease in waist: 4 inches

Sleep

Are you sleeping more soundly after the first fourteen days on the program? Do you find you're more rested and peaceful? In Phase 2, continue to refine your pre-sleep routine according to your needs, so that it becomes naturally incorporated into your life. Remember that sufficient high-quality sleep is one of the best things you can do to tune up your metabolism and safeguard your health.

Stress Relief

Has the 5-minute stress reduction practice helped you to feel more peaceful throughout the day? Stress reduction works with sleep, physical activity, and diet to help fat cells calm down, open up, and release their excess store of calories back into the body—making weight loss virtually automatic. In Phase 2, it's time to add a second session. Space them out through the day, one in the morning or early afternoon and one in the evening, for sustained benefits.

If you're having trouble being consistent with this practice, experiment with a different method. Stress reduction doesn't have to involve sitting cross-legged in silent meditation. Consider listening to recorded guided imagery, reading inspirational poetry, or taking a short walk in nature during the most stressful time of day. Anything to disconnect from the frenetic outside world and soothe your nervous system. No matter how busy your day is, you deserve a few moments for yourself.

Other Supports

Connect with Your Big Why. Have you already experienced some benefits from the program, such as increasing energy level, more stable mood, and weight loss? If so, you're probably already feeling motivated! However, to make lifestyle changes stick for the long term, continue to connect with the most important reasons for losing weight and becoming healthier—your Big Why. If you haven't found your Big Why amulet yet, take a moment to do so now. You might simply write a few words on a sticky note and post it on your bathroom mirror. Keeping your Big Why front and center will help you avoid self-defeating behaviors and keep you on track to your goals.

Assess Your If-Then Plans. How are your if-then plans working? Take a few moments to analyze any obstacles you've encountered and create additional if-then plans for those scenarios.

My Always Hungry Story

We had an unprecedented snowy winter and I had to sleep four days at the hospital where I work. I found that if you stick to simple foods, then you could find things to eat in the cafeteria: cheese, hummus, carrots, fruit, and things like that. I actually found it to be quite easy. So while people were gaining weight because of the hard winter we had, I was consistently dropping a little bit every week.

—Renee B., 49, West Roxbury, MA
Weight loss: 13 pounds. Decrease in waist: 6 inches

Keep on Trackin'. Have the Daily Tracker and Monthly Progress Chart helped you notice patterns in your response to the program? Are your hunger, cravings, energy level, and weight beginning to tick in the right direction? Don't stop tracking now. These tools play an increasingly important role as you continue through Phase 2 and enter Phase 3.

Embrace the Teaching Moment. Nobody's perfect. There will inevitably come a time when you overindulge, eat too much of the wrong foods, and have a negative reaction. Perhaps you splurged at a party on cake and ice cream. Or just grabbed a bagel for breakfast in a rush, instead of something more balanced and nourishing. Soon thereafter, you might feel physically uncomfortable, experience a fall-off in energy level, become irritable, or maybe even develop a headache. A couple of hours later, you might get excessively hungry and battle food cravings. At these times, it's important not to be too hard on yourself. Don't engage in self-blame. Remember— getting back on track is just one meal away. Instead of judging yourself severely, think of these small slips as natural experiments— opportunities to learn about how your body responds to variations in food quality and discover more about what your body actually needs. (The Daily Tracker and Monthly Progress Chart are intended to help you do this.) With mindfulness, these teaching moments can be powerful guides on the path to optimal health.

My Always Hungry Story

I have stopped wondering what is "wrong" with me and started thinking that "next time I will make a better choice," which is far healthier and makes me much happier than beating myself up for not being able to fight what felt like an addiction.

—Pat M., 66, Maple Grove, MN
Weight loss: 4 pounds. Decrease in waist: 0.5 inch

THE PHASE 2 TOOLS

In this section, you'll find a complete 7-day meal plan to help you shift easily to the new protein (25 percent), fat (40 percent), and carbohydrate (35 percent) ratios of Phase 2. You'll also find detailed guides and other tools, as you begin creating meals for yourself and negotiating the challenges of eating out.

Building a Phase 2 Meal

In this phase, the carbohydrates go up a bit, fat goes down a bit, and food choices become more flexible. In addition to the carbohydrates in Phase 1, you can add whole-kernel grains (see the Guide to Cooking Whole Grains, Appendix C, page 317) and starchy vegetables (except white potato). Phase 2 meals follow this general design.

START WITH A HIGH-QUALITY PROTEIN...	BULK UP THE PROTEIN IF NEEDED...	POUR ON THE FAT...	INCLUDE NONSTARCHY CARBOHYDRATES...	THEN ADD A STARCHY VEGETABLE OR WHOLE-KERNEL GRAIN
Higher protein/ higher fat: -fatty meat or fish, poultry with skin (4 to 6 ounces) *Higher protein/ lower fat:* -lean meat or fish, poultry without skin (4 to 6 ounces) -cold cuts (4 to 6 ounces) -protein powder (about 1 ounce) *Lower protein/ higher fat:* -tempeh, tofu (4 to 6 ounces) -eggs (3) -cheese (3 ounces)	*For lower-protein items, add another source of protein:* -Greek yogurt (½ cup) -beans (½ cup) -cheese (1 to 2 ounces) -nuts or nut butter (2 to 3 tablespoons)	*For lower-fat items, add a larger portion of fat:* -dressings and sauces (1 to 2 tablespoons) -oils (2 to 3 teaspoons) -heavy cream or canned coconut milk (1 to 3 tablespoons) -nuts or nut butter (1 to 2 tablespoons) -⅓ avocado *For higher-fat items, add a smaller portion of fat:* -dressing and sauces (2 to 4 teaspoons) -oils (1 to 2 teaspoons) -heavy cream or canned coconut milk (2 to 4 teaspoons) -nuts or nut butter (2 to 3 teaspoons) -avocado, few slices	*If your meal doesn't already have a carbo-hydrate, add one serving of the following:* -beans or bean soup (½ cup) -vegetable soup (e.g., carrot) (1 cup) -fruit (non-tropical) (1 cup) **Note:** Include as many extra nonstarchy vegetables as you like (e.g., salad or cooked vegetables).	-whole-kernel grain (brown rice, wheat berries, qui-noa, barley, steel-cut oats,* etc.) -sweet potato or yams (but not white potato) -winter squash (acorn, butter-nut, buttercup, kabocha) **Note:** Serving size is about ½ cup.

* Steel-cut oats (in contrast to rolled oats) have much of the grain structure preserved, and are considered an acceptable option.

My Always Hungry Story

My taste buds changed to where the plan's foods are delicious and the old processed foods are not that appealing. I wouldn't have believed it, but now it's a fact of life for me.

—Dan B., 45, Lehi, UT
Weight loss: 15 pounds. Decrease in waist: 1 inch

Make Your Own Snacks

In Phases 2 and 3, snacks are optional, based on individual needs. Some people will do best continuing with one or two a day, whereas others may need them only occasionally. As always, let your hunger be your guide. Dependable options include:

- Full-fat (4%) cottage cheese with fruit
- Full-fat Greek yogurt, berries, and a dollop of peanut butter (a personal favorite!)
- 2 hard-boiled eggs and a few grapes
- Cold cuts (regular or vegetarian) and mayo wrapped in lettuce, with carrots
- A handful of roasted nuts

Or choose from these snack recipes, appropriate for all program phases. (These items also work as side dishes or appetizers.)

- Cucumber Boats with Turkey and Feta (page 294)
- Cold-Cut Lettuce Boats (page 294)
- Smoked Salmon and Dill Cream Cheese on Cucumber Rounds (page 295)
- Basic Hummus (page 290)
- Edamame (page 296)
- Trail Mix (page 291)
- Handful of Spicy Pumpkin Seeds (page 292)
- Herb-Roasted Chickpeas (page 293)

- Cheesy Pinto Bean Dip (page 290)
- Slice of leftover Dr. Ludwig's Favorite Frittata (page 225)

Restaurant and Grab-and-Go Recommendations

When you're traveling or too busy to prepare a home-cooked meal, follow these suggestions to help stay on track.

What to Order...at a General American Bistro

- Protein (meat, fish, chicken, eggs, tofu—4 to 6 ounces)
- Veggies cooked in olive oil
- Salad with full-fat dressing
- Beans and/or small serving of whole grains
- Soup (optional)
- Dessert: fresh berries with dark chocolate and nuts

What to Order...at a Mediterranean/Greek/Italian Restaurant

- Fresh fish, chicken, or meat (not breaded)
- Vegetable side dishes cooked or dressed in olive oil
- Hummus or lentil salad (no pita—eat with fresh carrots, celery, radishes, sliced red pepper, or other "snappy" vegetable)
- Olive tapenade
- Olives and feta
- Greek salad
- Tabbouleh (with bulgur wheat)
- Caprese salad (with fresh mozzarella)
- Dessert: fruit with unsweetened Greek yogurt and a touch of honey (optional)

What to Order at...an Asian Restaurant

- Curry with tofu, meat, chicken, or fish (no rice!)
- Sashimi (rather than sushi, which includes sweetened white rice)
- Vegetable stir-fry

- Miso or coconut milk–based soup
- Sautéed greens
- Brown rice (if available)
- Dessert: fruit

What to Order at...a Mexican Restaurant

- Fajitas, using lettuce leaves instead of tortillas
- "Deconstructed burrito"—a bowl with beans, chicken, veggies, cheese, guacamole, lettuce, tomatoes, sour cream
- Chili or black bean soup topped with sour cream and/or cheese
- Guacamole with radishes, fennel, cucumbers, jicama, or any other "snappy" vegetable
- Brown rice (if available)

What to Order at...Salad Bars

Over a bed of romaine, spinach, or other greens, add:
- Chicken, tuna, tofu
- Sardines (or stash a can in your bag for emergencies)
- Smoked salmon
- Boiled egg
- Any and all nonstarchy vegetables
- Nuts
- Beans (chickpeas, hummus, lentils, black beans)
- Avocado
- Olives
- Shredded cheese
- Cottage cheese
- Whole grains (e.g., wheat berries or quinoa)
- Full-fat dressings (without added sugar)
- Soups (not potato based)
- Dessert: fruit (pour cream from the coffee station on top)

What to Order at...a Convenience Store/Deli

- Mixed nuts
- Cold cuts *or* hard-boiled egg, full-fat cheese stick, and apple

- Smoked salmon on lettuce leaf with cream cheese, tomato, and onion
- Unsweetened Greek yogurt, blueberries, and package of cashews
- Hummus (topped with olive oil), with carrots, celery, cherry tomatoes, and/or bell peppers

Tips for Phase 2 Success

Depending on your starting weight and other individual factors (see page 101), you might remain on Phase 2 for a significant amount of time. Once you become comfortable with the basic approach, experiment as much as possible with new ingredients and recipes to keep things fresh. (Check out www.alwayshungrybook.com for regularly updated recipes.)

Enjoy intact whole grains. Have up to three servings daily, but no more than one per meal. A serving is about ½ cup cooked whole grains, such as brown rice, steel-cut oats, or quinoa. Until Phase 3, avoid processed grains like bread, pasta, white rice, and crackers (including products made from whole-grain flour).

Serve up starchy vegetables (if you'd like). You can enjoy a serving of about ½ cup cooked corn (technically a grain), yams, or sweet potatoes a day. Hold off on white potatoes until Phase 3. Beans don't count as starchy vegetables and you can have them as often as you like.

But don't combine starchy vegetables and grains. Have *either* ½ cup grains or ½ cup starchy vegetables at a meal, but not both. (Or have half portions of each, such as ¼ cup peas mixed with ¼ cup cooked quinoa.)

Use a touch of honey or maple syrup (if you'd like). Have up to 3 teaspoons daily in Phase 2. These sweeteners have a stronger flavor—so you don't need to use as much—and they also contain a few beneficial phytonutrients. Avoid white sugar and the other highly processed sweeteners for now. Stevia, a non-calorie herbal extract, is OK in small amounts, but the effects of high doses on metabolism haven't been adequately examined. And any high-intensity sweetener might interfere with the process of getting unhooked from sugar.

My Always Hungry Story

I had pineapple over the weekend and it was almost too sweet! I couldn't believe my taste buds had changed that much in such a short time.

—Lynn B., 33, Southborough, MA
Weight loss: 11.5 pounds. Decrease in waist: n/a

Make "like" substitutions. As in Phase 1, you can substitute foods with similar content of the major nutrients: apples for pears, quinoa for brown rice, tofu for chicken, etc. (See Program Foods Phase-by-Phase on page 110 for more specifics.)

To start, follow the 1-week Phase 2 meal plan closely. You might even repeat the meal plan an extra time, to learn how to hit the right combinations of nutrients and foods.

Then, begin to branch out. After following the meal plans for a week or two, start to create your own meals, as described on page 184. You can always return to the meal plan—for a single meal or an entire day—whenever you like.

Experiment with portions. In Phase 2, practice paying attention to your body's key feedback signals of hunger, satiety, and energy level. As we saw in chapter 5, young children register and respond naturally to these internal signals. But in our modern, supersized food environment, we seem to lose touch with them over time. Experiment with portion sizes to achieve just the right balance—satisfied but not over-full after eating. In this way, you'll rediscover how much food your body actually needs, and how to adjust this amount for differing circumstances (for example, if you've been especially active one day). Ask yourself:

- Am I pleasantly hungry before each meal? Am I satisfied afterward?
- Am I eating regular meals, or are my mealtimes chaotic and throwing my body off track? Am I hungry late at night?

- If I find myself thinking about specific foods, what am I craving, and what is that craving telling me? (*For example:* If I'm craving crunchy foods, do I need more fresh vegetables in my diet?)
- Do I develop carbohydrate cravings when sleep deprived, at times of stress, or if my diet has fallen a bit off track?

My Always Hungry Story

I had an "aha" about hunger today: When I think of chocolate, I could consider it a signal that my body requires food. So, instead of being at the mercy of my cravings, I can use them to let me know it is time for a positive action, like finding decent food. Nothing like a paradigm shift to give a girl hope that her life will no longer be controlled by chocolate cravings.

—*Pat M., 66, Maple Grove, MN*
Weight loss: 4 pounds. Decrease in waist: 0.5 inch

Remember, you can always go back to Phase 1 meals. Phase 1 meals are fine to enjoy in Phase 2. And some people may do best staying close to this nutrient combination (for instance, if you have prediabetes). However, Phase 2 meals offer greater flexibility, especially when eating out, and will be the easiest to follow for most people over the long term.

PHASE 2 MEAL PLAN

Start Phase 2 by following the Meal Plan on page 192. As with Phase 1, at the start of this week, take a look at the Meal Plans or the Menus At-A-Glance chart (online) and modify according to your individual preferences. Then download the Phase 2 Shopping Lists from www.alwayshungrybook.com. These lists can be used for one (such as Sunday) or two (Sunday and Wednesday) shopping trips each week. Feel free to modify this recommendation as needed. In subsequent weeks, you will build your own meal plan using the blank Meal Planning Worksheet and Weekly Prep Worksheet (online).

For the Phase 2 meal plan, you choose your own snacks if hungry between meals. Select higher-protein options for days with main meals that average less than 25 percent protein and vice versa. As with Phase 1, the Meal Plan is designed for two people and described per serving, but can be easily scaled up for families of any size. If you're cooking just for yourself, either reduce recipes accordingly or refer to the Simplified Meal Plan online.

PHASE 2 MEAL PLAN

MONDAY (DAY 1)

Breakfast

Strawberry Fig Yogurt with Nuts

1 cup plain whole-milk Greek yogurt, 1 cup strawberries, halved, 2 dried figs, cut into small pieces, 1 teaspoon honey, and 2 tablespoons peanuts or other nuts

Protein: 24%	Fat: 41%	Carbohydrate: 35%	Calories: 432*

Prep: Assemble and pack today's snacks.

Lunch

Cobb Salad

*Cobb Salad*** (page 255); 1 cup berries or other seasonal fruit

Protein: 26%	Fat: 41%	Carbohydrate: 33%	Calories: 544*

Dinner

Lamb Shanks, Baked Sweet Potato, and Asparagus

Melt-in-Your-Mouth Lamb Shanks (page 233) (from Phase 1, Day 14 Dinner); *Roasted Sweet Potatoes* (page 279—use baked whole potato variation) (from Phase 1, Day 14 Additional Cooking Prep); 6 to 10 spears asparagus (roasted, blanched, or steamed—page 313—Guide to Cooking Vegetables)

Additional Cooking Prep:

Make *Red Lentil Soup* (page 283) for Day 4 Lunch (make a full recipe, and freeze extra portions for future meals).

Dessert

1 medium pear

Protein: 27%	Fat: 40%	Carbohydrate: 33%	Calories: 673*

Prep: Assemble tomorrow's lunch—*Shrimp over Cracked Wheat Salad* (page 256).

---

* Calorie content provided for descriptive purposes only—not as a measure to limit food intake.
** To serve two people, make a full recipe and store reserved portions to be used in subsequent meals as directed in prep notes.
*** To serve two people, make ½ recipe.

TUESDAY (DAY 2)

Breakfast

Black Bean Tofu Hash

Black Bean Tofu Hash*** (page 222) with ¼ cup *Ranchero Sauce* (page 272), 3 tablespoons shredded cheddar cheese, and 1 tablespoon guacamole or a large slice of avocado. Serve with 1 cup fresh fruit.

| Protein: 21% | Fat: 42% | Carbohydrate: 37% | Calories: 528* |

Prep: Assemble and pack today's snacks.

Lunch

Shrimp over Cracked Wheat Salad

Shrimp over Cracked Wheat Salad** (page 256)

| Protein: 23% | Fat: 46% | Carbohydrate: 31% | Calories: 539* |

Dinner

Marinara Primavera

Marinara Primavera** (tempeh version—page 234); ½ cup cooked quinoa

Additional Cooking Prep:

Make ¾ cups dry quinoa per person (page 317—Guide to Cooking Whole Grains). Yields about 2¼ cups. (Use ½ cup cooked quinoa per person for tonight's dinner. Reserve ½ cup per person for tomorrow's lunch, and ⅓ cup per person for Day 5 Breakfast. Use the remainder to make *Quinoa Salad with Pecans and Cranberries* (page 277) for Day 4 Dinner and Day 5 Lunch.

Dessert

1 cup chai with 1 to 2 tablespoons soy milk or whole milk and 1 teaspoon honey

| Protein: 21% | Fat: 46% | Carbohydrate: 33% | Calories: 560* |

Prep: Pack tomorrow's lunch—*Marinara Primavera* (tempeh version); ½ cup quinoa.

Store remaining quinoa for Day 4 *Quinoa Salad with Pecans and Cranberries* and Day 5 Breakfast Scramble.

Start *Overnight Steel-Cut Oats**** (page 226).

---

* Calorie content provided for descriptive purposes only—not as a measure to limit food intake.

** To serve two people, make a full recipe and store reserved portions to be used in subsequent meals as directed in prep notes.

*** To serve two people, make ½ recipe.

WEDNESDAY (DAY 3)

Breakfast

Overnight Steel-Cut Oats

Warm the *Overnight Steel-Cut Oats**** (page 226). Top with 2 tablespoons nuts and ½ cup blueberries per serving. Serve with 2 eggs scrambled in ½ teaspoon olive oil.

Protein: 22%	Fat: 44%	Carbohydrate: 34%	Calories: 523*

Prep: Assemble and pack today's snacks.

Lunch

Marinara Primavera

Marinara Primavera (tempeh version—from previous night's dinner); ½ cup cooked quinoa (from previous night's Additional Cooking Prep)

Protein: 21%	Fat: 47%	Carbohydrate: 32%	Calories: 540*

Dinner

Mexican Shredded Chicken and Soft Millet-Corn Polenta

Mexican Shredded Chicken** (page 241); *Soft Millet-Corn Polenta**** (page 275); 1 cup blanched kale or other green vegetable topped with 2 tablespoons *Creamy Lime-Cilantro Dressing* (page 271)

Dessert

1 cup strawberries topped with ⅓ cup plain whole-milk Greek yogurt mixed with 1 teaspoon honey

Protein: 25%	Fat: 40%	Carbohydrate: 35%	Calories: 618*

Prep: Assemble tomorrow's lunch—Mexican Shredded Chicken and Corn Salad (see Day 4 Lunch) using reserved portion of *Mexican Shredded Chicken*; store lettuce separately and add tomorrow before serving.

Freeze additional two portions of *Mexican Shredded Chicken* for future meals.

---

   * Calorie content provided for descriptive purposes only—not as a measure to limit food intake.
  ** To serve two people, make a full recipe and store reserved portions to be used in subsequent meals as directed in prep notes.
*** To serve two people, make ½ recipe.

THURSDAY (DAY 4)

Breakfast

Phase 2 Power Shake

Peanut Butter Banana Power Shake (page 221).

Protein: 25%	Fat: 41%	Carbohydrate: 34%	Calories: 442*

Prep: Assemble and pack today's snacks.

Lunch

Red Lentil Soup, Mexican Shredded Chicken and Corn Salad with Chipotle Mayonnaise

About 1½ cups *Red Lentil Soup* (page 283) (from Day 1 Additional Cooking Prep). For the salad, combine ½ cup *Mexican Shredded Chicken* (from previous night's dinner), ⅓ cup corn, ½ cup diced tomatoes, ½ cup chopped red pepper, tossed with 2 tablespoons *Chipotle Mayonnaise* (page 268) or *Creamy Lime-Cilantro Dressing* (page 271). Toss with 1 cup salad greens.

Protein: 26%	Fat: 38%	Carbohydrate: 36%	Calories: 586*

Dinner

Broiled Salmon, Quinoa Salad, and Steamed Butternut Squash

Broil 9 ounces salmon per person—use *Broiled Fish with Garlic and Lemon*** (page 232—follow Salmon Variation). Serve 5 ounces for dinner and reserve 4 ounces for tomorrow's lunch. *Quinoa Salad with Pecans and Cranberries*** (page 277), using reserved portion of quinoa from Day 2 Dinner Additional Cooking Prep; ¾ cup steamed butternut squash (make an extra ⅔ cup for tomorrow's lunch).

Additional Cooking Prep:

Make *Coconut Cashew Clusters*** (page 284) follow directions for 6 clusters and set aside for tomorrow night's dessert.

Dessert

Poached Seasonal Fruit (page 288) (Poached pear goes nicely with this meal.)

Protein: 22%	Fat: 42%	Carbohydrate: 36%	Calories: 628*

Prep: Pack tomorrow's lunch—reserved portion of salmon, *Quinoa Salad with Pecans and Cranberries*, and steamed butternut squash; ½ cup fruit.

Soak 1 cup dry brown rice per person (page 317—Guide to Cooking Whole Grains). Optional: Soak more to use in future recipes.

---

* Calorie content provided for descriptive purposes only—not as a measure to limit food intake.
** To serve two people, make a full recipe and store reserved portions to be used in subsequent meals as directed in prep notes.
*** To serve two people, make ½ recipe.

FRIDAY (DAY 5)

Breakfast

Scrambled Eggs with Spinach, Tomato, and Quinoa

Scramble 2 eggs in 1 teaspoon olive oil with 1 cup baby spinach leaves, 1 medium tomato, diced, $\frac{1}{3}$ cup cooked quinoa; top with 1 to 2 tablespoons shredded cheddar cheese. Serve with 1 cup fresh fruit topped with ½ cup plain whole-milk Greek yogurt and optional 1 teaspoon honey.

Additional Cooking Prep:

Optional: Cook brown rice to be ready for dinner tonight.

Protein: 24%	Fat: 42%	Carbohydrate: 34%	Calories: 520*

Prep: Assemble and pack today's snacks.

Lunch

Broiled Salmon with Garlic and Lemon

Broiled Salmon, *Quinoa Salad with Pecans and Cranberries* (page 277), and $\frac{2}{3}$ cup steamed butternut squash. Serve with ½ cup fruit.

Protein: 24%	Fat: 43%	Carbohydrate: 33%	Calories: 557*

Dinner

Chicken Stir-Fry with Brown Rice

Chicken or Tofu Stir-Fry** (page 230)—Follow the Phases 2 and 3—Brown Rice Variation
Dessert

Coconut Cashew Clusters (made last night) Serve 1 and reserve remainder for future meals or snacks

Protein: 28%	Fat: 38%	Carbohydrate: 34%	Calories: 644*

Prep: Pack tomorrow's lunch—Lettuce Wrap (see Day 6 Lunch) using reserved portion of Chicken Stir-Fry with Brown Rice; store lettuce and dressing separately; pack a tangerine.

* Calorie content provided for descriptive purposes only—not as a measure to limit food intake.
** To serve two people, make a full recipe and store reserved portions to be used in subsequent meals as directed in prep notes.
*** To serve two people, make ½ recipe.

SATURDAY (DAY 6)

Breakfast

Grain-Free Waffles with Turkey Bacon

Grain-Free Waffles or Pancakes with Fruit Sauce (reheat reserved portion from Phase 1, Day 13 breakfast) topped with 1 tablespoon *Whipped Cream* (page 230); 1 slice turkey bacon

Protein: 26%	Fat: 43%	Carbohydrate: 31%	Calories: 428*

Prep: Assemble and pack today's snacks.

Lunch

Chicken Stir-Fry Lettuce Wrap with Ginger-Soy Vinaigrette

Divide a lunch-size portion of *Chicken or Tofu Stir-Fry with Brown Rice* (from previous night's dinner) evenly among 3 or 4 large lettuce leaves, leaving plenty of room to fold and wrap each leaf around the filling. Place 1 to 2 tablespoons *Ginger-Soy Vinaigrette* (page 267) in a shallow container. Dip the wraps in the sauce; serve with a tangerine.

Protein: 25%	Fat: 40%	Carbohydrate: 35%	Calories: 459*

Dinner

Beef, Bean, and Barley Stew

Beef or Tofu, Bean, and Barley Stew (page 235)*

Dessert

Pear Strawberry Crisp (page 285)

Protein: 25%	Fat: 34%	Carbohydrate: 41%	Calories: 617*

Prep: Pack tomorrow's lunch—*Beef or Tofu, Bean, and Barley Stew* with handful of spinach leaves on the side, ½ ounce dark chocolate, and 1 tablespoon of peanuts (from Sunday's prep).

---

* Calorie content provided for descriptive purposes only—not as a measure to limit food intake.
** To serve two people, make a full recipe and store reserved portions to be used in subsequent meals as directed in prep notes.
*** To serve two people, make ½ recipe.

SUNDAY (DAY 7)

Breakfast

Dr. Ludwig's Favorite Frittata

Dr. Ludwig's Favorite Frittata*** (page 225—follow Phase 2 Variation). Serve with ½ cup black beans topped with 1 tablespoon sour cream, and 1 cup fruit mixed with 2 tablespoons plain whole-milk Greek yogurt.

Protein: 23%	Fat: 41%	Carbohydrate: 36%	Calories: 438*

Prep: Assemble and pack today's snacks.

Lunch

Beef, Bean, and Barley Stew

Beef or Tofu, Bean, and Barley Stew (page 235) with handful of raw spinach; ½ ounce dark chocolate, and 1 tablespoon of peanuts

Protein: 27%	Fat: 37%	Carbohydrate: 36%	Calories: 566*

Dinner

Honey Balsamic Marinated Cod, Roasted Sweet Potatoes, and Kale with Carrots and Currants

5 ounces *Honey Balsamic Marinated Fish**** (page 251); *Roasted Sweet Potatoes*** (page 279); *Kale with Carrots and Currants**** (page 276)

Dessert

Poached Seasonal Fruit*** (page 288) with 3 tablespoons *Chocolate Sauce**** (page 289)

Protein: 23%	Fat: 41%	Carbohydrate: 36%	Calories: 672*

Prep: Pack tomorrow's lunch.

Store reserved portion *Roasted Sweet Potatoes* for future meals.

---

* Calorie content provided for descriptive purposes only—not as a measure to limit food intake.

** To serve two people, make a full recipe and store reserved portions to be used in subsequent meals as directed in prep notes.

*** To serve two people, make ½ recipe.

After one or two weeks following the Phase 2 meal plan, it's time to take off the training wheels! It's your turn to plan meals, using everything you've learned on the program so far. Once a week, on your regular prep/shopping day, fill in the blank Meal Planning Worksheet (download it from www.alwayshungrybook.com), selecting as many meals as possible for the days ahead. (Consider keeping this tool on your refrigerator to note ideas you'd like to try the following week.) Choose from any items on the Phase 1 or 2 Meal Plans. Or design your own meals, referring as needed to the make-your-own meals charts (Phase 1, page 152, or Phase 2, page 184), Lettuce Wrap (page 153), the Restaurant and Grab-and-Go options (page 186), and the Program Foods Phase-by-Phase (page 110). Once you've completed this blueprint for your week, use the blank Weekly Prep Worksheet (online) to note which sauces, snacks, and roasted seeds/nuts you'll make, which key ingredients to prep in advance, and which casseroles or other meals you intend to make ahead and freeze. Then record which foods you'll need to buy on the Shopping List Template (online).

A Few Favorites for the Weekly Rotation

Here are a few Always Hungry Solution staples that can help make meal preparation easy and the results delicious. Modify this list according to your (and your family's) preferences.

Sauces:
- Chipotle Mayonnaise
- Creamy Dill Sauce
- Ginger-Soy Vinaigrette
- Lemon Olive Oil Dressing
- Mustard Vinaigrette
- Ranchero Sauce
- Tartar Sauce
- Other _____

Nuts/Seeds:

Roasted Nuts

- almonds
- cashews
- pecans
- walnuts

Roasted Seeds
- pumpkin seeds
- sunflower seeds

Trail Mix

WHAT IF I DON'T REACH
MY GOAL WEIGHT?

The aim of Phase 2 is to reach a new, lower set point that's right for your body. For some people, the results will speak for themselves, with progressive weight loss until reaching a personal weight goal in the optimal range for BMI. But for others, weight loss may slow down or stop short of a personal goal. If that happens for you, consider the following questions:

Am I especially sensitive to all carbohydrate? As we will consider in more detail in chapter 8, people vary in their ability to handle highly processed carbohydrate. (Phase 3 is designed to help you find your individual tolerance level for those foods.) But some people—perhaps related to a strong family history of diabetes or other individual factors—may do best limiting all high–glycemic load carbohydrates (see Appendix A, page 305), even unprocessed whole grains. Did you respond really well in Phase 1 without any starchy foods or added sugar? Have your hunger and food cravings increased with addition of these items in Phase 2? If so, reduce or eliminate grains, potatoes, and added sugar for a while and instead increase fat intake (e.g., nuts, olive oil, etc.). Make sure to have protein at every meal and most snacks. Then see if your rate of weight loss picks up again.

Have I listened to my body's weight control signals? A fundamental goal of the Always Hungry Solution is to shift focus away from arbitrary external measures (calories) to the body's internal weight control system. If you give it the right combination of foods, your body can let you know more accurately how much food it needs, and when enough is enough. But it's important to pay attention. Eat mindfully, aiming to find just the right point at every meal when you feel pleasantly satisfied but not uncomfortably over-full—then stop. Savor a cup of coffee or tea to be sociable (if others are still eating) and help end the meal on a nice note. Some people have lost touch with the body's weight control signals through the years, so it may take practice. Listen to your body between meals as well. If you feel hungry and the next meal is still a ways away, have a healthy snack. Ignoring hunger for too long sets the stage for overeating later.

My Always Hungry Story

I'm the type of person, like most, who wants instant gratification. In the past when I began a diet program, I never followed through past a couple of months. This program has had me more mindful and focusing more on how I am feeling before and after I eat. Intuitive eating.

—Elizabeth R., 39, Boston, MA
Weight loss: 8 pounds. Decrease in waist: 0.5 inch

Do I have low lean body mass? Most people with high body fat actually have increased lean body mass, as their muscles undergo regular workouts carrying around the extra weight. But some may have unusually low muscle mass for various reasons—very low birth weight, a lifetime of physical inactivity, certain chronic diseases, or long-term use of steroid medications. If you're in this category, you may tend to have a slow metabolism and, as a result, more difficulty losing weight. Consider increasing physical activities beyond the general recommendation in Phase 2, especially including strength training (body-building exercises) and aerobic exercises.

Am I getting too little sleep or under too much stress? Sleep deprivation can cause stress, excess stress can affect sleep, and both can undermine metabolism and interfere with weight loss. Recommit yourself to the Phase 2 sleep and stress-relief practices. If you've experienced any personal or professional life challenges that feel too big to handle on your own, consider seeking help from a trusted friend or a mental health professional.

Am I consuming too much alcohol? Do you drink alcoholic beverages most days of the week, or frequently have more than 1 to 2 drinks per day? Do you rely on alcohol to manage stress? Consider abstaining for a few weeks, and incorporate other ways to unwind and relax into your daily life.

Do I have an underlying medical problem? Consistently poor energy level, excessive daytime sleepiness, extreme sensitivity to the cold, chronic constipation, very dry skin or hair, and (for women) unexplained changes in menstrual cycle can be signs of a medical problem like hypothyroidism or sleep apnea. If you've been unable to lose weight despite following the program closely and experience any concerning changes in health, discuss the situation with your health care provider.

Is my personal weight goal realistic? Even under ideal circumstances, of course, some people will always be heavier than others. And norms of beauty have been grossly distorted, through incessant images of ultrathin fashion models in the media (images that have also been distorted by computer manipulation). In addition to weight, consider other changes that may have occurred since starting the program—in energy level, overall well-being, waist size (a better measure of body fat than weight), and chronic disease risk factors. If these are improving, perhaps your current weight is the right weight for your body, at least for this stage of your life.

My Always Hungry Story

Yesterday, I had a Phase 2 Power Shake for breakfast and left the house for a swim and some errands. I thought I'd be out for a couple hours, so I didn't bother bringing a snack—big mistake. Two hours turned into six. While getting my haircut, I could feel my blood sugar drop by the second. I was annoyed about how long my errands had taken, and stress and hunger aren't a good mix for me. Normally at this point, I'd look for the quickest, most unhealthy food option, and eat way more than I needed, very fast. Bad eating would lead to guilt, which would lead to more eating. Taco Bell with an extra-large Dr Pepper was my go-to, but wouldn't rule out a family-size bag of Doritos dipped in queso, or a pint of Ben & Jerry's with a Tastycake on the side. (Sounds like exaggeration, but my wife could tell you it's not.)

Instead, I did something I would have never done before starting the program. I walked over to the grocery story, got some almonds and an apple, and—surprisingly enough—the snack held me over until dinner. Now I know that when you are 10/10 on a hungry scale, you don't have to eat until you get to 0/10. I will keep a can of almonds in my car because that feeling was not one that I missed. This was a big step for me in changing my mind-set about food (my major goal of this whole thing).

—*Matthew F., 36, Roslindale, MA*
Weight loss: 31 pounds. Decrease in waist: 5.5 inches

CHAPTER 8

Phase 3—Lose Weight Permanently

By now, you've been on the program for anywhere from one or two months to six months or more. Your weight has decreased to a new, lower set point. Perhaps you've experienced other benefits, like more energy and lower heart disease risk factors. And if you accomplished this without hunger and troublesome food cravings, congratulations— you've mastered the Always Hungry Solution! Now, the key is to tailor the program to your body's specific needs and your personal preferences, allowing you to maintain all these benefits easily...and for good. And that's the purpose of Phase 3.

In Phase 3, you'll mindfully reintroduce some of the more pro- cessed carbohydrates—breads and other refined grains, white potato products, and sweets—as mini experiments, to see how your body responds. After a few months of optimal eating, improved sleep, stress reduction, and regular physical activities, some people can begin again with a clean slate and tolerate moderate amounts of these foods. If you're one of them, why not enjoy a fresh-baked pastry when visiting Paris, some fettuccine in Little Italy, or the occasional slice of ice cream cake at a party? Others may find that any amount of processed carbohydrates triggers cravings or other symptoms, setting the stage for weight regain. For them, the rewards of good health will more than make up for any momentary pleasures missed.

My Always Hungry Story

I feel a lot trimmer and healthier, and ready to stay on Phase 3 for the rest of my life (with a few drop-off points for vacations and special events).
—Roshni T., 51, Norfolk, MA
Weight loss: 15 pounds. Decrease in waist: n/a

But regardless of which category you're in now, your body may change over time—toward greater flexibility with continuing improvements in metabolism the longer you stay on the program; or in the opposite direction at times of stress. During Phases 1 and 2, you've reconnected with your body and its weight control signals of hunger and satiety. Don't tune out now! Compare your eating and lifestyle habits with your physical symptoms and body weight regularly, so that you can adjust the program to your needs in the months and years ahead. The Daily Tracker and Monthly Progress Chart are designed to help you do this.

The ratios of protein to fat to carbohydrate in Phase 3 are individualized and will vary between people, but typically 20 percent of your calories will come from protein, 40 percent from fat, and 40 percent from carbohydrate, as shown in the figure on page 109. (Total protein intake doesn't actually change from Phase 2, but the percentage decreases slightly as the amount of other food you eat increases.) These proportions resemble those of the U.S. diet in the mid-twentieth century, before the low-fat craze, and typical Mediterranean diets consumed today. With approximately equal contributions from fat and carbohydrate, you won't have to restrict any major nutrient and can enjoy freedom in food choices. As with the other phases of the program, let your hunger be your guide. Eat until you feel pleasantly satisfied but not uncomfortably full, and maintain your focus on food quality.

PHASE 3 LIFE SUPPORTS

The goal of Phase 3 is to create a personalized prescription for long-term success, not only for diet, but also for movement, sleep, and stress relief—the other key components of healthy living. To accomplish this, consider which practices will be most enjoyable, practical, and rewarding for you—and integrate them deeply into your life.

Movement

If you've enjoyed the evening *passeggiata*, make it a permanent practice. Perhaps the habit will catch on, and entire communities will turn off the TV to head outdoors after dinner for a chance to move, relax, and socialize together. What about your moderate to vigorous physical activities three to four times a week? Have you found options that you enjoy and can continue indefinitely? Consider connecting with friends around these activities for group support—commuting together to a regular dance class or meeting at a designated time each week to shoot hoops. Have you lost weight, become fitter, and gained physical confidence? If so, activities that might have seemed intimidating before, like roller skating or rock climbing, may now be within your easy reach! And look for opportunities to add movement throughout your day: Walk rather than drive when feasible; take the stairs rather than the elevator; stand while talking on the phone; or hold a walking business meeting if the weather permits.

My Always Hungry Story

I'd like to do my joyful exercise *with* my children. I tend to view exercising as something I need to do by myself at the gym. I still do want to keep that up, but have started taking the kids to the pool in the evenings after dinner. They love it—and so do I. The "informal" fun things burn calories too. And build memories.

—Monica M., 45, Great Falls, VA
Weight loss: 11 pounds. Decrease in waist: 2 inches

Sleep

Increased movement and stress reduction will help you fall asleep more easily in the evening. Try setting bedtime half an hour earlier. Do you wake up feeling more rested and need less caffeine to get through the day? Continue to refine your pre-sleep routine and protect your sleep sanctuary.

Stress Relief

If you've found benefits from the two brief stress-relief sessions in Phase 2, consider expanding the total time to 20 to 30 minutes a day. But keep in mind that maintaining a daily practice, not achieving a time target, is most important here. In what other ways can you protect yourself from the toll of modern life on your nervous system? For many people, there is no substitute for regular time in nature—be it a stroll in the park, a swim in the ocean, or a hike in the mountains.

Other Supports

Rewrite Your If-Then Plans. Perhaps you've successfully used your if-then strategies to deal with recurring obstacles. Or maybe you've never gotten into the habit of using them. Either way, consider rewriting your if-then plans as you continue into Phase 3. Obstacles that seemed daunting in Phase 1 may no longer present problems, whereas new ones may emerge. Many of us are used to staying on a "diet" for a specified period of time. But what happens when we try to make the changes permanent? Your if-then plans will help you stay (and get back) on track for the long journey.

Reimagine a Bigger Why. Perhaps your Big Why—the defining reason you started the Always Hungry Solution—remains unchanged: to avoid getting diabetes or to feel as good as possible day after day. But if your Big Why involved something more short term, such as getting in shape for summer, maybe you've already achieved

My Always Hungry Story

> If we're going to do ice cream or go out to a local place, about half the time I skip it altogether, and the other half the time, I'll have just a smaller amount than I would have had previously. So it's not about deprivation—just about more moderation, which I really appreciate.
>
> —*Eric F., 42, Needham, MA*
> *Weight loss: 17 pounds. Decrease in waist: 3 inches*

your goal. If so, it's time for a new one. What specific vision will help you align your daily behaviors with your highest aspirations in life? Take this opportunity to reflect on the big picture of your life (refer to page 128 for guidance).

THE PHASE 3 TOOLS

Phase 3 does not have a specific meal plan, but is instead built upon Phase 2. Use the charts, tips, and meal suggestions that follow, the recipes in chapter 9, and the meal planning worksheets online at www.alwayshungrybook.com for guidance.

After several months of conscientious eating, you can now begin to reintroduce some processed carbohydrates into your diet (see Program Foods Phase-by-Phase, page 110). Have a piece of bread with an omelet at breakfast, a tortilla with a Mexican dish at lunch, pasta for dinner, or a sweet dessert. Start with just one such food a few times a week, and increase slowly as tolerated. (Even with foods made with milled flour, whole-grain products are preferable, but not mandatory.)

As you make these changes to your diet, pay special attention to your hunger level, food cravings, energy level, mood, general sense of well-being, weight, and waist circumference (as recorded in the Daily Tracker and Monthly Progress Chart). If you begin to experience setbacks, dial back the processed carbohydrates and/or refocus on your life supports related to movement, sleep, and stress reduction. You can return to Phase 2 anytime, or even Phase 1 to clean the slate again.

Many people find they don't do well with too many processed carbohydrates, but even if you don't experience obvious negative effects, I recommend limiting yourself to two modest portions of processed carbohydrates per day as a general rule. Highly processed carbohydrates are among the lowest-quality components of the food supply, accounting for the majority of diet-related disease in the United States today—they're highly concentrated in calories but devoid of real nutrition. One size definitively doesn't fit all. With a developing awareness of your body's biological signals and needs, you'll be well equipped to find the right balance for you. And if you're among the sizable group of people who can't tolerate much processed carbohydrate, simply making the decision that "these foods don't work for me" can be liberating, especially since you know how satisfying a higher-fat, whole foods diet can be without them!

My Always Hungry Story

I used to feel so low energy in the afternoon, but now I feel much better. I'm very satisfied with the food, did not have any cravings so I could stay on the program even with lots of company eating at home and going out to eat. I have had food allergies for years, and I have never felt this good. My son came over the other day and said how good I looked and that my color was so much better. This is the first eating plan on which I have felt completely satisfied.

—*Betty T., 76, Garland, TX*
Weight loss: 17 pounds. Decrease in waist: 3 inches

Convert Phase 1, Phase 2, and Phase 3 Meals

With just a few simple modifications, you can adapt familiar favorites to Phase 3 meals. Here are a few examples to get you started. Remember, including more processed carbohydrates in Phase 3 is entirely optional. Have them in moderation, only if your body can handle them. If not, stick with the Phase 2 eating plan.

PHASE 1 MEAL	PHASE 2 VARIATION	PHASE 3 VARIATION
BREAKFAST		
Omelet 2 eggs 1 egg white Olive oil, 2 teaspoons Spinach Cheese, 3 tablespoons Berries, 1 cup Greek yogurt, ½ cup	*Same as Phase 1, except:* Omit the egg white Decrease olive oil to 1 teaspoon Include tomato with spinach Decrease cheese to 2 tablespoons Add ¼ cup cooked quinoa Add 1 teaspoon honey to berries and yogurt	*Same as Phase 2 except:* Serve with 1 slice of bread instead of quinoa
Black Bean Tofu Hash *Black Bean Tofu Hash* (page 222) Top with: Cheddar cheese, 2 tablespoons Sour cream, 1 to 2 tablespoons Avocado, ½ sliced	*Same as Phase 1, except:* Mix ⅓ cup brown rice into *Black Bean Tofu Hash* Top with: Cheddar cheese, 2 tablespoons Sour cream, 1 tablespoon Avocado, ¼ sliced	*Same as Phase 2 except:* Wrap *Black Bean Tofu Hash* in 1 wheat or 2 corn tortillas and omit brown rice
Smoked Salmon Smoked salmon, 3 ounces Cheese, 1 ounce Tomato, 1 medium, sliced Cucumber, 1 small, sliced Top with: *Creamy Dill Sauce* (page 270), 3½ tablespoons Blueberries, 1 cup	*Same as Phase 1 except:* Decrease *Creamy Dill Sauce* to 2 tablespoons Decrease blueberries to ½ cup Serve with: Steel-cut oats, ½ cup cooked	*Same as Phase 2 except:* Make open-faced salmon sandwiches with 2 slices bread (Mestemacher pumpernickel especially recommended for this meal) Omit oats
LUNCH		
Taco Salad *Mexican Shredded Chicken* (page 241) Mix with salad (chopped lettuce, tomato, carrots, etc.) *Creamy Lime-Cilantro Dressing* (page 271)	*Same as Phase 1 except:* Reduce *Creamy Lime-Cilantro Dressing* by ⅓ Add whole corn kernels, ½ cup	*Same as Phase 2 except:* Use shredded vegetables (e.g., cabbage) instead of salad Wrap in 1 or 2 corn tortillas instead of adding corn Top each wrap with dressing
Steak Salad *Steak Salad with Blue Cheese Dressing* (page 253) Tangerine, 1	*Same as Phase 1 except:* Reduce *Blue Cheese Dressing* by ⅓ Serve with *Roasted Sweet Potatoes* (page 279), fries variation	*Same as Phase 2 except:* Add 1 cup croutons to salad and omit fries

PHASE 1 MEAL	PHASE 2 VARIATION	PHASE 3 VARIATION
DINNER		
Curry *Coconut Curry Shrimp* (page 248) Serve over a bed of spinach	*Same as Phase 1 except:* Serve over brown rice instead of spinach	*Same as Phase 2 except:* Serve over brown or white rice
Roasted Chicken *Creamy Cauliflower Soup* (page 280) *Herb-Roasted Chicken Thighs* (page 241) Broccoli, 1 cup Carrot, small, ½ Serve vegetables with *Lemon Olive Oil Dressing* (page 269), 1 tablespoon	*Same as Phase 1 except:* Substitute a squeeze of lemon for *Lemon Olive Oil Dressing* Add small baked sweet potato	*Same as Phase 2 except:* Add small baked potato of any kind
Thai Peanut Tempeh *Thai Peanut Tempeh* (page 258) Sliced raw vegetables (cucumbers, carrot, red bell pepper) with a squeeze of lemon	*Same as Phase 1 except:* Reduce portion of *Thai Peanut Tempeh* by ¼ Serve over a bed of brown rice (½ cup)	*Same as Phase 2 except:* Serve *Thai Peanut Tempeh* over a bed of Asian noodles (½ cup)
DESSERT		
Berries and Cream Berries, 1 cup Heavy cream, 2 tablespoons	*Same as Phase 1 except:* Add optional drizzle of honey	*Same as Phase 2 except:* Top with *Homemade Granola* (page 229) instead of honey

Tips for Phase 3 Success

Phase 3 is for life. You'll need inspiration and new ideas to keep things fresh. Experimentation is the name of the game. Check out www.alwayshungrybook.com for updated recipes. If you have one you love, please consider submitting it to mail@alwayshungry book.com.

The amount of protein you choose will not change. Have 4 to 6 ounces of protein per meal, including vegetarian options.

Continue to emphasize fats. Rich sauces and spreads, nuts and nut butters, seeds, avocado, and olive oil—these remain basic staples, making meals delicious, nutritious, and satisfying. The total amount you'll use stays about the same as in Phase 2.

Enjoy the full range of nonstarchy vegetables and fruits. Aim to fill half of every meal with these health-promoting natural foods.

Continue to include ½ cup grains or starchy vegetables up to three times a day. Unlike in Phase 2, you can include white potatoes, white rice, rolled oats, breads and other flour products, popcorn, and the like as part of your total (see Program Foods Phase-by-Phase, page 110). Aim for the majority of the grains you eat to be either milled "whole-grain" (processed into flour but with the bran and germ present) or, even better, unmilled "whole-kernel" options.

Find your sweetener "sweet spot" (if desired). You can now have a small amount of white sugar, based on your individual tolerance, but aim to limit total added sweetener (including honey, maple syrup,

GRAIN PROCESSING CHART

Choose intact whole-kernel options for most of your grains. Highly processed whole-grain products are preferable to refined grain products (from which the fiber and germ have been removed). This chart provides a few examples to illustrate differences among types of grain products.

MINIMALLY PROCESSED/ WHOLE-KERNEL GRAINS	HIGHLY PROCESSED WHOLE GRAINS	HIGHLY PROCESSED REFINED GRAINS
Recommended total grain intake: 0 to 3 servings/day		
Phases 2 and 3*	Phase 3 Only	
0 to 3 servings/day	Up to 2 servings/day may be included as part of the daily total	
Wheat berries	Bread, whole grain**	Bread, white
Oats, whole groats or steel cut	Pasta or couscous, whole wheat	Pasta or couscous, white
Rice, brown		Rice, white
Buckwheat (kasha)	Crackers, whole grain	Crackers, white
Millet	Tortilla, corn or whole wheat	Chips
Quinoa	Oats, rolled	

 * Phase 1 has no grains of any kind
 ** "Flourless," sprouted, and "stone-ground" breads are less processed than conventional products made from finely milled flours and resemble whole-kernel grains in nutritional value. Food for Life Baking Company (Ezekiel bread) and Mestemacher offer such product lines.

and all other types—see page 85) to 6 teaspoons a day. Having spent several months on the program so far, it's likely your taste threshold will have changed, so that you don't need so much sugar to enjoy the experience of sweetness. With an ability to appreciate the taste of a perfectly ripe strawberry, you can have a small slice of cake at an office party without feeling out of control.

My Always Hungry Story

We traveled to New Orleans and tried not to eat bread or dessert (which was unbelievable for me and my husband)—but we did have fried shrimp and oysters and some French fries. I did not feel good eating it—I craved my home salad! Can you believe that! My body is gradually getting used to this way of eating and now does not want to eat differently. I never thought I would say this.

—Jyoti A., 59, Muskogee, OK
Weight loss: 7 pounds. Decrease in waist: 4 inches

Alcohol and caffeine. It's OK to have up to 2 alcoholic drinks a day as tolerated. Enjoy coffee and tea according to your tolerance, but for many people, 2 to 3 caffeinated beverages a day is a reasonable limit. Higher amounts can produce insulin resistance—an underlying cause of weight-related complications (see page 56)—and have other negative effects.

Mindful eating. With highly processed carbohydrates, it's easy to go from too hungry to too full too quickly. The transition from hunger to satiety occurs more slowly with whole, natural foods, leaving you more time to adjust the amount you eat for your body's needs. You can make this adjustment most precisely by eating mindfully. As you sit down for a meal, turn off the TV and put away the newspaper. Relax and turn your focus to the food. If you're with others, steer the conversation away from stressful topics. This isn't the time to resolve a political debate or a personal misunderstanding. Eat slowly. Pay attention to your sensory experience of smells, tastes, textures, chewing, and swallowing. Every few minutes, consider how the food feels in your stomach, as your appetite becomes satisfied. Look for that moment when you've had just enough food, but not too much. The Japanese call this point *hara hachi bu*, which translates as "stomach 80 percent full." Paradoxically, eating beyond this point lessens overall enjoyment of the meal, as discomfort displaces pleasant feelings. When you have had just enough food, savor a cup of tea or coffee, to help bring the meal to a satisfying close.

The five-hour rule. One of the best ways to fine-tune your eating habits is to tune into your body in the five hours after any meal.

- Do you feel completely satisfied but not over-full after eating?
- Do you experience stable energy level and mood over the next few hours?
- Do you develop a healthy appetite (but not ravenous hunger) in time for the next meal, about five hours later?

If not, consider what and how much you ate at the last meal, and make adjustments. With practice, you'll deeply associate eating right with feeling great—an invaluable skill in navigating our modern food environment. In time, you'll become your own best guide.

My Always Hungry Story

Our big family dinners used to be mashed white potatoes, gravy, and other heavy foods. Last time we all got together, I did an Asian shabu-shabu type dinner that we still talk about—it was as much fun to cook at the table as it was to eat so abundantly and to feel so good instead of all bogged down and sluggish. The kitchen is fun again!

—Kim S., 47, South Jordan, UT
Weight loss: 25 pounds. Decrease in waist: 3.5 inches

PHASE 3 MEAL SUGGESTIONS

In place of a meal plan, use the Meal Planning Template, Weekly Prep Template, and Weekly Shopping List Template (all three online) for support as you fine-tune and follow your diet. Here are a few meal suggestions to get you into the swing of Phase 3.

BREAKFASTS

Breakfast Burrito

Heat one 8-inch sprouted or whole-grain tortilla in a cast-iron skillet. Transfer the warmed tortilla to a plate and top with with 1½ cups Black Bean Tofu Hash (page 222), 1 tablespoon shredded cheddar cheese, 2 tablespoons guacamole, 1 tablespoon sour cream, 1 teaspoon salsa, or to taste. Fold one side of the tortilla over the filling by about an inch, then fold the other two sides together, overlapping over the middle, and roll into a burrito wrap. Serve as a quick, grab'n'go breakfast.

Spinach Omelet and Toast

Heat 1 teaspoon olive oil in a skillet. Whisk 2 eggs and 1 egg white together and add 1 cup baby spinach leaves. Season with salt and pepper. Pour into the skillet. Top with 2 tablespoons shredded cheddar cheese. Fold over and cook until done. Serve with 1 slice whole-grain bread and 1 tablespoon nut butter.

Yogurt and Granola

Top 1 cup plain whole-milk Greek yogurt with ¼ cup Homemade Granola (page 229) and 1 cup blueberries.

Whole-Grain Pancakes with Fruit Sauce

Whole-Grain Pancakes with Fruit Sauce and Whipped Cream Topping (page 227) and 2 slices turkey bacon.

Chicken or Tofu Quesadilla with Guacamole and Sour Cream

Top a Chicken Quesadilla (page 246) (of six slices—serve two for breakfast or lunch, one for snack, and three for dinner) with 1 to 2 tablespoons guacamole, 1 tablespoon salsa, and 1 to 2 teaspoons sour cream. Serve with ¼ cup black beans.

LUNCHES/DINNERS

Chipotle Fish or Chicken Tacos

Heat 2 or 3 small to medium corn tortillas in a cast-iron skillet. Fill them each with about 2 ounces cooked fish or chicken, some shredded vegetables like cabbage, carrots, and cilantro, and a dollop of Chipotle Mayonnaise (page 268). Fold in half and eat immediately. (*Note:* This is best assembled immediately prior to eating so the tortillas don't get soggy.)

Salmon Salad with Soup and Crackers

Salmon (or Tofu) Salad (page 254) on a few 100% whole-grain crackers such as thin rye crisps. Serve with a vegetable soup like Creamy Cauliflower Soup (page 280) or Carrot-Ginger Soup (page 282), and an orange.

Melted Open-Faced Tomato, Basil, and Mozzarella Sandwiches

Top two slices of 100% whole wheat bread with sliced fresh basil (about 2 teaspoons), ¼ teaspoon dried basil, or a thin layer of basil pesto, a few slices of fresh tomato, 3 to 4 ounces mozzarella slices (total). Heat in a toaster oven or oven until the cheese has melted. Serve open-faced, with a green salad with chopped vegetables tossed with 1 tablespoon Mustard Vinaigrette (page 264) or another dressing of your choice.

Pasta Primavera

Spoon 1 to 1½ cups Marinara Primavera (page 234) over ½ to 1 cup cooked whole wheat pasta. Top with grated Parmesan (about 1 teaspoon). Serve with 1 cup blanched green beans or another green vegetable.

Herb-Roasted Chicken, Rice, and Broccoli

Serve Herb-Roasted Chicken Thighs (page 241) with ½ cup cooked white or brown rice (see the Guide to Cooking Whole Grains, page 317) and steamed or blanched broccoli, snap peas, carrots, or other vegetables with a spritz of lemon juice and salt and pepper to taste. *Variation:* Remove the chicken skin, stir the meat together with the broccoli, rice, and cheese, and bake into a broccoli rice casserole.

Sloppy Joes with Coleslaw and Fries

Serve a Modern Day Sloppy Joe (page 239) on ½ whole-grain bun with Tangy Coleslaw (page 279) and Roasted Sweet Potatoes (page 279), made using the variation for fries.

DESSERTS

Fruit and Granola Dessert

Top 1 cup fresh or cooked fruit with ¼ cup Homemade Granola (page 229) and 2 tablespoons heavy cream or canned coconut milk.

Apple Crisp

Enjoy Apple Crisp (page 287).

THE ROAD AHEAD

Though we've come to the end of the program, I hope you'll find the Always Hungry Solution a good companion as you continue along your path to optimal health. And please join me in another journey—to make the world a healthier place for all of us. Having brought healing into our personal lives, let's now work together so that this generation of children won't face the prospect of having shorter, less healthful lives than their parents. I invite you to read the Epilogue (page 297) for a road map.

My Always Hungry Story

I have struggled with my weight since I was a young child, but now it's my time in life to dedicate effort to stop struggling and start taking control of my health. I have fears that in twenty years my joints and digestive system will have only further deteriorated and prevent me from living a full life. I am learning that I do deserve to be healthy and it *is* possible for me—I just need help!

The program has helped me not be a stress eater. I have very, very limited cravings and improved control over impulsive eating by simply not desiring the sweet, processed foods. In fact, I only notice slight cravings if I did not properly eat a well-rounded meal or had a lack of sleep. Otherwise, none.

I'm less irritable and I have more energy most days than I would have on any other diet—normally, I would be dragging by now. My internal works feel less bloaty and inflamed, my knee joints are much less irritated, and my skin appears healthier and more hydrated. I just feel *decompressed*. An amazing feeling!

This program has changed my life. I have never stuck to a program, let alone turned one into my way of life. I feel better, look better, sleep better, and I am genuinely happier. I cannot believe how much processed food I used to eat. The freedom from nagging, negative thoughts surrounding food and self-image, every minute of the day, is in itself a reward. Not only to have lost weight and inches, but to have the knowledge of how to stay with it and prevent it coming back? No amount of thank-yous could cover it.

—Dominique R., 40, St. Paul, MN
Weight loss: 28 pounds. Decrease in waist: 6.5 inches

CHAPTER 9

Recipes

BREAKFASTS

Phase 1 Power Shake

Because the body registers calorie density as luscious, this shake satisfies cravings without even having to add sweetener. The Phase 1 Power Shake fits the Phase 1 profile perfectly, all in just one little power-packed glass.

Preparation time: 5 minutes

Total time: 5 minutes

Makes 1 serving

- 3 tablespoons heavy cream or canned coconut milk
- ⅓ cup unsweetened almond or soy milk or whole milk
- 1½ tablespoons almond butter or peanut butter
- 5 tablespoons 100% whey protein powder (one serving, no sugar, flavors, or artificial ingredients added)
- ½ cup frozen blueberries, cherries, or strawberries
- ½ ripe pear, or substitute another ½ cup frozen berries

Place all the ingredients in a blender and blend until smooth, about 30 seconds. Serve immediately.

Tip: If the shake is too thick, try adding the cream at the end, after the other ingredients are well blended.

Calories: 500*   Carbohydrate: 32 g   Total Fat: 31 g
Protein: 29 g   Dietary Fiber: 8 g

Peanut Butter Banana Power Shake (Phases 2 and 3)

This is a variation on the Phase 1 Power Shake. The classic combination of banana and peanut butter with a touch of nutmeg is sure to satisfy. With exactly the right combination of nutrients, you'll feel satiated all morning!

Preparation time: 5 minutes

Total time: 5 minutes

Makes 1 serving

- 1 fresh or frozen banana
- 2 to 3 tablespoons no-sugar-added peanut butter or other nut butter
- 1 cup unsweetened soy or almond milk
- 2½ tablespoons 100% whey protein powder (½ serving, no sugar, flavors, or artificial ingredients added)
- Dash of ground or freshly grated nutmeg

Place all the ingredients in a blender and blend until smooth, about 30 seconds. Serve immediately.

Tip: Prep frozen bananas by peeling and cutting ripe bananas into slices and freezing them in a zip-top plastic freezer bag.

Calories: 442   Carbohydrate: 37 g   Total Fat: 20 g
Protein: 28 g   Dietary Fiber: 5 g

*Nutrient data are approximations and will vary to some degree according to the specific products used.

Black Bean Tofu Hash (All Phases)

Tofu is a blank canvas: It takes on the flavor of your favorite seasoning. If you've never been a tofu enthusiast, give it another try. With the right blend of seasonings, you'll be surprised at how versatile and delicious this high-protein plant food can be.

Preparation time: 3 minutes

Total time: 10 minutes

Makes 4 servings (about 6 cups)

- 1 tablespoon extra-virgin olive oil
- 1 clove garlic, minced
- 14 to 16 ounces extra-firm tofu, drained, gently pressed with an absorbent towel
- 1 tablespoon chili powder
- ½ teaspoon ground cumin
- Dash of cayenne pepper, or more to taste
- 1 teaspoon salt
- ¼ teaspoon ground black pepper
- 2 tablespoons water
- 1¾ cups cooked black beans, drained (one 15-ounce can)
- ½ cup chopped fresh cilantro

Heat the oil in a large skillet over medium heat. Add the garlic. Crumble in the tofu and sprinkle with the chili powder, cumin, cayenne, salt, and pepper. Sauté for 2 to 3 minutes. Add the water, stirring to allow the tofu to absorb the seasonings and water. Stir in the black beans and sauté for 2 to 3 minutes more. Add the cilantro and adjust the seasoning to taste.

Serve with sliced avocado, sour cream, salsa, Ranchero Sauce (page 272), or your favorite sauce.

Tip: This is also great served in a lettuce wrap, in a Taco Salad (see Phase 1 Meal Plan Day 4 Lunch), or with cheese as filling in a Quesadilla (page 246) for Phase 3.

Calories: 243   Carbohydrate: 21 g   Total Fat: 10 g
Protein: 22 g   Dietary Fiber: 10 g

Grain-Free Waffles or Pancakes with Fruit Sauce (All Phases)

There is no sugar added to these waffles, highlighting the sweetness of the fruit topping. Make a batch to eat immediately, or cool and store in a large zip-top plastic bag in the fridge or freezer. Reheat the waffles in the toaster or toaster oven—a breakfast treat for any Phase!

Preparation time: 15 minutes

Total time: 30 minutes

Makes 4 waffles

Waffles
- 1 cup garbanzo-fava or garbanzo bean flour
- ⅛ teaspoon salt
- ¾ teaspoon baking soda
- 1 egg, separated
- ¾ cup plain whole-milk Greek yogurt
- ¼ cup unsweetened soy or almond milk or whole milk
- ¼ cup neutral-tasting oil, such as high-oleic safflower or avocado oil, plus more for brushing waffle pan
- ½ teaspoon pure vanilla extract (no sugar added)

Fruit Sauce
- 3 cups frozen blueberries, strawberries, or cherries
- 1 tablespoon water
- *For Phases 2 and 3:* 3 tablespoons pure maple syrup

Whipped Cream Topping
Phase 1: ¾ cup Whipped Cream (page 230; start with about 6 tablespoons heavy cream)

Phases 2 and 3: ¼ cup Whipped Cream (page 230; start with about 2 tablespoons heavy cream)

Make the waffles: Preheat a waffle iron. Combine the flour, salt, and baking soda in a large bowl. In another bowl, whisk together the egg yolk, yogurt, milk, oil, and vanilla. Stir the wet ingredients into the dry ingredients until well combined. Batter should be thick like a muffin or cake batter.

Beat the egg white with a whisk or the whisk attachment of an immersion blender until it forms soft peaks. Gently fold the egg white into the batter.

Brush the waffle iron with oil. Spoon ½ cup of batter per waffle into the waffle iron (or follow the manufacturer's instructions).

Cook until the waffles are golden, about 2 minutes or according to the manufacturer's instructions. Serve immediately, or keep warm in the oven on the lowest temperature until the rest of the waffles are done. Cover with a kitchen towel to prevent them from drying out.

Make the fruit sauce: Place the fruit and water in a small saucepan. For Phases 2 and 3 only, add the maple syrup (if using). Cover and cook over medium-low heat until soft and warm. Pour the mixture into a wide-mouthed glass mason jar or deep cup. Using an immersion blender, gently puree the berries.

Serve each hot waffle with about ⅓ cup fruit topping and 3 tablespoons whipped cream per serving for Phase 1 or 1 tablespoon whipped cream per serving for Phases 2 and 3.

Tip: Gluten-free batters like this one need to be thick in order to hold their structure when cooked. Adding liquid to make it look more like a typical, pourable pancake batter will make the center soggy and undercooked.

Variations

Make pancakes instead of waffles by pouring the batter onto a hot skillet (brushed with oil) and turning once to brown on both sides.

Phase 1 version (with no maple syrup in the fruit topping and 3 tablespoons whipped cream)

Per serving: Protein: 12 g   Dietary Fiber: 5 g
Calories: 406   Carbohydrate: 29 g   Total Fat: 28 g

Phase 2 version (with maple syrup in the fruit topping and 1 tablespoon whipped cream)

Per serving: Protein: 12 g   Dietary Fiber: 5 g
Calories: 393   Carbohydrate: 38 g   Total Fat: 22 g

Dr. Ludwig's Favorite Frittata (All Phases)

This is a staple brunch in the Ludwig household. It is easy to make and easy to reheat leftovers in a toaster oven. You can even have a leftover slice for a quick snack.

Preparation time: 8 minutes

Total time: 25 minutes

Makes 4 servings

- 3 teaspoons extra-virgin olive oil
- 5 eggs
- 3 egg whites
- 1 or 2 cloves garlic, minced
- ½ teaspoon salt
- ¼ teaspoon ground black pepper
- 1 small zucchini, cut in thin rounds
- 1 small tomato, thinly sliced
- 1 teaspoon dried Italian herb mix
- ½ cup shredded cheddar cheese
- 1 cup packed kale leaves (in bite-size pieces)
- ½ avocado, pitted, peeled, and sliced, for garnish

Preheat the oven to 400°F.

Heat 2 teaspoons of the oil in a 12-inch cast-iron skillet or ovenproof nonstick skillet over low heat. In a bowl, whisk together the eggs, egg whites, garlic, salt, and pepper until frothy. Pour the egg mixture into the skillet. Turn off the heat. Arrange the zucchini slices in a single layer over the eggs. Arrange the tomato slices in a layer over the zucchini. Sprinkle with the herbs. Top evenly with the cheese.

Transfer to the oven and bake for 5 minutes, or until the cheese melts. Toss the kale with the remaining 1 teaspoon oil. Arrange the kale on top of the frittata and bake for 8 to 10 minutes more, or until the eggs are fluffy and the kale begins to get crispy.

Serve garnished with fresh avocado slices.

Variations

Instead of tomatoes, spread on a few dollops of marinara sauce (no added sugar).

For Phase 1, drizzle the finished frittata with 1 tablespoon extra-virgin olive oil.

For Phase 2, use 4 eggs plus 4 egg whites.

Calories: 238	Carbohydrate: 7 g	Total Fat: 17 g
Protein: 16 g	Dietary Fiber: 2 g	

Overnight Steel-Cut Oats (Phases 2 and 3)

Try these oats as a cold pudding or heated—it's delicious both ways. For a complete breakfast, serve each portion with a couple of eggs, boiled, scrambled, or fried. Make a to-go breakfast in a jar by layering oats with nuts, fruit, and some Greek yogurt, and bring a hard-boiled egg on the side.

Preparation time: 10 minutes

Total time: Overnight plus 10 minutes

Makes 4 servings

- 4 cups unsweetened soy or almond milk
- 1 cup steel-cut oats
- Pinch of salt
- Dash of ground cinnamon, cardamom, or nutmeg (optional)
- ½ cup slivered almonds (or other roasted nuts, chopped)

Place the milk, oats, and salt in a medium saucepan with a lid. Bring to a boil, uncovered, over medium heat, stirring occasionally. (Watch the pot toward the end, as this mixture tends to froth up and over the edge when it comes to a full boil.) Reduce the heat to low and cook for 2 minutes. Turn off the heat and cover. Leave on the counter or cool the oats and place in the refrigerator overnight.

In the morning, serve as a cold pudding or reheat the oats over medium heat, stirring often, until warmed through. Sprinkle spices on top, if desired. Divide the oatmeal into four portions and top each with 2 tablespoons nuts.

Variations

Fresh fruit: Top each serving with ½ to 1 cup berries, diced apples, or other fruit of your choice.

Dried fruit: Cook the oats with ¼ cup (about 2 ounces) raisins, dried plums, dried apricots, or other dried fruit.

Calories: 318	Carbohydrate: 34 g	Total Fat: 14 g
Protein: 16 g	Dietary Fiber: 11 g	

Whole-Grain Pancakes (Phase 3)

These pancakes make an ideal brunch dish combined with a protein of your choice. Serve with fruit topping and whipped heavy cream. Making your own pancake mix is a lot less expensive than buying premade mix. Double or triple the dry pancake mix recipe. Store it in an airtight jar in your cupboard, then just add the wet ingredients for a quick batch of pancakes. Or, make a full batch and freeze them to pop in the toaster for a quick breakfast.

Preparation time: 5 minutes

Total time: 20 minutes

Makes 6 servings (ten to twelve 5-inch pancakes)

Pancake Mix

- 1 cup whole wheat pastry flour or white whole wheat flour
- 1 cup buckwheat flour or whole wheat pastry flour
- 2 teaspoons baking powder
- ¼ teaspoon salt

Pancake Batter

- ½ cup chopped pecans or other favorite nuts
- 2 cups whole milk, soy milk, or almond milk plus more as needed
- 2 eggs
- 1 tablespoon neutral-tasting oil, such as high-oleic safflower or avocado oil, plus more for brushing the skillet
- 1 teaspoon pure maple syrup

Fruit Sauce and Whipped Cream Topping
- 2 cups frozen blueberries, strawberries, or cherries
- 1 tablespoon water
- 1 tablespoon pure maple syrup (optional)
- ¼ cup Whipped Cream (page 230; start with about 2 tablespoons heavy cream)

Preheat a nonstick griddle or a cast-iron skillet.

Make the pancake mix: Combine the pancake mix ingredients in a bowl.

Make the pancakes: Add the nuts to the bowl with the pancake mix.

In a separate bowl, combine the milk, eggs, oil, and maple syrup. Whisk until well combined. Pour the wet ingredients into the dry ingredients, stirring gently until all the flour is moist. If needed, add more milk to create a thick, pourable batter. Make sure not to overmix.

Brush the skillet lightly with oil. Pour batter into 5-inch circles onto the hot skillet. Flip the pancakes when the edges are golden brown and small bubbles rise in the center. (If bubbles don't rise, more milk may be needed in the batter, or the batter may have been overmixed.) Cook until the second side is lightly browned and the pancake is cooked through. Serve immediately or keep warm in the oven on the lowest setting until ready to serve.

Make the fruit sauce: Place the berries and water in a small saucepan. Add the maple syrup (if using). Cover and cook over medium-low heat until soft and warm. Pour the mixture into a wide-mouthed glass mason jar or deep cup. Using an immersion blender, puree the berries in the jar.

Serve the pancakes hot, with ¼ cup fruit topping and 1 tablespoon whipped cream per serving. The pancakes can also be cooled and placed in a zip-top plastic bag in the refrigerator or freezer. Reheat in the toaster or toaster oven.

Variations
Sprinkle the nuts on top of the pancakes instead of mixing them into the batter.

Add more or less milk for thicker or thinner pancakes, depending on your preference.

Play with different types of whole-grain flours. Remember that different flours will soak up different amounts of milk, so you will have to adjust based on the flour you are using. Experiment to find the right amount for your perfect pancakes.

Calories: 337   Carbohydrate: 42 g   Total Fat: 16 g
Protein: 10 g   Dietary Fiber: 7 g

Homemade Granola (Phase 3)

No need to buy expensive granola mixes: This one is more nutritious, simple to make at home, and easy to store until you are ready to use it. Serve with full-fat Greek yogurt for a delicious treat.

Preparation time: 5 minutes

Total time: 25 minutes

Makes 4 to 6 servings (about 1½ cups)

- 2 tablespoons neutral-tasting oil, such as high-oleic safflower or avocado oil
- 2 tablespoons pure maple syrup
- ¾ cup rolled oats (not instant)
- ½ tablespoon sesame seeds
- ¾ cup coarsely chopped nuts (pecans, cashews, almonds, peanuts, etc.)
- 2 tablespoons unsweetened shredded coconut

Preheat the oven to 350°F.

Whisk together the oil and maple syrup in a bowl.

In a separate bowl, combine the oats, seeds, and nuts. Add the wet ingredients and stir until the granola is well coated.

Spread the mixture in a shallow baking pan. Bake for 15 to 20 minutes, or until bubbling and golden brown, stirring every 5 to 10 minutes to ensure even browning. Remove from the oven and add the shredded coconut. Mix well. Let cool and serve, or store in an airtight jar in the cupboard.

Per ¼-cup serving: Protein: 7 g   Dietary Fiber: 3 g
Calories: 266   Carbohydrate: 19 g   Total Fat: 20 g

Whipped Cream (All Phases)

You won't believe how simple and quick it is to make your own whipped cream. This luscious topping makes any recipe delicious, and you won't miss the added sugar!

Preparation time: 3 minutes

Total time: 3 minutes

Makes 4 to 8 servings (about ½ cup)

- ¼ cup heavy cream

Pour the heavy cream into a deep bowl. Whip with the whisk attachment on an immersion blender until the cream forms soft peaks. Serve immediately or store in the refrigerator until ready to use.

| Per 1 tablespoon: | Protein: 0 g | Dietary Fiber: 0 g |
| Calories: 13 | Carbohydrate: 0 g | Total Fat: 1 g |

ENTRÉES

Chicken Stir-Fry (All Phases)

This is a go-to recipe when you want something fresh, quick, and delicious. Use precut vegetables and this meal will be done in a flash. It also tastes great in a lettuce wrap the next day.

Preparation time: 10 minutes

Total time: 20 minutes

Makes 4 servings

- 1 tablespoon neutral-tasting oil, such as sesame (untoasted), high-oleic safflower, or avocado oil
- 6 boneless, skinless chicken thighs (about 1½ pounds), cut into bite-size pieces
- 1 recipe Stir-Fry Sauce (page 260)
- 4 ounces shiitake, cremini, or white button mushrooms
- 1 head of broccoli, cut into small florets, stem peeled and cut into small pieces

- 2 medium carrots, cut into matchsticks or coarsely shredded (about 1 cup)
- 2 cups shredded cabbage
- 8 ounces snow peas or snap peas (15 to 20 pods)
- 3 cups packed spinach
- Freshly ground black pepper and salt

Heat the oil in a large skillet over medium heat. Add the chicken and sauté until it begins to brown, about 5 minutes.

Add the Stir-Fry Sauce and mushrooms. Sauté until the chicken is no longer pink in the middle, 5 to 7 minutes. Stir in the broccoli, carrots, cabbage, and snow peas. Reduce the heat to medium-low, cover, and simmer, stirring a few times, until the vegetables are tender but still bright, 3 to 5 minutes. Add water as needed to keep the mixture from burning or sticking.

Spread the spinach on a serving tray or divide among individual bowls. Spoon the hot chicken and vegetables on top of the spinach, leaving any excess liquid in the skillet. The spinach should begin to wilt under the heat of the chicken. Bring the liquid in the skillet to a boil, then reduce the heat to medium-low and simmer until the sauce thickens. Pour the thickened sauce over the stir-fry. Serve immediately while the vegetables are still bright. Garnish with freshly ground black pepper and salt to taste.

Tip: Serve with a higher-fat dessert like Coconut Cashew Clusters (page 284) or for Phase 2, Pear Strawberry Crisp (page 285)

Variations

Add or substitute other vegetables of your choice.

For Phases 2 and 3—Brown Rice Variation: Add the spinach with the other vegetables. After the vegetables and chicken are removed from the skillet, add ½ cup cooked brown rice or cooked quinoa per serving to the remaining sauce (2 cups total for the full recipe). Sauté until all the sauce has been absorbed into the grain. Serve the vegetables and chicken on top of the grain.

For a vegetarian version, substitute 1½ pounds extra-firm tofu, drained, gently pressed with an absorbent towel, and cut into bite-size pieces for the chicken, and season with additional salt or soy sauce to taste.

Substitute 16 to 20 ounces peeled and deveined shrimp for the chicken.

For a version of Pepper Steak, substitute 1¼ pounds steak strips for the chicken, and onions with red, yellow, and green bell peppers for the vegetables.

Calories: 371	Carbohydrate: 22 g	Total Fat: 15 g
Protein: 40 g	Dietary Fiber: 8 g	

Broiled Fish with Garlic and Lemon (All Phases)

This quick, easy recipe works with almost every kind of white-fleshed fish, as well as salmon. A perfect weeknight meal—you can have it on the table in twenty minutes with all the sides.

Preparation time: 5 minutes

Total time: 15 minutes

Makes 4 servings

- 1¼ to 1½ pounds white-fleshed fish fillet (cod, scrod, hake, or other white fish)
- ½ teaspoon salt, or more to taste (fillets thicker than 1 inch may need more salt)
- 2 tablespoons extra-virgin olive oil
- 1 to 2 cloves garlic, minced
- ½ lemon, cut in thin slices
- Chopped fresh parsley, cilantro, or scallions, for garnish

Set the oven to broil.

Rinse the fish, pat dry, and sprinkle lightly with the salt. Heat the oil in a cast-iron skillet or ovenproof skillet over medium-high heat. Add the garlic and sauté for a few seconds. Place the fish in the pan and sear for a few seconds on each side. Remove the fish from the skillet and turn off heat.

In a single layer, arrange the lemon slices in the pan. Place the fish on top of the lemon. It is best if the fish is covering most of the lemon slices so that the lemon doesn't burn in the broiler, but still makes a nice sauce.

Place the skillet in the oven and broil until the fish is opaque and begins to brown on top, 8 to 10 minutes per inch of fillet thickness. Transfer the fish to a serving plate. If liquid still remains, heat the skillet on the stovetop for 3 to 5 minutes to thicken the sauce. Pour the sauce over the fish and arrange the lemon slices on top. Garnish with chopped parsley. Serve immediately.

Variations

Salmon Variation: Use skin-on salmon and broil skin-side up until the skin is crispy.

Calories: 205   Carbohydrate: 2 g   Total Fat: 8 g
Protein: 31 g   Dietary Fiber: 0 g

Melt-in-Your-Mouth Lamb Shanks (All Phases)

The name says it all!

Preparation time: 5 minutes

Total time: 1 hour and 45 minutes

Makes 4 servings

- 4 medium lamb shanks (about 2½ pounds total)
- 1 cup red wine
- ½ cup water
- 1 bay leaf
- 10 whole black peppercorns
- ½ to ¾ teaspoon salt

Place the lamb shanks in a deep skillet or saucepan. Add the red wine, water, bay leaf, and peppercorns. Sprinkle with the salt and bring to a boil over medium heat. Reduce the heat to medium-low, cover, and simmer, turning the shanks every 20 minutes, for 90 minutes or more, until the meat is tender and easily comes off the bone. Reduce the heat further or add a little water as necessary to keep the shanks from burning. Transfer the shanks to a serving plate. Cook the sauce over medium heat for 3 to 5 minutes more to thicken. Pour the sauce over the shanks and serve.

Variations

Sprinkle with your favorite dried herbs like thyme or oregano.

Cook in a slow cooker according to the manufacturer's instructions.

Substitute a pork loin roast or shanks for the lamb.

Calories: 442   Carbohydrate: 1 g   Total Fat: 30 g
Protein: 41 g   Dietary Fiber: 0 g

Marinara Primavera (All Phases)

This reimagined standard satisfies those Italian cravings and is a great way to get extra vegetables into a meal. Serve as a main dish in Phase 1, over quinoa or fluffy millet in Phase 2, or tossed with whole wheat pasta in Phase 3.

Preparation time: 10 minutes

Total time: 30 minutes

Makes 4 servings

- 1 teaspoon extra-virgin olive oil
- 1 small onion, diced
- 1 clove garlic, minced
- 1 large zucchini, cut into bite-size pieces
- ⅛ teaspoon salt
- ¼ teaspoon ground black pepper
- 2 to 3 cups marinara sauce (no sugar added)
- 1 recipe Crumbled Tempeh (page 244)
- 1 to 2 cups packed leafy greens (kale, collards, spinach, arugula, beet greens, chard, etc. in bite-size pieces)

Heat the oil in a large skillet or pot over medium heat. Add the onion, garlic, zucchini, salt, and pepper. Cook until the onion is soft, about 5 minutes. Stir in the marinara sauce.

Reduce the heat to medium-low, cover, and simmer for 10 minutes, or until the zucchini is soft. Stir in the Crumbled Tempeh and greens. Cover and simmer until the greens are tender but still bright, 3 to 5 minutes for kale or collards and 1 to 2 minutes for softer greens like spinach or arugula.

Adjust the seasoning to taste. Serve as is for Phase 1, with whole grains for Phase 2, or on whole-grain pasta for Phase 3.

Variations

To keep the tempeh crispy, add 3 to 4 ounces Crumbled Tempeh (page 244) as a garnish on top of each serving instead of mixed in with the sauce.

Add or substitute other vegetables of your choice like mushrooms, eggplant, bell peppers, broccoli, roasted garlic, artichoke hearts, or fresh herbs.

Substitute 1¼ pounds ground turkey, ground beef, ground lamb, or 1½ pounds boneless skinless chicken thighs for the tempeh. Cook the meat with the vegetables until done and increase the salt to ½ teaspoon, or to taste, depending on the salt content of the marinara sauce.

Calories: 429   Carbohydrate: 25 g   Total Fat: 28 g
Protein: 25 g   Dietary Fiber: 12 g

Beef, Bean, and Barley Stew (All Phases)

This mellow soup takes a bit of cooking time, but the reward for your patience will be ultra-tender meat and a rich broth. You can eat it right away, but the flavors will improve after twenty-four hours in the refrigerator.

Preparation time: 20 minutes

Total time: 1 hour

Makes 4 servings

- 1 tablespoon extra-virgin olive oil
- 1 pound beef chuck or other stew meat, cut into ½-inch cubes
- 1 teaspoon salt
- ¼ teaspoon ground black pepper, plus more for garnish
- 1 medium onion, sliced
- 1 stalk celery, diced
- 4 cups water
- 1¾ cups canned diced tomatoes (one 14.5-ounce can)
- ½ cup barley, uncooked
- 1¾ cups cooked kidney beans, drained and rinsed (one 15-ounce can)
- 8 cups chopped chard or other leafy greens
- 2 teaspoons finely chopped fresh rosemary, or 1 teaspoon dried
- 1 teaspoon dried thyme, or more to taste
- Fresh parsley or scallions, chopped, for garnish

Preheat the oven to 325°F.

Heat the oil in a large ovenproof pot with a lid or Dutch oven over medium heat. Add the beef, salt, and pepper. Cook until browned. Add the onion, celery, water, tomatoes, barley, kidney beans, half the chard, the rosemary, and the thyme. Bring to a boil. Cover, place in the oven, and bake for 1 hour.

Remove from the oven and stir the remaining chard into the hot soup. Adjust the seasoning to taste. Garnish with freshly ground black pepper and parsley. Serve hot. Refrigerate any leftovers for up to 3 days, or freeze in individual portions.

Variations

Simmer on the stovetop or in a slow cooker instead of baking.

For a gluten-free version, use brown rice instead of barley.

Add other herbs or spices like cayenne, curry, or other seasonings to your taste.

For a vegetarian version, substitute 14 to 16 ounces extra-firm tofu, drained, gently pressed with an absorbent towel, and cut into ½-inch cubes for the beef.

Calories: 423   Carbohydrate: 43 g   Total Fat: 13 g
Protein: 35 g   Dietary Fiber: 13 g

Cabbage Casserole (All Phases)

This is a no-fuss variation on a traditional stuffed cabbage recipe. With this recipe, you get all the satisfaction of cabbage rolls in a sweet-and-savory sauce without the bother of stuffing individual cabbage leaves.

Preparation time: 15 minutes

Total time: 1 hour and 25 minutes

Makes 4 servings

- 1 medium onion, quartered
- 4 cloves garlic
- 1 red bell pepper, cored and seeded
- 1¼ pounds 90% lean ground beef

- 1 teaspoon salt
- ¼ teaspoon ground black pepper
- 3½ cups canned diced tomatoes (about two 14.5-ounce cans)
- 2 to 4 tablespoons apple cider vinegar
- 1 apple, quartered and cored
- ¼ teaspoon ground cinnamon
- 5 to 6 cups shredded cabbage (from about ½ small cabbage, cored)

Preheat the oven to 375°F. In a medium saucepan, bring a few inches of water to a rolling boil over high heat.

In a food processor, combine the onion, garlic, and bell pepper. Pulse until finely chopped. (If you don't have a food processor, finely dice the vegetables.) Transfer to a medium bowl. (Set the food processor container aside for next ingredients, no need to wash.) Stir the beef, ½ teaspoon of the salt, and ⅛ teaspoon of the black pepper into the onion mixture.

In the food processor or in a jar that fits the immersion blender without splashing, combine the tomatoes, vinegar, apple, cinnamon, remaining ½ teaspoon salt, and remaining ⅛ teaspoon black pepper. Pulse until the apple is finely chopped.

Blanch the cabbage by immersing it in the boiling water for about 30 seconds, 1 to 2 cups at a time. Remove from the water with a mesh skimmer or slotted spoon. Place on a large plate to drain.

Cover the bottom of a 9 x 12-inch ovenproof baking dish with 1 cup of the tomato mixture. Layer with half of the cabbage, then half of the beef mixture. Layer with a second cup of the tomato mixture, the remaining cabbage, and the remaining beef mixture. Finish with the remaining tomato mixture. Cover with aluminum foil and bake for 45 minutes. Remove the foil and cook for 30 minutes more.

Variations

For a vegetarian version, substitute 1 recipe Crumbled Tempeh (page 244) for the beef and reduce the salt by half.

Substitute 1¼ pounds ground turkey for the beef.

Use less vinegar for a milder-tasting casserole.

Calories: 366	Carbohydrate: 26 g	Total Fat: 14 g
Protein: 32 g	Dietary Fiber: 6 g	

Shepherd's Pie with Cauliflower Topping (All Phases)

This recipe was a huge hit with our pilot participants. The dish's cauli-flower and white bean topping is arguably richer and tastier than the traditional potato topping...and the kids won't know it doesn't have potatoes unless you tell them! Consider making these in individual por-tions and freezing extra servings for a last-minute heat-and-serve meal. For a fantastic vegetarian meal, try the tempeh variation.

Preparation time: 15 minutes

Total time: 45 minutes

Makes 6 servings

- 1 small to medium head cauliflower, cut into large pieces (about 4 to 6 cups)
- 1 large onion, quartered
- 2 cloves garlic
- 1 medium fennel bulb (or substitute 4 small carrots), cut into large pieces
- 1 teaspoon plus 2 tablespoons extra-virgin olive oil or butter
- 8 ounces sliced button or cremini mushrooms
- 1½ pounds 90% lean ground beef
- 1¼ teaspoons salt
- ⅛ teaspoon plus ¼ teaspoon ground black pepper
- 6 ounces canned tomato paste
- ½ cup water
- Dash of cayenne pepper (optional)
- 1¾ cups cooked cannellini or other white beans, drained and rinsed

Place the cauliflower in a pot and add water just to cover. Bring to a boil over high heat, reduce the heat to medium, and cook until tender, about 10 minutes.

While cauliflower is cooking, preheat the oven to 375°F.

Place the onion, garlic, and fennel in a food processor and pulse until finely chopped.

Heat 1 teaspoon of the olive oil in a large skillet over medium heat. Add the onion mixture, mushrooms, beef, ½ teaspoon of the salt, and ⅛ teaspoon of the pepper. Cook, stirring often, until the beef is browned, 5 to 10 minutes.

Stir the tomato paste and water together in a small bowl and add the mixture to the skillet with the beef. Add the cayenne (if using) and turn off the heat.

Drain the cauliflower, return it to the pot, and add the remaining 2 tablespoons oil, ¾ teaspoon salt, ¼ teaspoon pepper, and the white beans. Puree with an immersion blender until smooth.

Transfer the beef mixture to a 9 x 12-inch baking dish (or six individual 4- or 5-inch ramekins). Top with the cauliflower mixture. Bake for 20 to 30 minutes, or until the casserole is bubbling.

Serve immediately. Cool and refrigerate or freeze extra portions. If you refrigerate assembled pies, then reheat in a preheated 375°F oven until warm throughout, about 20 minutes. Serve hot.

Variations

For a vegetarian version, substitute 1 recipe Crumbled Tempeh (page 244) for the beef, increase water to 1 cup, and reduce salt by ½ teaspoon or to taste.

Substitute 1½ pounds ground turkey or ground lamb for the beef.

Calories: 400	Carbohydrate: 31 g	Total Fat: 17 g
Protein: 32 g	Dietary Fiber: 8 g	

Modern Day Sloppy Joe (Phases 2 and 3)

Who doesn't love a sloppy joe? Even your pickiest eaters will love this reinvented favorite. Even better, pair it with Tangy Coleslaw (page 279) and Roasted Sweet Potato Fries (page 279) for a complete meal.

Preparation time: 10 minutes

Total time: 20 minutes

Makes 4 servings

- 2 tablespoons extra-virgin olive oil
- 1 onion, diced
- 1 red bell pepper, cored, seeded, and diced
- 1¼ pounds 90% lean ground beef
- 1 teaspoon salt
- 1¾ cups canned diced tomatoes (one 14.5-ounce can)
- 1 tablespoon honey
- ¼ cup apple cider vinegar
- ¼ teaspoon ground cloves
- ¼ teaspoon ground cinnamon
- ¼ teaspoon mustard powder
- ⅛ teaspoon ground black pepper
- Cayenne pepper, to taste
- *For Phase 3:* 2 whole wheat hamburger buns (use sprouted-grain buns, if available)

Heat the oil in a large skillet over medium heat. Add the onion and bell pepper and cook for 3 minutes, stirring often. Add the beef and salt and cook, stirring often, until the beef is browned, about 5 minutes.

In a blender or in a large wide-mouthed mason jar using an immersion blender, blend the tomatoes, honey, vinegar, cloves, cinnamon, mustard powder, black pepper, and cayenne. Stir the tomato mixture into the beef mixture. Bring to a simmer over medium-low heat and cook for 5 to 10 minutes. Serve as a main dish in Phase 2, or serve each portion open-faced on half a bun in Phase 3.

Variations

For a vegetarian version, substitute 14 to 16 ounces extra-firm tofu, drained, gently pressed with an absorbent towel, and crumbled for the beef, and increase the salt to taste.

Phase 2

Calories: 377   Carbohydrate: 13 g   Total Fat: 23 g
Protein: 28 g   Dietary Fiber: 2 g

Phase 3 (with Sprouted Whole-Grain Burger Buns)

Calories: 462   Carbohydrate: 30 g   Total Fat: 23 g
Protein: 28 g   Dietary Fiber: 5 g

Herb-Roasted Chicken Thighs (All Phases)

You can't find an easier way to make chicken. Get creative and add your favorite dried herb blends. Leftover thighs are great in a salad or wrapped in a lettuce leaf with a creamy sauce over them.

Preparation time: 5 minutes

Total time: 50 minutes

Makes 4 servings

- 6 to 8 bone-in, skin-on chicken thighs (about 2 pounds)
- 1 tablespoon extra-virgin olive oil
- 1 to 2 teaspoons dried Italian herb mix (or substitute your favorite dried herb blend)
- ½ to ¾ teaspoon salt
- ¼ teaspoon ground black pepper

Preheat the oven to 350°F. Place the chicken skin-side up in a 9-inch square baking dish. Drizzle with the oil and sprinkle with the dried Italian herb mix, salt, and pepper. Bake for 45 minutes, or until the chicken is well cooked and no longer pink. Baste occasionally by spooning the juices in the baking dish over the thighs.

Variations

Substitute ⅓ cup Mustard Vinaigrette (page 264) for the olive oil

Calories: 350   Carbohydrate: 1 g   Total Fat: 24 g
Protein: 32 g   Dietary Fiber: 0 g

Mexican Shredded Chicken (All Phases)

Use as a filling for taco salads, or casseroles, or serve rolled in a tortilla, or in Quesadillas (page 246), and topped with guacamole or sour cream. The extra servings will keep well in the refrigerator for up three days, or freeze them for longer storage.

Preparation time: 5 minutes

Total time: 10 to 25 minutes

Makes 6 servings (about 3 cups)

- 3 tablespoons extra-virgin olive oil
- 6 to 8 boneless, skinless chicken thighs (about 1¾ pounds)
- ¼ teaspoon garlic powder
- 1 teaspoon ground cumin
- ¼ teaspoon powdered red chile such as New Mexican, ancho or chile de arbol
- Dash of cayenne pepper, or to taste
- ½ teaspoon salt
- ⅛ teaspoon ground black pepper

Heat the oil in a large skillet over medium heat. Add chicken, spices, salt, and pepper.

Cover and cook, turning regularly, especially in the beginning, until the oil and juices from the chicken begin to make a sauce. Add water as needed, 1 tablespoon at a time, to keep the mixture from burning or sticking. Cook until the chicken is cooked throughout, 15 to 20 minutes. Using two forks, shred the chicken in the pan, pulling along the grain to create thin strands. Continue to heat the shredded chicken, stirring frequently, until the liquid and spices have been absorbed and the chicken is fully cooked, 3 to 5 minutes.

Variations

For a vegetarian version, substitute 1½ pounds extra-firm tofu, drained, gently pressed with an absorbent towel, and crumbled for the chicken. Increase the salt to 1 teaspoon and the cumin to 2 to 3 teaspoons. Cook for about 10 minutes. The final mixture should look like scrambled eggs.

Calories: 220	Carbohydrate: 0 g	Total Fat: 12 g
Protein: 26 g	Dietary Fiber: 0 g	

Pan-Fried Tempeh or Tofu Strips (All Phases)

Cooking tempeh and tofu might seem mysterious at first—but once you get the hang of it, you may find yourself substituting them for meat often. This recipe provides an easy way to prepare tempeh or tofu for use in your favorite recipes. Serve it in place of any of the meats used in the meal plans, like Herb-Roasted Chicken Thighs (page 241) or Melt-in-Your-Mouth Lamb Shanks (page 233). If you are choosing the vegetarian version of any meal plan recipe, add this recipe to your regular prep day activities. Make enough to use for the week, and store it in the refrigerator to create a quick meal anytime.

Preparation time: 3 minutes

Total time: 20 minutes

Makes 4 servings

- 2 tablespoons extra-virgin olive oil
- 1 pound soy tempeh, cut lengthwise into ¼-inch-wide strips, or 14 to 16 ounces extra-firm tofu, drained, gently pressed with an absorbent towel, and cut into ¼-inch slices
- 1 tablespoon soy sauce
- 3 tablespoons water
- ¼ teaspoon garlic powder

Heat the oil in a large cast-iron skillet or griddle over medium to medium-high heat. Arrange the tempeh in a single layer in the skillet and cook until browned and crispy on the first side, 5 to 7 minutes. Turn the strips over and brown on the other side. Reduce the heat to low. In a small bowl, combine the soy sauce, water, and garlic powder. Pour the sauce over the browned tempeh.

For tempeh: Cover and simmer for about 3 minutes more. Turn the tempeh strips and cook, uncovered, for 3 minutes more to ensure even distribution of flavors.

For tofu: Cook, uncovered, for about 1 minute on each side.

Serve or refrigerate to use in other recipes.

Variations
Add fresh ginger or other herbs or spices to the sauce.

Marinate the tempeh overnight or tofu for a few hours in the sauce. Remove from the marinade, cook as directed, then add the liquid at the end to simmer and absorb.

Tofu Version:

Calories: 169	Carbohydrate: 2 g	Total Fat: 13 g
Protein: 16 g	Dietary Fiber: 2 g	

Tempeh Version:

Calories: 251	Carbohydrate: 14 g	Total Fat: 13 g
Protein: 22 g	Dietary Fiber: 5 g	

Crumbled Tempeh (All Phases)

Cooking tempeh like this before using it in a recipe will produce a rich flavor and meaty texture. Substitute Crumbled Tempeh for any ground meat in your favorite recipes. You might be surprised by how satisfying this protein-packed bean can be. Tempeh keeps well after it is cooked, too. Add this recipe to your regular prep-day activities. Make enough to use for the week, and store it in the refrigerator to create a quick meal anytime.

Preparation time: 5 minutes

Total time: 25 minutes

Makes 4 servings

- 3 tablespoons extra-virgin olive oil
- 1 teaspoon salt
- 1 pound tempeh, minced or crumbled

Preheat the oven to 375°F.

Stir the oil and salt into the tempeh until well distributed. Transfer the tempeh to a 9 x 12-inch baking pan. Bake for 20 to 30 minutes, stirring regularly, until the tempeh is brown and crispy on all sides.

Variations

Heat the oil in a large cast-iron or heavy-bottomed skillet over medium heat. Add the tempeh and salt. Sauté, stirring frequently and breaking up larger pieces into smaller crumbles with a spatula, until the tempeh is browned and fully cooked, about 20 minutes. Add water as needed to keep from burning or sticking.

Calories: 279   Carbohydrate: 13 g   Total Fat: 16 g
Protein: 22 g   Dietary Fiber: 5 g

Mediterranean Chicken (All Phases)

This hearty, one-pot meal is a big hit at family dinners, as it suits many ages and palates. Bring it to your next potluck party as an creative alternative to chili.

Preparation time: 10 minutes

Total time: 30 minutes

Makes 4 servings

- 3 tablespoons extra-virgin olive oil
- 6 boneless, skinless chicken thighs (about 1½ pounds), cut into 1-inch pieces
- ¼ to ½ teaspoon salt, depending on the salt content of the olives and feta cheese
- ¼ teaspoon ground black pepper
- 1 medium onion, sliced into half-moons
- 4 cloves garlic, minced
- 3½ cups canned diced tomatoes (about two 14.5-ounce cans)
- ¾ cup Kalamata olives
- 1⅓ cups cooked garbanzo beans (chickpeas), drained and rinsed
- ½ pound green beans (about 2 cups, or a large handful)
- ¼ cup (about 10 ounces) feta cheese, for garnish

Heat the oil in a large skillet or pot over medium heat. Add the chicken, salt, and pepper and sauté for about 5 minutes. Add the onion and garlic and sauté until the onion is soft, about 5 minutes. Add the tomatoes, olives, and garbanzo beans. Bring to a boil, then reduce the heat to medium-low and simmer for 10 to 15 minutes, or until the chicken is fully cooked. Stir in the green beans. Cover and simmer for 3 to 5 minutes, until the green beans are tender but still bright green. Serve immediately, garnished with the feta cheese.

Variations

For a vegetarian version, substitute 1½ pounds extra-firm tofu, drained, gently pressed with an absorbent towel, and cut into bite-size pieces for the chicken.

For Phases 2 and 3, reduce the oil to 1 to 2 tablespoons.

Calories: 495	Carbohydrate: 28 g	Total Fat: 24 g
Protein: 41 g	Dietary Fiber: 8 g	

Chicken Quesadillas (Phase 3)

Who doesn't love quesadillas? One of the quickest, easiest ways to feed the whole family, these quesadillas keep well, are easily portable, and taste fantastic when reheated the next day for breakfast, lunch, or a quick snack. Make a double batch and save the extras for the next day.

Preparation time: 5 minutes

Total time: 10 minutes

Makes 4 servings (2 full quesadillas)

- 4 (8-inch) whole wheat or sprouted-wheat tortillas
- 6 tablespoons shredded Monterey Jack or cheddar cheese
- 1 cup Mexican Shredded Chicken (page 241)
- ½ cup chopped fresh cilantro
- 2 tablespoons salsa

Heat a cast-iron skillet or griddle over medium-high heat. Warm one tortilla on one side, about 15 seconds, then flip.

Lower the heat to medium. Sprinkle 1½ tablespoons of the cheese over the whole tortilla. Top the cheese with ½ cup of the chicken and ¼ cup of the cilantro, spreading them evenly over the tortilla. Top with an additional 1½ tablespoons of the cheese and cover with a second tortilla.

Cook on the first side until browned, 1 to 2 minutes. Turn carefully with a large spatula so that the filling does not fall out, then cook on the second side until browned, 1 to 2 minutes. Carefully remove from the skillet and place on a large wooden cutting board to cool, 2 to 3 minutes. Repeat with the remaining tortillas, cheese, chicken, and cilantro.

Cut each quesadilla into six wedges. Serve warm, topped with salsa.

Tip: Nothing browns a tortilla better than a cast-iron skillet: It heats them as though they're fresh off the griddle.

Variations

Add the salsa to the center of the tortilla with the cilantro.

Top with guacamole or sliced avocado and sour cream.

For a vegetarian version, substitute ¾ cup Black Bean Tofu Hash (page 222) or Mexican Shredded Chicken—Tofu Variation (page 241) for the chicken.

Calories: 455   Carbohydrate: 49 g   Total Fat: 17 g
Protein: 28 g   Dietary Fiber: 10 g

Eggplant Parmesan (All Phases)

Another favorite with the pilot participants, this dish is the ultimate in comfort food. If you are short on time, assemble the dish in advance, cover, refrigerate, and cook it just before serving.

Preparation time: 15 minutes

Total time: 45 minutes

Makes 4 servings

- 1 medium eggplant (about 1 pound), cut into ¼-inch-thick rounds
- 4 teaspoons extra-virgin olive oil
- ¾ teaspoon salt (adjust based on the saltiness of marinara sauce)
- 14 to 16 ounces extra-firm tofu, drained and gently pressed with an absorbent towel
- ⅛ teaspoon ground black pepper
- 1 cup grated mozzarella cheese
- 1 cup ricotta cheese
- 1 large zucchini, cut into ¼-inch rounds
- 2 cups marinara sauce (no added sugar)
- ¼ cup fresh basil leaves
- ¼ cup grated Parmesan cheese

Preheat the oven to 425°F.

Brush the eggplant with the oil and arrange the rounds in a single layer, or slightly overlapping at the edges, on a large baking sheet (or two, if necessary). Sprinkle with ¼ teaspoon of the salt. Roast until tender, 12 to 15 minutes. Remove from the oven but leave the oven on.

Meanwhile, crumble the tofu into a large bowl with the remaining ½ teaspoon salt and the pepper. Combine well. Stir in the mozzarella and ricotta until well mixed.

Cover the bottom of a 9 x 12-inch baking dish with ¾ cup of the marinara sauce. Top with half the basil, then half the roasted eggplant, half the zucchini, and half the mozzarella mixture. Repeat by topping with another ¾ cup of the marinara sauce and the remaining basil, eggplant, zucchini, and mozzarella mixture. Top with the remaining tomato sauce and sprinkle evenly with the Parmesan.

Roast until the eggplant is soft, the casserole is bubbling throughout, and the Parmesan is golden brown on top, about 30 minutes. Serve warm.

Variations

Add or substitute other vegetables of your choice like red bell peppers or onions.

For a quick shortcut, substitute frozen grilled vegetables for the eggplant and zucchini and omit precooking the eggplant.

For Phase 3: Add a layer of no-boil lasagna noodles

Calories: 485   Carbohydrate: 17 g   Total Fat: 34 g
Protein: 34 g   Dietary Fiber: 8 g

Coconut Curry Shrimp (All Phases)

The combination of shrimp, creamy coconut, and cashews with spicy curry—just one of the many mouthwatering uses of Coconut Curry Sauce (page 266)—makes this meal so rich and satisfying, you'll never miss the rice. (And after Phase 1, you won't have to!)

Preparation time: 5 minutes

Total time: 20 minutes

Makes 4 servings

- 1 teaspoon neutral-tasting oil, such as high-oleic safflower, or avocado oil
- 1½ pounds medium shrimp, peeled and deveined
- ¼ teaspoon salt
- 2 medium carrots, cut into matchsticks or coarsely shredded (about 1 cup)
- ½ red bell pepper, cored, seeded, and diced
- 2 cups shredded cabbage
- ¾ to 1 pound snow peas or snap peas (30 to 40 pods)
- 2½ cups Coconut Curry Sauce (page 266)
- ½ cup chopped fresh cilantro
- Curry powder
- 3 cups (packed) spinach, chopped

Heat the oil in a large skillet or pot over medium heat. Add the shrimp and sprinkle with the salt. Sauté until the shrimp are pink on all sides, 3 to 5 minutes.

Stir in the carrots, bell pepper, cabbage, snow peas, and Coconut Curry Sauce. Bring to a boil, then reduce the heat to medium-low, cover, and simmer, stirring frequently, until the vegetables are tender but still bright, and the sauce is thickened, 5 to 7 minutes. Stir in the cilantro. Adjust the seasoning with more curry powder or salt.

Spread the spinach on a serving tray or divide it among individual bowls. Place the hot vegetable curry mixture on top of the spinach. The spinach should begin to wilt under the heat of the sauce. Serve immediately, while the vegetables are still bright.

Variations

For a vegetarian version, substitute ¾ cup cooked garbanzo beans (chickpeas), drained and rinsed and 1 pound extra-firm tofu, drained, gently pressed with an absorbent towel, and cut into bite-size pieces for the shrimp. Increase the salt to ½ teaspoon, or to taste

Substitute 1½ pounds chicken or fish for the shrimp. If using chicken, cut it into bite-size pieces and sauté for 7 to 10 minutes, or until the chicken is no longer pink in the middle.

For Phases 2 and 3, serve a smaller portion over ¼ to ½ cup cooked brown rice or quinoa per serving.

Add or substitute other vegetables of your choice.

Add ½ to 1 cup cooked garbanzo beans (chickpeas) for a creamier sauce.

Calories: 421	Carbohydrate: 21 g	Total Fat: 25 g
Protein: 30 g	Dietary Fiber: 4 g	

Chipotle Mayonnaise Baked Fish (All Phases)

Here is another quick, easy fish recipe. It combines the smoky flavor of chipotle and the creamy lusciousness of mayo.

Preparation time: 5 minutes

Total time: 30 minutes

Makes 4 servings

- 1½ pounds white-fleshed fish fillets (haddock, cod, scrod, hake, or other white fish)
- ¼ teaspoon salt
- ⅔ cup Chipotle Mayonnaise (page 268)
- Fresh cilantro or scallions, chopped, for garnish

Preheat the oven to 425°F.

Rinse the fish and pat dry. Lightly salt the fish fillets and place them in a baking dish. Spread a layer of the Chipotle Mayonnaise over each fillet, until ⅔ cup is evenly distributed among the fillets. Bake for 20 to 25 minutes, or until the fish is opaque and flakes easily. It will take less time for thin fillets and more time for fillets over an inch thick. Garnish with cilantro and serve.

Calories: 293	Carbohydrate: 1 g	Total Fat: 18 g
Protein: 31 g	Dietary Fiber: 0 g	

Honey Balsamic Marinated Fish (Phases 2 and 3)

A touch of sweetness complements the savory with this dish—perfect for a summer night!

Preparation time: 2 minutes

Total time: 55 minutes

Makes 4 servings

- ½ cup Honey Balsamic Marinade (page 273)
- 1¼ to 1½ pounds white-fleshed fish fillets (cod, scrod, hake, or other white fish)
- Fresh parsley or scallions, chopped, for garnish

Rinse the fish, pat dry, and place the fillets in a baking dish. Cover with the marinade and place in the refrigerator for 30 minutes to 1 hour (shorter time for thin, flaky fish and longer time for thick, firm fish).

Preheat the oven to 425°F. Bake the fish, still in the marinade, for 20 to 25 minutes, or until the fish is opaque and flakes easily. It will take less time for thin fillets and more time for fillets over an inch thick.

If the marinade left in the baking pan is watery, transfer the fish to a serving platter and drain the marinade into a saucepan. Heat the marinade on the stovetop over medium heat, stirring regularly, until it thickens. Serve the fish with the thickened marinade poured over the top. Garnish with parsley.

Variations
For a Phase 1 recipe use the Ginger-Soy Vinaigrette (page 267), Mustard Vinaigrette (page 264) or Ranchero Sauce (page 272) as the marinade.

Calories: 237   Carbohydrate: 8 g   Total Fat: 8 g
Protein: 32 g   Dietary Fiber: 0 g

Chicken Salad with Grapes and Walnuts (All Phases)

This protein-packed salad has just the right mix of sweetness and crunch. The recipe gives you a range for the amount of mayonnaise to use. Start with 3 tablespoons, but feel free to add up to an additional 2 tablespoons if you like more sauce.

Preparation time: 5 minutes

Total time: 5 minutes

Makes 2 servings

- 8 ounces cooked chicken thigh or leg, skin discarded, meat cut into strips or bite-size pieces
- ½ cup cooked garbanzo beans (chickpeas), drained and rinsed
- 1 cup chopped celery (about 2 stalks)
- ½ to 1 cup shredded carrots (1 to 2 medium carrots)
- 2 cups grapes, halved (about 1 pound)
- 2 tablespoons chopped roasted walnuts (page 319)
- 3 to 5 tablespoons Basic Mayonnaise (page 259), or substitute store-bought mayonnaise (no added sugar)
- 2 teaspoons fresh lemon juice
- ¼ teaspoon salt
- 2 to 3 cups chopped romaine lettuce
- Freshly ground black pepper

In a medium bowl, combine the chicken, garbanzo beans, celery, carrots, grapes, walnuts, mayonnaise, lemon juice, and salt. Toss until thoroughly combined. Gently toss in the lettuce. Garnish with freshly ground black pepper.

Tip: Make sure the chicken is seasoned before you add it to the salad (which can be leftover chicken from dinner or store-bought rotisserie chicken). This salad is better made ahead to allow the flavors to fully develop for an hour or more before adding the lettuce. Add the romaine just before serving.

Variations

For a vegetarian version, substitute 4 ounces Pan-Fried Tempeh or Tofu Strips (page 243), cut into bite-size pieces, or Crumbled Tempeh (page 244) for the chicken.

For Phase 2: Use quinoa instead of chickpeas.

For Phase 3: Use croutons in place of chickpeas.

Calories: 572	Carbohydrate: 35 g	Total Fat: 34 g
Protein: 34 g	Dietary Fiber: 8 g	

Steak Salad with Blue Cheese Dressing (All Phases)

This beloved recast of a classic is one of those dishes that caused many pilot participants to ask, "This is diet food?" The recipe gives you a range for the amount of blue cheese dressing to use: Start with 6 tablespoons, but feel free to add up to 2 additional tablespoons if you like more dressing on your salad.

Preparation time: 5 minutes

Total time: 10 minutes

Makes 2 servings

- 8 ounces beef tenderloin steak
- 1 teaspoon extra-virgin olive oil
- ¼ teaspoon salt
- ¼ teaspoon ground black pepper, plus more for garnish
- 2 to 3 cups chopped romaine lettuce
- ½ cup cooked cannellini or other white beans, drained and rinsed
- 1 cup shredded carrots (about 1 large carrot)
- 2 small tomatoes, diced, or other raw vegetables of your choice
- 6 to 8 tablespoons Blue Cheese Dressing (page 263)

Heat a heavy-bottomed skillet over medium-high heat. Rub the steak with the oil and season with the salt and pepper. Place the steak in the hot pan and cook until browned on one side, about 90 seconds or longer for steak thicker than 1 inch. Flip the steak and cook for 90 seconds more, or until the meat is cooked to your desired doneness. Remove the meat from the pan and let rest on a cutting board.

With a sharp knife, thinly slice the steak. In a large bowl, combine the lettuce, beans, carrots, tomatoes, and steak. Toss with the Blue Cheese Dressing. Garnish with freshly ground black pepper.

Variations

For a vegetarian version, substitute 8 ounces Pan-Fried Tempeh or Tofu Strips (page 243), cut into bite-size pieces, or Crumbled Tempeh (page 244) for the steak.

Substitute leftover cooked chicken (with the skin removed) from a store-bought rotisserie chicken, or Herb-Roasted Chicken Thighs (page 241).

For Phase 2: Use quinoa instead of cannellini beans.

For Phase 3: Use croutons in place of cannellini beans.

Calories: 525	Carbohydrate: 27 g	Total Fat: 30 g
Protein: 38 g	Dietary Fiber: 7 g	

Salmon Salad (All Phases)

Using salmon as an alternative to the traditional tuna is a great way to get heart-protective omega-3 fats in your diet, reduce mercury exposure, and enjoy a delicious and easy dish. To mix things up, use this recipe as a base with other proteins: Substitute hard-boiled eggs to make an egg salad, or try the tofu variation. Serve in a lettuce wrap, on top of a green salad, or as a snack with cucumbers.

Preparation time: 7 minutes

Total time: 7 minutes

Makes 2 servings (about 1¾ cups)

- 1 (7.5-ounce) can sockeye or red salmon
- 1 stalk celery, diced (about ½ cup)
- ¼ cup shredded carrots (about ½ medium carrot)
- 3 to 4 sprigs fresh parsley, lower stems removed, upper stems and leaves finely chopped

- ½ to ¾ cup Tartar Sauce (page 261)
- ½ to 2 teaspoons fresh lemon juice
- ¼ teaspoon garlic powder
- Salt and freshly ground black pepper to taste

Combine all the ingredients except the salt and pepper in a large bowl. Add salt, as needed (depending on the saltiness of the salmon), and garnish with freshly ground black pepper.

Variations

For a vegetarian version, substitute 7 to 8 ounces extra-firm tofu, drained, gently pressed with an absorbent towel, crumbled, and seasoned with ½ teaspoon salt and ½ teaspoon paprika for the salmon.

Calories: 475   Carbohydrate: 5 g   Total Fat: 34 g
Protein: 39 g   Dietary Fiber: 1 g

Cobb Salad (All Phases)

Our version of the classic, invented at the Brown Derby restaurant in Los Angeles in the 1930s.

Preparation time: 5 minutes

Total time: 5 minutes

Makes 2 servings

2 to 3 cups salad greens
2 hard-boiled eggs, sliced
1 cup cooked kidney beans, drained and rinsed
2 slices turkey bacon, cooked and crumbled (about 2 ounces)
4 ounces chicken or turkey cold cuts, cut into small pieces
1 large tomato, diced
2 to 4 tablespoons Mustard Vinaigrette (page 264)
2 tablespoons crumbled Roquefort or blue cheese (about ⅔ ounce)
Freshly ground black pepper

Toss together all the ingredients except the pepper in a large bowl. Garnish with freshly ground black pepper. Serve.

Variations

For a vegetarian version, substitute 6 ounces Pan-Fried Tempeh or Tofu Strips (page 243), cut into bite-sized pieces, or Crumbled Tempeh (page 244) for the cold cuts and turkey bacon.

Calories: 460   Carbohydrate: 25 g   Total Fat: 25 g
Protein: 35 g   Dietary Fiber: 10 g

Shrimp over Cracked Wheat Salad (Phases 2 and 3)

This refreshing salad makes a perfect one-dish lunch. It also keeps well in the refrigerator if you want to make it in advance. Add additional cumin, lemon juice, or even a dash of cayenne pepper if you prefer more spice.

Preparation time: 10 minutes

Total time: 15 minutes

Makes 2 servings

- ½ cup cracked wheat (bulgur wheat), uncooked
- ½ cup boiling water
- 2 teaspoons extra-virgin olive oil
- 2 cloves garlic, minced
- 12 ounces shrimp, peeled and deveined
- ½ teaspoon salt
- ¼ cup Lemon Olive Oil Dressing (page 269)
- ½ teaspoon ground cumin
- ¼ cup cooked garbanzo beans (chickpeas), drained and rinsed
- 1 medium tomato, chopped
- ½ cup shredded carrots (about 1 medium carrot)
- 1 cup chopped fresh parsley
- 2 tablespoons minced onion
- Freshly ground black pepper
- ¼ avocado, pitted, peeled, and sliced, for garnish

Place the cracked wheat in a medium bowl and pour the boiling water over it. Cover and set aside for at least 5 minutes, or until it has absorbed the water.

Heat 1 teaspoon of the oil in a heavy-bottomed skillet over medium heat. Add the garlic, shrimp, and salt and sauté for 3 to 5 minutes, or until the shrimp are pink on all sides and firm. Remove from the pan and set aside.

In a large bowl, combine the Lemon Olive Oil Dressing and cumin. Add the garbanzo beans, tomato, carrot, parsley, onion, and shrimp. Combine well. Stir in the cracked wheat and garnish with freshly ground black pepper. Top with the sliced avocado and serve.

Variations

For a vegetarian version, substitute 8 to 10 ounces Pan-Fried Tempeh or Tofu Strips (page 243), cut into bite-size pieces, or Crumbled Tempeh (page 244) for the shrimp.

For a whole-grain, gluten-free version, cook millet (fluffy millet variation) or quinoa according to the Guide to Cooking Whole Grains (page 317). Use 1 cup cooked fluffy millet or quinoa in place of the cracked wheat and omit the boiling water.

Calories: 540   Carbohydrate: 44 g   Total Fat: 28 g
Protein: 32 g   Dietary Fiber: 12 g

Ranchero Chicken (All Phases)

Add some South of the Border zip to your week! As with so many of the Always Hungry Solution recipes, make the sauce ahead of time to prepare this fabulous meal in a flash.

Preparation time: 1 minute

Total time: 25 to 45 minutes

Makes 4 servings

- 6 boneless, skinless chicken thighs (about 1½ pounds)
- ¼ teaspoon salt
- 1½ cups Ranchero Sauce (page 272)

Preheat the oven to 350°F.

Place the chicken in an 8- or 9-inch baking dish. Sprinkle with the salt. Pour the Ranchero Sauce over the top.

Bake for 30 to 45 minutes, or until cooked through.

Variations

Substitute 1½ pounds white-fleshed fish fillets (cod, scrod, hake, or other white fish) for the chicken and reduce the cooking time to 25 minutes.

Substitute 1½ pounds extra-firm tofu, drained, gently pressed with an absorbent towel, and cut into ¼-inch slices for the chicken and reduce the cooking time to 25 minutes.

Calories: 272	Carbohydrate: 6 g	Total Fat: 12 g
Protein: 34 g	Dietary Fiber: 1 g	

Thai Peanut Tempeh (All Phases)

A vegetarian version of the classic Asian favorite.

Preparation time: 10 minutes

Total time: 20 minutes

Makes 4 servings

- 1 teaspoon extra-virgin olive oil
- 1 medium onion, diced
- 1 large carrot, cut into matchsticks or coarsely shredded (about 1 cup)
- 1 large bunch kale, cut into bite-size pieces (4 to 5 cups)
- 2 tablespoons water
- 1 recipe Crumbled Tempeh (page 244)
- 1 recipe Thai Peanut Sauce (page 262)
- 3 cups (packed) spinach
- 1 cup packed sprouts (sunflower, alfalfa, bean, or any other), for garnish
- ¼ to ½ cup chopped roasted peanuts (page 319), for garnish
- 1 lime, cut into slices, for garnish

Heat the oil in a large skillet or pot over medium heat. Add the onion and sauté until translucent, 3 to 5 minutes. Add the carrot, kale, and water. Cover and steam for 1 minute. Uncover and stir in the tempeh and Thai Peanut Sauce. Cook until the sauce and tempeh are hot, 1 to 2 minutes.

Spread the spinach on a serving tray or divide it among individual bowls. Place the hot Thai Peanut Tempeh on top of the spinach. The spinach should begin to wilt under the heat of the sauce. Garnish with the sprouts, peanuts, and a squeeze of lime. Serve immediately while the vegetables are still bright.

Variations

Add or substitute other vegetables of your choice.

For Phase 2, serve with rice or quinoa.

For Phase 3, serve over Asian noodles.

Substitute 1 to 1½ pounds chicken, shrimp, or fish for the tempeh.

| Calories: 659 | Carbohydrate: 41 g | Total Fat: 42 g |
| Protein: 38 g | Dietary Fiber: 18 g | |

SAUCES

Basic Mayonnaise (All Phases)

Almost all commercial mayonnaise has added sugar. Fortunately, making your own is extremely easy. Double, triple, or even quadruple the recipe to make a large batch, and use it in any recipes that call for mayonnaise.

Preparation time: 5 minutes

Total time: 5 minutes

Makes about ¾ cup

- ¼ cup unsweetened soy milk or whole milk
- ½ teaspoon salt
- 1 teaspoon fresh lemon juice
- ¼ teaspoon white wine vinegar or unseasoned rice vinegar
- ¼ cup neutral-tasting oil, such as high-oleic safflower or avocado oil
- ⅓ cup additional neutral-tasting oil, for a classic mayonnaise taste, or extra-virgin olive oil, for a zippier taste

Place all the ingredients in a wide-mouthed mason jar or cup that will fit an immersion blender without splashing. Blend with the immersion blender until thick and creamy, about 2 minutes. Place a lid on the jar. Allow the flavors to develop for 1 hour or more in the refrigerator. The mayonnaise will keep for 1 to 2 weeks in the refrigerator.

Tip: Almond or other milk substitutes don't set up as well as soy milk or whole milk for this recipe. Add more oil or blend more if the mayo is not thick enough.

| Per 1 tablespoon: | Protein: 0 g | Dietary Fiber: 0 g |
| Calories: 80 | Carbohydrate: 0 g | Total Fat: 9 g |

Stir-Fry Sauce or Marinade (All Phases)

You can use this versatile sauce with any protein. Add Asian vegetables with chicken or tofu; red, orange, or green bell peppers with steak strips for pepper steak; or use it as a marinade with tofu or fish to be baked or cooked on the stovetop.

Preparation time: 5 minutes

Total time: 5 minutes

Makes about ⅓ cup

- 1 (1-inch) piece fresh ginger, peeled
- 1 clove garlic
- ¼ cup water
- ½ teaspoon salt
- 1 tablespoon neutral-tasting oil, such as sesame (not toasted), high-oleic safflower, or avocado oil

Combine all the ingredients in a wide-mouthed mason jar. Puree with an immersion blender until the ginger is finely minced.

Tip: Peel ginger by scraping it with a spoon. This removes the skin without losing any of the ginger flesh. For thicker skin, use a vegetable peeler or knife.

Variations

Double the ginger and garlic for a more intense flavor.

Use 1 tablespoon soy sauce in place of salt for a more Asian-style stir-fry sauce.

Use toasted sesame oil for more depth of flavor.

Increase the salt by ¼ teaspoon, or to taste, if using tofu as the protein.

Per 1 tablespoon:	Protein: 0 g	Dietary Fiber: 0 g
Calories: 26	Carbohydrate: 1 g	Total Fat: 3 g

Tartar Sauce (All Phases)

As with mayonnaise, almost all commercial tartar sauce has added sugar. Making your own using the Basic Mayonnaise recipe is a snap, and the sauce keeps in the fridge just as long as mayonnaise.

Preparation time: 5 minutes

Total time: 5 minutes

Makes about ¾ cup

- 1 medium dill pickle
- ⅛ small red onion
- 1 small clove garlic, or ⅛ teaspoon garlic powder
- ½ teaspoon fresh lemon juice
- ½ teaspoon Dijon or brown mustard (optional)
- Dash of salt
- ½ cup Basic Mayonnaise (page 259), or substitute store-bought mayonnaise (no added sugar)

Place the pickle, onion, and garlic in a food processor and pulse until finely chopped. Add the remaining ingredients and pulse just until combined. Transfer to a jar with a lid. For best results, allow the flavors to develop for 1 hour or more in the refrigerator. The sauce will keep for 1 to 2 weeks in the refrigerator.

Variations

Mix in the garlic that comes in the bottom of the dill pickle jar for a little extra zing.

Per 1 tablespoon:	Protein: 0 g	Dietary Fiber: 0 g
Calories: 49	Carbohydrate: 0 g	Total Fat: 5 g

Thai Peanut Sauce (All Phases)

Commercial peanut sauces are also notorious for added sugar, along with other artificial ingredients. Use for the Thai Peanut Tempeh (page 258) recipe or whenever you want a sweet and spicy dip.

Preparation time: 5 minutes

Total time: 5 minutes

Makes about 1¾ cups

- 1 large orange, 4 small clementines, or 2 large tangerines, peeled, seeded, and cut into 1-inch pieces
- 1 (½-inch) piece fresh ginger, peeled
- 1 teaspoon fresh lime juice
- ½ cup peanut butter (no sugar added)
- 2 teaspoons unseasoned rice vinegar
- 2 tablespoons water
- 1 tablespoon soy sauce
- ¼ teaspoon salt
- ¼ to ½ teaspoon cayenne pepper, or to taste

Place all the ingredients in a wide-mouthed mason jar or cup that will fit an immersion blender without splashing. Blend with the immersion blender until the orange is fully blended and the sauce is thick and creamy. Adjust the seasoning to taste. Place a lid on the jar. Allow the flavors to develop for 1 hour or more in the refrigerator. The sauce will keep for about a week in the refrigerator.

Tip: Peel ginger by scraping it with a spoon. This removes the skin without losing any of the ginger flesh. For thicker skin, use a vegetable peeler or knife.

Variations

Optional for Phases 2 and 3: Reduce the orange by half and add 1 tablespoon honey.

Per 1 tablespoon:	Protein: 1 g	Dietary Fiber: 1 g
Calories: 33	Carbohydrate: 1 g	Total Fat: 3 g

Blue Cheese Dressing (All Phases)

This dressing turns simple salad greens into a satisfying side dish. You'll also use it in a Phase 1 lunch recipe, Steak Salad with Blue Cheese Dressing (page 253). Different varieties of blue cheese vary greatly in taste, from strong to mild. Experiment with different varieties until you find your favorite.

Preparation time: 5 minutes

Total time: 5 minutes

Makes about ½ cup

- 2 ounces crumbled blue cheese
- 1 teaspoon finely chopped fresh chives or scallions
- 2 tablespoons sour cream
- 2 tablespoons Basic Mayonnaise (page 259), or substitute store-bought mayonnaise (no added sugar)
- 1½ teaspoons fresh lemon juice
- 1 tablespoon water
- Dash of salt, if needed
- Dash of ground black pepper

Place 1 ounce of the blue cheese, the chives, sour cream, mayonnaise, lemon juice, water, salt, and pepper in a wide-mouthed mason jar or cup that will fit an immersion blender without splashing. Blend with the immersion blender until combined. Stir in the remaining 1 ounce blue cheese, as this dressing is best if it remains a bit chunky. Place a lid on the jar. Allow the flavors to develop for 1 hour or more in the refrigerator. The dressing will keep for 1 to 2 weeks in the refrigerator.

Tip: Blue cheese varies greatly in saltiness and texture, so taste the dressing before adding salt and choose a variety that is crumbled or dry enough to crumble easily.

Variations

Substitute feta cheese for the blue cheese.

| Per 1 tablespoon: | Protein: 2 g | Dietary Fiber: 0 g |
| Calories: 52 | Carbohydrate: 0 g | Total Fat: 5 g |

Mustard Vinaigrette (All Phases)

This vinaigrette is so versatile, you may want to make a double batch as a go-to for salads, or over vegetables, meat, poultry, or fish. It even works as a marinade for baked fish or chicken.

Preparation time: 3 minutes

Total time: 3 minutes

Makes about 1 cup

- ¾ cup extra-virgin olive oil
- ¼ cup red wine vinegar
- 2 tablespoons Dijon mustard
- ⅛ teaspoon salt
- ⅛ teaspoon ground black pepper

Combine all the ingredients in a jar with a tight-fitting lid. Cover and shake until thoroughly combined.

Tip: Mustard Vinaigrette can be stored in the refrigerator for months or in the cupboard for 1 to 2 weeks. Store in the cupboard to keep the extra-virgin olive oil soft and liquid, or remove from the refrigerator at least an hour before using, as extra-virgin olive oil solidifies when refrigerated. If your olive oil does not solidify, check the quality—it might have other oils added.

Variations

Add dried herbs like thyme, oregano, basil, or other favorites.

Optional for Phases 2 and 3, replace half or all the red wine vinegar with balsamic vinegar.

Per 1 tablespoon: Protein: 0 g   Dietary Fiber: 0 g
Calories: 92   Carbohydrate: 0 g   Total Fat: 10 g

Tangy Coleslaw Dressing (All Phases)

This very rich and thick dressing turns shredded lettuce or cabbage into a treat! It serves as the dressing for the Tangy Coleslaw recipe on page 279.

Preparation time: 5 minutes

Total time: 5 minutes

Makes about 1 cup

- 1 tablespoon Dijon mustard
- 1 tablespoon apple cider vinegar
- 1 tablespoon fresh lemon juice
- ¼ teaspoon salt
- ½ cup Basic Mayonnaise (page 259)
- ¼ cup sour cream
- ⅛ teaspoon ground black pepper

Combine all the ingredients in a wide-mouthed mason jar or cup that will fit an immersion blender without splashing. Stir or blend with the immersion blender until smooth. Place a lid on the jar. Allow the flavors to develop for 1 hour or more in the refrigerator. The dressing will keep for 1 to 2 weeks in the refrigerator.

Variations

For a dairy-free version, substitute Basic Mayonnaise (page 259) for the sour cream.

Per 1 tablespoon: Protein: 0 g   Dietary Fiber: 0 g
Calories: 59   Carbohydrate: 0 g   Total Fat: 6 g

Coconut Curry Sauce (All Phases)

Curry is a mixture of spices that will vary widely depending on the brand you choose. Try a few different brands until you find one that you love, and feel free to add some extra red pepper flakes or a dash of cayenne to spice it up. Use this recipe to make a variety of vegetables and protein choices more hearty and satisfying. Add it to your favorite vegetables and tofu, fish, shrimp, chicken, or tempeh.

Preparation time: 5 minutes

Total time: 5 minutes

Makes about 2½ cups

- ¾ cup raw cashews
- ¾ cup hot water
- 1¼ cups canned coconut milk (about three-quarters of a 14-ounce can, well combined before measuring)
- 1 (½- to 1-inch) piece fresh ginger, peeled and cut into ¼-inch rounds
- 1 small clove garlic
- 1½ to 2 tablespoons curry powder, or more, to taste
- Red pepper flakes (optional)
- 1 teaspoon salt

Place all the ingredients in a high-speed blender or into a large jar or deep bowl that will fit an immersion blender without splashing. Blend until smooth. If using an immersion blender, work the blender into the thicker pieces of vegetables and nuts until they are smooth and creamy. Place a lid on the jar. Allow the flavors to develop for 1 hour or more in the refrigerator. The dressing will keep for 1 to 2 weeks in the refrigerator.

Tip: Peel ginger by scraping it with a spoon. This removes the skin without losing any of the ginger flesh. For thicker skin, use a vegetable peeler or knife.

Variations

Soak cashews in the hot water for 1 hour, then drain, to create a creamier texture.

Per 1 tablespoon: Protein: 1 g   Dietary Fiber: 0 g
Calories: 28   Carbohydrate: 1 g   Total Fat: 2 g

Ginger-Soy Vinaigrette (All Phases)

This flavorful recipe is great served over tofu or chicken, shredded cabbage as an Asian slaw, salad greens, or baked fish as a marinade. For Phase 3, add it to soba noodles and vegetables for a refreshing Asian noodle salad.

Preparation time: 5 minutes

Total time: 5 minutes

Makes ¾ cup

- 1 (1-inch) piece fresh ginger, peeled and cut into ¼-inch rounds
- 1 clove garlic
- ¼ cup water
- 1 tablespoon soy sauce
- 2 tablespoons unseasoned rice vinegar
- 1 tablespoon sweet white miso
- 3 tablespoons toasted sesame oil
- 3 tablespoons neutral-tasting oil, such as sesame (not toasted), high-oleic safflower, or avocado oil

Place all the ingredients in a wide-mouthed mason jar or cup that will fit an immersion blender without splashing. Blend until smooth, working the blender into the thicker pieces of ginger until they are finely chopped. Place a lid on the jar. Allow the flavors to develop for at least 1 hour or more in the refrigerator. The vinaigrette will keep for 1 to 2 weeks in the refrigerator.

Tip: Peel ginger by scraping it with a spoon. This removes the skin without losing any ginger. For thicker skin, use a vegetable peeler or knife.

Per 1 tablespoon: Protein: 0 g   Dietary Fiber: 0 g
Calories: 66   Carbohydrate: 1 g   Total Fat: 7 g

Chipotle Mayonnaise (All Phases)

Depending on the amount of spice you like, add more or less chipotle powder. This favorite spices up beans, tofu, or chicken for a more interesting leftover meal, and is great as a dip for vegetables. Spread it in a thick layer on white-fleshed fish, and bake for a quick and delicious fish entrée.

Preparation time: 5 minutes

Total time: 5 minutes

Makes 1¼ cups

- ¼ cup unsweetened soy milk or whole milk
- 2 teaspoons tomato paste
- 2 teaspoons fresh lime juice
- ¼ teaspoon apple cider vinegar (or substitute white wine or distilled white vinegar for a milder taste)
- ¼ cup neutral-tasting oil, such as high-oleic safflower or avocado oil
- ⅓ cup extra-virgin olive oil
- 1 small clove garlic
- ¼ teaspoon chipotle powder, or more to taste
- ½ teaspoon salt

Place all the ingredients in a wide-mouthed glass mason jar or cup that will fit an immersion blender without splashing. Blend with the immersion blender until creamy. Adjust the seasoning to taste. Place a lid on the jar. Allow the flavors to develop for 1 hour or more in the refrigerator. The mayonnaise will keep for 1 to 2 weeks in the refrigerator.

Per 1 tablespoon: Protein: 0 g   Dietary Fiber: 0 g
Calories: 58   Carbohydrate: 0 g   Total Fat: 6 g

Lemon Olive Oil Dressing (All Phases)

This sunny combination enhances the flavor of blanched or steamed vegetables, and makes a flavorful topping for grain salads or lettuce wraps.

Preparation time: 3 minutes

Total time: 3 minutes

Makes 6 tablespoons

- 2 tablespoons fresh lemon juice
- ¼ cup extra-virgin olive oil
- Pinch of salt
- Dash of ground black pepper

Place all the ingredients in a wide-mouthed glass mason jar. Place a lid on the jar and shake. The dressing will keep for 1 to 2 weeks in the refrigerator. Shake well just before using.

Tip: Remove the dressing from the refrigerator at least an hour before using, as extra-virgin olive oil solidifies when refrigerated. If your olive oil does not solidify, check the quality—it might have other oils added.

Variations

Add herbs or spices like ground cumin, cayenne, thyme, oregano, or dried Italian herb mix.

Per 1 tablespoon:	Protein: 0 g	Dietary Fiber: 0 g
Calories: 81	Carbohydrate: 0 g	Total Fat: 9 g

Lemon Tahini Sauce (All Phases)

Enjoy this refreshing sauce on blanched vegetables, salads, falafel, hummus, or quinoa.

Preparation time: 5 minutes

Total time: 5 minutes

Makes ¾ cup

- 2 tablespoons fresh lemon juice
- 1 small clove garlic
- Leaves from 2 to 3 sprigs fresh parsley
- ¼ cup tahini
- 2 tablespoons extra-virgin olive oil
- ½ teaspoon salt
- ¼ cup water, as needed

Place all the ingredients except the water into a wide-mouthed mason jar or cup that will fit an immersion blender without splashing. Blend with the immersion blender to create a thick paste. Slowly add the water while blending to create a creamy, pourable dressing. Place a lid on the jar. Allow the flavors to develop for 1 hour or more in the refrigerator. The sauce will keep for 1 to 2 weeks in the refrigerator.

Variations
Add less water and use as a dip.

Per 1 tablespoon: Protein: 1 g   Dietary Fiber: 0 g
Calories: 50   Carbohydrate: 1 g   Total Fat: 5 g

Creamy Dill Sauce (All Phases)

The fresh dill, yogurt, and dash of paprika in this sauce bring back memories of a cool, creamy, ranch-style dressing that pairs perfectly with almost anything. Pour it over smoked salmon, cucumbers, and tomatoes for a delicious breakfast. Use it as a sauce or dip to make simple vegetables more interesting.

Preparation time: 5 minutes

Total time: 5 minutes

Makes 1¼ cups

- ¼ cup unsweetened soy milk or whole milk
- ⅓ cup plain unsweetened whole-milk Greek yogurt
- ½ small clove garlic
- 1 teaspoon fresh lemon juice

- ½ teaspoon white wine vinegar or unseasoned rice vinegar
- ¼ cup neutral-tasting oil, such as high-oleic safflower or avocado oil
- ¼ cup extra-virgin olive oil
- ¼ to ½ cup coarsely chopped fresh dill stems and leaves, or 1 to 2 tablespoons dried dill
- Dash of paprika
- ½ teaspoon salt
- ⅛ teaspoon ground black pepper

Place all the ingredients in a wide-mouthed mason jar or cup that will fit an immersion blender without splashing. Blend with the immersion blender to create a creamy, pourable dressing. Place a lid on the jar. Allow the flavors to develop for 1 hour or more in the refrigerator. The sauce will keep for 1 to 2 weeks in the refrigerator.

| Per 1 tablespoon: | Protein: 0 g | Dietary Fiber: 0 g |
| Calories: 53 | Carbohydrate: 0 g | Total Fat: 6 g |

Creamy Lime-Cilantro Dressing (All Phases)

The lime and cilantro add a Mexican flair to this simple, creamy dressing—great served over salads, cooked vegetables, tacos, or burritos.

Preparation time: 5 minutes

Total time: 5 minutes

Makes ½ cup

- 2 tablespoons water
- ½ teaspoon salt
- 1½ teaspoons fresh lime juice
- 1 small clove garlic
- ½ avocado, pitted and peeled
- ¼ cup packed fresh cilantro, leaves and stems coarsely chopped
- 2 tablespoons flax oil or extra-virgin olive oil
- Dash of ground black pepper

Place all the ingredients in a wide-mouthed mason jar or cup that will fit an immersion blender without splashing. Blend using the immersion blender to create a thick, creamy sauce. Place a lid on the jar. Allow the flavors to develop for an hour or more in the refrigerator. Serve immediately or use within 3 to 4 days so that the avocado doesn't turn brown.

Variations
Substitute parsley for cilantro.

Per 1 tablespoon:	Protein: 0 g	Dietary Fiber: 1 g
Calories: 45	Carbohydrate: 1 g	Total Fat: 5 g

Ranchero Sauce

Although this recipe uses spicy chile peppers, like jalapeños, they become milder when cooked. Get creative with different chiles to create a milder or spicier sauce that you love. Serve with eggs, tacos, or lettuce wraps for any meal of the day or pour over chicken, tofu, or fish and cook on the stovetop or bake as in Ranchero Chicken (page 257).

Preparation time: 5 minutes

Total time: 25 minutes

Makes 4½ cups

- 1 yellow bell pepper, cored and seeded
- 1 Anaheim or poblano pepper, stemmed and seeded
- 2 to 4 jalapeños, stemmed and seeded
- 1 large clove garlic
- 1 large onion, cut into large chunks
- ¼ cup extra-virgin olive oil
- 1 teaspoon salt
- ½ teaspoon ground black pepper
- 1 tablespoon dried Mexican oregano or regular dried oregano
- ½ teaspoon powdered red chile, such as New Mexican, ancho, or chile de arbol (optional)
- Dash of cayenne pepper (optional)
- 4 ounces canned mild green chiles
- 3½ cups canned diced fire-roasted tomatoes or diced tomatoes (about two 14.5-ounce cans)

Place the bell pepper, Anaheim pepper, jalapeños, garlic, and onion in a food processor and process until finely minced.

Heat the oil in a deep skillet or pot over medium heat. Add the pepper and onion mixture, the salt, black pepper, oregano, and powdered chili and cayenne (if using). Sauté until the onion is soft, about 5 minutes. Add the canned green chiles and tomatoes. Reduce the heat to medium-low and simmer for 10 to 15 minutes. If desired, add more cayenne for a spicier sauce.

Blend with an immersion blender until the sauce is still a bit chunky, but well combined. Simmer for 5 minutes more. Serve immediately, refrigerate in a jar, or let cool and freeze in a zip-top plastic freezer bag. The sauce will keep for 1 to 2 weeks in the refrigerator and up to 1 month in the freezer.

Per ¼ cup:	Protein: 1 g	Dietary Fiber: 1 g
Calories: 47	Carbohydrate: 4 g	Total Fat: 3 g

Honey Balsamic Marinade (Phases 2 and 3)

Cooking fish in a marinade or sauce keeps it moist and delicious. Using this marinade demystifies the process and leaves you with a luscious meal every time.

Preparation time: 5 minutes

Total time: 5 minutes

Makes ½ cup

- 1 (2-inch) piece fresh ginger, peeled and cut into ¼-inch rounds
- 1 clove garlic
- 2 tablespoons water
- 1 tablespoon sweet white miso
- 1 tablespoon honey
- 1 tablespoon balsamic vinegar
- 2 tablespoons soy sauce
- 2 tablespoons extra-virgin olive oil

Place all the ingredients in a wide-mouthed mason jar or cup that will fit an immersion blender without splashing. Blend using the immersion blender until smooth, working the blender into the thicker pieces of ginger until they are finely chopped. Use immediately to marinate any protein of your choice, or place a lid on the jar and store in the refrigerator until ready to use. The marinade will keep for 1 to 2 weeks in the refrigerator.

| Per 1 tablespoon: | Protein: 1 g | Dietary Fiber: 0 g |
| Calories: 48 | Carbohydrate: 4 g | Total Fat: 3 g |

SIDES

Sautéed Greens with Garlic (All Phases)

Here's one for even the vegetable skeptics out there! Beet greens or chard are superb this way, but you can also use a bag of prechopped kale. It may seem like a lot of greens at first, but they cook down. Make extra—you'll be surprised how fast they go!

Preparation time: 5 minutes

Total time: 7 minutes

Makes 4 servings

- 1 tablespoon extra-virgin olive oil
- 2 small cloves garlic
- 1 bunch beet greens, chard, or kale, stems cut into thin rounds, leaves chopped into bite-size pieces (4 to 5 cups)
- ¼ teaspoon salt

Heat the oil in a large skillet over medium heat. Add the garlic and sauté for 30 seconds. Add the greens and sprinkle with the salt. Sauté until the greens are coated with oil, about 1 minute. Cover and allow the greens to gently steam, about 1 minute. Remove the lid and continue to sauté until the greens are wilted and tender but still bright in color. Chard and beet greens will be done faster than kale or other hearty greens.

| Calories: 53 | Carbohydrate: 5 g | Total Fat: 4 g |
| Protein: 2 g | Dietary Fiber: 1 g | |

Soft Millet–Corn Polenta (Phases 2 and 3)

This variation on the classic polenta is easy to make and great for leftovers.

Preparation time: 5 minutes

Total time: 25 minutes

Makes 4 servings

- 2½ cups water
- ⅔ cup millet, rinsed
- 3 tablespoons frozen or canned corn kernels, drained
- ¼ to ½ teaspoon salt
- Soy sauce or salt, for serving (optional)

Bring the water to a boil in a medium pot. Stir in the millet, corn, and salt and return the water to a boil. Stir briefly, reduce the heat to low, cover, and simmer until water has been fully absorbed, about 20 minutes. Scoop a portion onto each plate and serve immediately with a splash of soy sauce or light sprinkle of salt.

Alternatively, spread the hot millet into an 8- or 9-inch baking dish. Let cool, slice into squares, and serve like traditional polenta.

Variations

Pan-fry the cooled millet squares in a cast-iron skillet with 1 to 2 tablespoons extra-virgin olive oil until brown and crispy on one side, then turn and brown on the other side.

Top with Parmesan or other cheese.

Add your favorite herbs or spices when you add the salt.

Add vegetables like cauliflower in place of the corn and puree with an immersion blender to a mashed potato consistency.

Calories: 132   Carbohydrate: 26 g   Total Fat: 1 g
Protein: 4 g   Dietary Fiber: 3 g

Kale with Carrots and Currants (Phases 2 and 3)

The sweetness of the currants and carrots with the zesty lemon dressing make this an irresistible dish—a great way to get the family to eat greens.

Preparation time: 5 minutes

Total time: 5 minutes

Makes 4 servings

- 1 large bunch kale (4 to 5 cups)
- 1 small carrot, cut into matchsticks or coarsely shredded (about ¼ cup)
- 1 tablespoon currants or raisins, chopped
- 3 to 4 tablespoons Lemon Olive Oil Dressing (page 269)

Bring 3 to 5 inches of water to a rolling boil in a medium pot.

Blanch the kale by immersing it in the boiling water for 1 minute, or until tender but still bright green. Remove from the water with a mesh skimmer or slotted spoon. Place on a large plate to drain.

Blanch the carrots in the boiling water for 15 to 30 seconds. Remove from the water with a mesh skimmer or slotted spoon. Place on a plate to drain.

In a large bowl, combine the blanched kale and carrots, currants, and Lemon Olive Oil Dressing.

Toss gently until the dressing coats the vegetables, and serve.

Tip: This quick blanching technique does not require immersing the vegetables in ice water after cooking. Leaving them in the boiling water only a very short time then spreading them out on a plate to drain will keep them from overcooking and will allow them to retain their full flavor. Quick-blanched vegetables should be warm, crisp, and bright in color when served. See Appendix C—Guide to Cooking Vegetables (page 313) for a comprehensive list of vegetable blanching times.

| Calories: 104 | Carbohydrate: 9 g | Total Fat: 7 g |
| Protein: 2 g | Dietary Fiber: 2 g | |

Garlic Herb Zucchini Rounds (All Phases)

This savory side dish goes with just about anything.

Preparation time: 2 minutes

Total time: 15 minutes

Makes 4 servings

- 1 tablespoon extra-virgin olive oil
- 1 clove garlic, minced or pressed in garlic press
- 2 large zucchini, cut into 1-inch rounds
- ½ to 1 teaspoon dried Italian herb mix
- ¼ teaspoon salt

Heat the oil in a large skillet over medium heat. Add the garlic and sauté for 5 to 10 seconds. Arrange the zucchini rounds in a single layer in the skillet. Sprinkle with the dried Italian herb mix and salt. Cover and cook until the zucchini slices are browned on the bottom, 6 to 8 minutes. Flip, cover, and cook until browned on the second side, about 5 minutes. Serve hot.

Calories: 59	Carbohydrate: 6 g	Total Fat: 4 g
Protein: 2 g	Dietary Fiber: 2 g	

Quinoa Salad with Pecans and Cranberries (Phases 2 and 3)

Looking for a dish to introduce intact whole grains to any crowd? Quinoa is light, with a pleasant, nutty flavor. The tangy dressing combines well with the sweet tartness of the cranberries. This recipe works best with leftover quinoa. Make a large pot of quinoa ahead of time and use it for recipes like this one—or just serve it with any sauce on top.

Preparation time: 10 minutes

Total time: 10 minutes

Makes 4 servings (about 3 cups)

Dressing

- 1 tablespoon extra-virgin olive oil
- 1½ teaspoons fresh lemon juice
- ⅛ teaspoon salt
- ½ teaspoon unseasoned rice vinegar
- ⅛ teaspoon ground black pepper

Salad

- 2 tablespoons finely chopped dried cranberries
- 1¾ cups cooked quinoa, cooled completely
- ½ stalk celery, diced (about ¼ cup)
- ½ small carrot, diced (about ¼ cup)
- 3 tablespoons chopped parsley
- 1 or 2 scallions, chopped
- 5 to 6 tablespoons coarsely chopped roasted pecans (page 319)
- Freshly ground black pepper

Make the dressing: Combine all the dressing ingredients in a small bowl or cup. Add the cranberries. Set aside.

Make the salad: In a large bowl, toss together the quinoa, celery, carrot, parsley, scallions, and pecans. Mix in the dressing until the quinoa is evenly coated. Garnish with freshly ground black pepper. Cover and refrigerate for at least an hour to allow the flavors to develop. Serve cool or at room temperature. This keeps well in the refrigerator for a few days.

Tip: Wash and rinse quinoa well before cooking to remove saponin, its bitter natural coating.

Variations

Add leftover chicken, Pan-Fried Tempeh or Tofu Strips (page 243), Crumbled Tempeh (page 244), or other protein of your choice, cut into small squares.

Calories: 232	Carbohydrate: 24 g	Total Fat: 14 g
Protein: 5 g	Dietary Fiber: 4 g	

Roasted Sweet Potatoes (Phases 2 and 3)

Cooking sweet potatoes this way caramelizes them, so it's almost like eating dessert. Try one of the variations, and make plenty to use as leftovers in other meals.

Preparation time: 5 minutes

Total time: 50 minutes

Makes 4 servings

- 2 medium sweet potatoes, skin on, cut into 1-inch chunks
- 2 tablespoons extra-virgin olive oil
- ¼ teaspoon salt

Preheat the oven to 425°F.

Toss the sweet potatoes with the oil and salt until evenly coated. Transfer to a 9 x 12-inch baking dish. Bake until tender on the inside and a bit crispy on the outside, about 45 minutes. Stir every 15 minutes for even baking.

Variations

For a whole potato: Wash, scrub, and wrap each whole medium sweet potato in foil (omit the oil and salt). Bake at 425°F for 45 to 60 minutes, or until tender when pierced with a fork.

For fries: Cut the sweet potatoes into strips and toss with 1 tablespoon oil. Spread in a single layer on a large baking sheet, salt, and bake at 425°F for 25 to 30 minutes, turning once after about 15 minutes. Cook until tender on the inside and crispy on the outside.

| Calories: 81 | Carbohydrate: 12 g | Total Fat: 3 g |
| Protein: 1 g | Dietary Fiber: 2 g | |

Tangy Coleslaw (All Phases)

The carrots in this tangy slaw add some extra crunch and sweetness. Done in five minutes or less, this dish is easy to make often. The taste and texture pairs beautifully with most main dishes.

Preparation time: 5 minutes

Total time: 5 minutes

Makes 4 servings

- 2 cups shredded cabbage
- ¼ cup shredded carrots (about 1 small carrot)
- ¼ to ⅓ cup Tangy Coleslaw Dressing (page 265)

In a medium bowl, combine all the ingredients and mix thoroughly.

This can be served immediately, but for best results, cover and refrigerate for an hour or more before serving.

Variations

Add 2 tablespoons chopped dry-roasted salted peanuts.

Add other vegetables or herbs of your choice, such as red onion, scallions, parsley, or dill.

Calories: 71	Carbohydrate: 3 g	Total Fat: 6 g
Protein: 1 g	Dietary Fiber: 1 g	

SOUPS

Creamy Cauliflower Soup (All Phases)

You'll be surprised how delicious a few simple ingredients can be. This creamy soup is a perfect way to bring balance, interest, and extra flavor to any higher-protein or high-fat meal. Check out the many variations and play with the seasonings to create a soup that is just right for your family.

Preparation time: 5 minutes

Total time: 20 minutes

Makes 4 servings (6 to 6½ cups)

- 1 medium head cauliflower, cut into large chunks
- 1 medium onion, diced

- 4 cups water, plus more as needed
- 1 teaspoon salt
- Freshly ground black pepper
- ¼ cup fresh parsley, chopped, for garnish
- Heavy cream, for garnish (optional, to increase fat content of a meal)

Place the cauliflower and onion in a pot. Add the water, adding more as needed just to cover the cauliflower. Add the salt and bring the water to a boil over high heat. Reduce the heat to medium-low, cover, and simmer until the cauliflower is very soft, 10 to 15 minutes. Puree the cauliflower, onion, and cooking water with an immersion blender. Add more water as needed to make a thick, creamy consistency. Adjust the seasoning to taste. Garnish with freshly ground black pepper, parsley, and heavy cream, if desired (use 1 to 2 tablespoons per serving). Serve hot.

Tip: The original recipe has no fat in it and is perfect to accompany a high-fat meal. If you're having a lower-fat meal, garnish the soup with heavy cream. This soup is great made a day ahead and served chilled or reheated before serving.

Variations

Add your favorite herbs or spices to create a variety of flavors. For example, add curry, herbes de Provence, or simple thyme or rosemary.

Garnish with basil pesto or another thick, flavorful paste or sauce.

Sauté the onion in oil before adding to the pot with the cauliflower.

Add other vegetables of your choice, such as celery, for added depth of flavor.

Substitute broccoli for cauliflower and garnish with cheddar cheese.

Serve chilled for a refreshing summer soup.

With 1 tablespoon heavy cream per serving:	Calories: 100 Protein: 4 g Carbohydrate: 11 g	Dietary Fiber: 4 g Total Fat: 6 g

Carrot-Ginger Soup (All Phases)

This zesty soup also complements higher-protein, higher-fat meals well. Make extra, refrigerate or freeze, and reheat for a delicious soup anytime. Depending on your preference, use more or less ginger, or change the seasonings altogether to suit your taste. This soup is a creamy base to which you can add a variety of flavors.

Preparation time: 5 minutes

Total time: 20 minutes

Makes 4 servings (6 to 6½ cups)

- 5 medium carrots, cut into chunks
- 1 medium onion, diced
- 4 cups water, plus more as needed
- 1 teaspoon salt
- 1 (½- to 1-inch) piece fresh ginger, peeled
- ¼ cup chopped scallions, for garnish
- Canned coconut milk, for garnish (optional, to increase fat content of a meal)

Place the carrots and onion in a pot. Add the water, adding more as needed just to cover. Add the salt and bring the water to a boil over high heat. Reduce the heat to medium-low, cover, and simmer until the carrots are soft, 10 to 15 minutes. Add the ginger.

Puree with an immersion blender until the ginger is well blended. Add more water as needed to create a thick, creamy consistency. Garnish with scallions and coconut milk, if desired (use 1 to 2 tablespoons per serving). Serve hot. This soup is also great made a day ahead and served chilled or reheated before serving.

Tip: If this soup will accompany a low-fat meal, garnish with a splash of canned coconut milk.

Variations

Instead of ginger, add your favorite herbs or spices to create a variety of flavors. For example, add curry, thyme, or even cinnamon and cardamom with a hint of nutmeg.

Sauté the onion in oil before adding it to the pot with the carrots and water.

Add celery or other vegetables.

Use butternut squash or other vegetables in place of the carrots.

Serve chilled for a refreshing summer soup.

| With 1 tablespoon canned coconut milk per serving: | Calories: 75 Protein: 1 g Carbohydrate: 11 g | Dietary Fiber: 3 g Total Fat: 3 g |

Red Lentil Soup (All Phases)

Lentils are well suited to a variety of flavors, so be creative with herbs and spices. Red lentils cook more quickly and have a creamier texture than other lentils. If you can't find red lentils, brown or green are acceptable substitutions. Make extra and refrigerate or freeze to reheat later. This thick, hearty soup is even better the second day, after the flavors have had time to fully integrate.

Preparation time: 5 minutes

Total time: 30 to 40 minutes

Makes 4 servings (6 to 6½ cups)

- 1 cup red lentils (or substitute brown or green lentils)
- 4 cups water
- 1 small onion, diced
- 2 stalks celery, sliced
- 1 medium carrot, cut into thick rounds
- 1 teaspoon dried thyme
- 1 bay leaf
- 1 teaspoon salt
- ¼ teaspoon ground black pepper, plus more for garnish
- ¼ cup fresh cilantro or scallions, finely chopped, for garnish
- Heavy cream or canned coconut milk, for garnish (optional, to increase the fat content of a meal)

Rinse the lentils in cold water a few times and drain. Transfer the lentils to a pot with the 4 cups water. Bring the water to a boil over medium-high heat. Skim off any foam that rises to the top with a mesh skimmer or spoon.

Stir in the onion, celery, carrot, thyme, and bay leaf. Reduce the heat to medium-low and simmer, stirring frequently, until the lentils are soft and the soup is thick and creamy, 25 to 40 minutes. Toward the end of the cooking time, season with salt and pepper and remove the bay leaf.

Garnish with freshly ground black pepper, chopped cilantro, and heavy cream, if desired (use 1 to 2 tablespoons per serving), and serve. Refrigerate any leftover soup; it will thicken in the refrigerator, so add a bit of water when reheating leftovers.

Tip: If this soup will accompany a low-fat meal, garnish with a splash of heavy cream or canned coconut milk.

Variations
Experiment with other fresh or dried herbs and spices. Curry works exceptionally well with red lentils.

Sauté the vegetables in oil before adding them to the pot with the lentils and water.

Without heavy cream garnish: Calories: 190	Protein: 14 g Carbohydrate: 33 g Dietary Fiber: 8 g	Total Fat: 1 g

DESSERTS

Coconut Cashew Clusters (All Phases)

Satisfy your craving for a baked chocolate treat in minutes! These clusters are much simpler and quicker to make than your average cookie. Prepare them ahead of time and take them along to the next children's party. The kids won't even miss the extra sugar.

Preparation time: 5 minutes

Total time: 15 minutes

Makes 4 to 6 servings

- ½ cup chopped raw unsalted cashew pieces or other nuts
- 3 ounces dark chocolate (at least 70% cocoa content), cut into small pieces
- 2 tablespoons unsweetened coconut flakes or shredded coconut

Preheat the oven to 375°F.

Line a baking sheet with parchment paper.

In a bowl, combine the cashews, chocolate, and coconut. Divide the mixture into four piles for larger clusters or six piles for smaller clusters on the lined baking sheet. Bake until the chocolate has melted, about 5 minutes. Slide the parchment, with clusters on it, off the baking sheet, and set aside to cool on the counter or in the refrigerator for a few hours, or until the chocolate is solid. The clusters will not hold together until they are fully cooled. Store in an airtight container on the counter or in the refrigerator.

Variations
Melt the chocolate in a double boiler. Stir in the nuts and coconut. Place on parchment paper in four large or six small clusters to cool.

Per large cluster:	Protein: 4 g	Dietary Fiber: 3 g
Calories: 245	Carbohydrate: 16 g	Total Fat: 19 g
Per small cluster:	Protein: 3 g	Dietary Fiber: 2 g
Calories: 163	Carbohydrate: 11 g	Total Fat: 13 g

Pear Strawberry Crisp (Phases 2 and 3)

A grain-free crisp? Believe it! This crisp is easy to make and so delicious your family won't notice what's missing. Get creative with seasonal fruits for a treat anytime of year.

Preparation time: 10 minutes

Total time: 25 minutes

Makes 6 servings

Topping

- ½ cup garbanzo flour or garbanzo-fava flour
- ¼ cup slivered almonds
- ½ cup chopped pecans
- 2 tablespoons neutral-tasting oil, such as high-oleic safflower or avocado oil
- 1 tablespoon honey
- 1 tablespoon pure maple syrup
- ⅛ teaspoon pure vanilla extract (no sugar added)

Filling

- ½ pound strawberries, cut in half (about 1½ cups)
- 1 medium pear, cored and diced (about 1 cup)

Preheat the oven to 375°F.

Make the topping: Stir together the flour and nuts in a bowl. In a separate bowl, stir together the oil, honey, maple syrup, and vanilla until well combined. Combine the wet and dry ingredients. Stir until evenly moist.

Make the filling: Place the strawberries and pear in an 8 x 4-inch loaf pan or six individual ovenproof ramekins. Cover the fruit filling evenly with the topping. Cover the pan with aluminum foil and bake for 7 to 10 minutes (less for ramekins). Remove the foil and bake until the topping is golden brown and the filling is bubbling, 7 to 10 minutes (less for ramekins). Serve warm from the oven, or let cool and store in the refrigerator.

Variations

Substitute 1 cup rhubarb plus ½ teaspoon honey for the pear.

Substitute 2 or 3 medium apples, peaches, or any other fruit of your choice.

Add spices like cinnamon, cardamom, nutmeg, or other favorite spices to the fruit or topping.

Calories: 208	Carbohydrate: 19 g	Total Fat: 14 g
Protein: 4 g	Dietary Fiber: 4 g	

Apple Crisp (Phase 3)

Pie crust can be frustrating and labor-intensive. This gluten-free treat is so much easier (and healthier, too). Use fruits that are in season for the most delicious combinations. Make the most of spring with strawberry rhubarb, summer with luscious peaches, or autumn with crisp apples and cinnamon.

Preparation time: 10 minutes

Total time: 30 minutes

Makes 4 to 6 servings

Topping
- ½ cup rolled oats (not instant)
- 6 tablespoons garbanzo flour or garbanzo-fava flour
- 2 tablespoons slivered almonds
- ¼ cup chopped pecans
- 8 teaspoons neutral-tasting oil, such as high-oleic safflower or avocado oil
- 1 tablespoon honey
- 1 tablespoon pure maple syrup
- ⅛ teaspoon pure vanilla extract (no sugar added)

Filling
- 2 or 3 medium apples, peaches, or any other fruit of your choice, chopped (about 2½ cups)

Preheat the oven to 375°F.

Make the topping: Stir together the oats, flour, and nuts in a bowl. In a separate bowl, stir together the oil, honey, maple syrup, and vanilla until well combined. Combine the wet and dry ingredients. Stir until evenly moist.

Making the filling: Place the fruit in an 8 x 4-inch loaf pan or four to six individual ovenproof ramekins. Cover the filling evenly with the topping. Cover the pan with aluminum foil and bake for 7 to 10 minutes (less for ramekins). Remove the foil and bake until the topping is golden brown and the filling is bubbling, about 10 to 15 minutes (less for ramekins). Serve warm from the oven, or let cool and store in the refrigerator.

Variations

Substitute ½ pound strawberries, cut in half (about 1½ cups), and 1 cup rhubarb plus ½ teaspoon honey for the fruit filling.

Substitute ½ pound strawberries, cut in half (about 1½ cups), and 1 medium pear, cored and diced (about 1 cup), for the fruit filling.

Substitute 2 or 3 medium peaches, pears, or any other fruit of your choice.

Add spices like cinnamon, cardamom, nutmeg, or other favorite spices to the fruit or topping.

Per ⅙ recipe:	Protein: 3 g	Dietary Fiber: 3 g
Calories: 195	Carbohydrate: 22 g	Total Fat: 11 g

Poached Seasonal Fruit (All Phases)

Get creative with any fruits that are piling up in the produce section. Late summer or early fall fruits are best, from peaches and nectarines to apples and pears. This year-round treat suits every phase of the plan.

Preparation time: 3 minutes

Total time: 15 minutes

Makes 4 servings

- 2 medium pears, apples, peaches, or apricots, halved and cored or pitted
- ½ cup water
- ¼ teaspoon ground cinnamon
- ¼ teaspoon ground cardamom
- ⅛ teaspoon ground or freshly grated nutmeg
- Pinch of salt

Arrange the fruit cut-side up in a single layer in a shallow skillet. Add the water. Sprinkle the spices and salt over the fruit. Bring to a boil over medium heat. Reduce the heat to medium-low, cover, and simmer for 10 to 15 minutes, or until the fruit is soft. Remove from the heat. Serve warm.

Variations

Add or substitute other spices of your choice.

Calories: 68   Carbohydrate: 18 g   Total Fat: 0 g
Protein: 0 g   Dietary Fiber: 4 g

Chocolate Sauce (All Phases)

Chocolate sauce that's allowed from day one of your plan—need we say more? This versatile sauce makes any fruit a special treat.

Preparation time: 3 minutes

Total time: 15 minutes

Makes 2 to 4 servings (about 6 tablespoons)

- ¼ cup unsweetened soy milk, almond milk, or whole milk
- 2 ounces dark chocolate bar or pieces (at least 70% cocoa content)

Pour the milk into a pan. Heat over medium-low heat until warm, then reduce the heat to low and add the chocolate. Heat, stirring regularly, until the chocolate is melted and smooth, 3 to 5 minutes. Be careful not to overcook. Chocolate should be smooth and creamy. If it starts to look grainy, it may be overcooked.

Spoon or drizzle the chocolate sauce over fruit on a tray or on individual plates. Serve warm.

Tip: The chocolate sauce can be refrigerated and reheated over low heat until soft. At room temperature, it will have the consistency of a thick frosting.

Per 1 tablespoon: Protein: 1 g   Dietary Fiber: 1 g
Calories: 60   Carbohydrate: 5 g   Total Fat: 4 g

SNACKS

Basic Hummus (All Phases)

Use this recipe as a base for creating a variety of hummus flavors. Serve it as is, or add Greek olives, roasted red peppers, garlic, or other favorite ingredients for a more richly flavored dish. Enjoy it with lightly blanched or raw vegetables like carrot sticks, broccoli, green beans, cauliflower, sliced red peppers, or cucumbers.

Preparation time: 5 minutes

Total time: 5 minutes

Makes 4 servings (about 1½ cups)

- 1½ cups cooked garbanzo beans (chickpeas), drained and rinsed
- 2 to 4 tablespoons fresh lemon juice
- 1 tablespoon tahini
- 2 tablespoons extra-virgin olive oil
- ½ teaspoon salt, or to taste
- ¼ to ½ cup water, or as needed
- Dash of paprika

Combine the garbanzo beans, lemon juice, tahini, oil, and salt in a food processor, high-power blender, or wide-mouthed mason jar or cup that will fit an immersion blender without splashing. Blend until creamy and smooth, adding the water as needed to reach a smooth consistency. Adjust the seasoning to taste. Garnish with the paprika.

Calories: 187	Carbohydrate: 19 g	Total Fat: 10 g
Protein: 6 g	Dietary Fiber: 5 g	

Cheesy Pinto Bean Dip (All Phases)

This snack is delicious at room temperature and even better when heated.

Preparation time: 5 minutes

Total time: 10 minutes

Makes 4 servings (about 1½ cups)

- 1 cup cooked pinto beans, drained and rinsed
- 4 teaspoons extra-virgin olive oil
- ¼ cup water
- ½ teaspoon chili powder
- ¼ to ½ teaspoon salt
- ¾ cup shredded cheddar cheese
- 2 red bell peppers, cut into strips

In a food processor or in a bowl that fits an immersion blender without splashing, combine the pinto beans, oil, water, chili powder, and salt. Blend until smooth, about 30 seconds. Mix in the cheese. Enjoy as is, or heat just until the cheese melts. Serve with red pepper strips for dipping.

Calories: 205   Carbohydrate: 15 g   Total Fat: 12 g
Protein: 9 g   Dietary Fiber: 5 g

Trail Mix (All Phases)

Trail mix can be expensive to buy in bulk but is actually quite easy to make at home—and you don't have to contend with any mystery additives or flavorings. Pack some for the office, car, or anywhere you might need a quick snack between meals. With healthy fats, protein, and slow acting carbohydrates, trail mix fits in perfectly with the meal plan any time.

Preparation time: 2 minutes

Total time: 15 minutes

Makes 8 servings (about 2 cups)

- 1 teaspoon neutral-tasting oil, such as high-oleic safflower or avocado oil
- ½ teaspoon salt
- 2 cups nuts, such as walnuts, pecans, cashews, or peanuts
- ¼ cup brown sesame seeds
- ¼ cup unsweetened shredded coconut

Preheat the oven to 350°F.

Mix the oil, salt, nuts, and seeds in a bowl. Spread the nuts on a large baking sheet and toast in the oven for 8 to 10 minutes, or until lightly browned. Remove from the oven, stir in the coconut, and let cool.

Variations

For Phase 3, add a small amount of dark chocolate chunks or unsweetened dried fruit at the end with the shredded coconut.

Get creative with this recipe by adding your favorite nuts and seeds. Sesame seeds are high in calcium, so we like to add them to many nut mixes.

Calories: 225   Carbohydrate: 7 g   Total Fat: 21 g
Protein: 5 g   Dietary Fiber: 3 g

Spicy Pumpkin Seeds (All Phases)

Crunchy, spicy, and salty—a terrific on-the-go snack. If you like spice, you can make these as hot as you'd like, but if you're not a fan of the heat, be careful with the cayenne!

Preparation time: 10 minutes

Total time: 10 minutes

Makes 4 servings (1 cup)

- 1 cup hulled pumpkin seeds
- 1 teaspoon extra-virgin olive oil
- ½ teaspoon chili powder, or to taste
- Cayenne pepper
- ¼ teaspoon salt

Preheat the oven to 350°F.

Place all the ingredients in a bowl and mix well. Take care to distribute the spices evenly. Arrange the seeds in a single layer on a baking sheet. Toast in the oven until the seeds begin to brown and puff up, 5 to 10 minutes. Remove from the oven, let cool, and enjoy. To store, transfer to a wide-mouthed mason jar with a tight-fitting lid or other airtight container.

Variations

Add or substitute curry powder or any other favorite spices.

Add or substitute dried herbs of your choice.

Calories: 192   Carbohydrate: 4 g   Total Fat: 17 g
Protein: 10 g   Dietary Fiber: 2 g

Herb-Roasted Chickpeas (All Phases)

A savory snack that feels like a meal, these chickpeas have lots of satisfying protein, made all the more luscious with extra-virgin olive oil and Parmesan.

Preparation time: 2 minutes

Total time: 22 minutes

Makes 4 servings

- 1¾ cups cooked garbanzo beans (chickpeas), drained and well rinsed (one 15-ounce can)
- 1 tablespoon extra-virgin olive oil
- 1 teaspoon dried oregano or dried Italian herb mix
- Dash of salt
- ¼ cup grated Parmesan cheese

Preheat the oven to 400°F.

Toss together the chickpeas, oil, oregano, and salt in a bowl.

Transfer the chickpeas to a baking dish or spread on a baking sheet. Roast, shaking the pan occasionally, until the chickpeas turn golden brown, 15 to 20 minutes. They should be soft on the inside and a bit crispy outside. Toss with the Parmesan immediately after removing from the oven.

Let cool and serve immediately, or store in a jar in the refrigerator.

Calories: 150   Carbohydrate: 15 g   Total Fat: 7 g
Protein: 8 g   Dietary Fiber: 5 g

SNACKS—HIGHER PROTEIN

Cold-Cut Lettuce Boats (All Phases)

This versatile snack lets you do away with the bread, but not the convenience.

Preparation time: 3 minutes

Total time: 3 minutes

Makes 2 servings

- 3 tablespoons dressing or sauce of your choice
- 8 romaine heart leaves or endive leaves
- 4 ounces sliced deli meat of your choice

Spread your favorite dressing evenly over the lettuce leaves. Roll half a slice of deli meat in the middle of each leaf, and enjoy!

Variations

Divide 2 teaspoons of mustard evenly among the lettuce or endive leaves. On each leaf, place ½ slice (about ½ ounce) sliced deli meat, and top with a small slice (about ¼ ounce) of Swiss cheese.

Experiment with your toppings: Substitute leftover Salmon or Tofu Salad (page 254), leftover Herb-Roasted Chicken Thighs (page 241), or store-bought smoked salmon for the deli meat.

| Calories: 140 | Carbohydrate: 4 g | Total Fat: 8 g |
| Protein: 14 g | Dietary Fiber: 2 g | |

Cucumber Boats with Turkey and Feta (All Phases)

Think of these as "portable Greek salad," especially when you toss in a couple of halved grape tomatoes.

Preparation time: 5 minutes

Total time: 5 minutes

Makes 2 servings

- 2 medium cucumbers
- 3 tablespoons feta cheese (about 1 ounce)
- 4 ounces turkey cold cuts or sliced deli meat of your choice

Cut each cucumber in half lengthwise. Scoop out the seeds, fill each half with 1½ tablespoons of the feta, and top with a rolled-up slice of turkey.

Variations

Experiment with your toppings: Use leftover Salmon or Tofu Salad (page 254), or leftover Herb-Roasted Chicken Thighs (page 241).

Substitute smoked salmon and cream cheese for the deli meat and feta.

Add grape tomatoes.

Calories: 170	Carbohydrate: 12 g	Total Fat: 6 g
Protein: 18 g	Dietary Fiber: 2 g	

Smoked Salmon and Dill Cream Cheese on Cucumber Rounds

This cocktail party favorite combines creamy, crunchy, and tangy.

Preparation time: 3 minutes

Total time: 3 minutes

Makes 2 servings

- 2 tablespoons cream cheese
- 1 tablespoon chopped fresh dill, or 1 teaspoon dried
- 1 medium cucumber, cut into ¼-inch rounds
- 4 ounces smoked salmon

Mix the cream cheese with the dill and spread on the cucumber slices. Evenly distribute the smoked salmon on top.

Variations

Add or substitute other fresh or dried herbs of your choice.

Add a squeeze of lemon to the cream cheese mixture.

Chop the salmon and mix it into the cream cheese with the dill.

Calories: 129   Carbohydrate: 3 g   Total Fat: 8 g
Protein: 12 g   Dietary Fiber: 1 g

Edamame

A fun finger food that's packed with nutrition, for adults and kids alike.

Preparation time: 5 minutes

Total time: 5 minutes

Makes 2 servings

- 1 cup frozen shelled edamame
- Dash of salt

Steam or boil the edamame according to the package directions. Season with the salt.

Variations

Use frozen edamame in the pods.

Calories: 120   Carbohydrate: 11 g   Total Fat: 4 g
Protein: 13 g   Dietary Fiber: 4 g

Ending the Madness

HEALTHY FOOD AS A
MATTER OF NATIONAL SECURITY

In ancient times, an invading army might poison the food or water supply in an effort to conquer the enemy's army. Now, suppose that a foreign power conspired to overpower America, economically and militarily, with a similar strategy. But instead of contaminating a water reservoir or food store—actions that would be easily identified and countered with modern public health surveillance systems— our adversary planned to gradually degrade the food supply. Teams of secret agents infiltrated key segments of society and worked insidiously to undermine the national diet so that the public would increasingly succumb to diabetes and other disabling obesity-related conditions. Their scheme targeted the following areas:

Government:

- Devise long-term agricultural policies that favor production of low-nutritional-quality commodity grains over nutrient-rich vegetables, fruits, legumes, and nuts[1]
- Provide free junk food and sugary beverages—amounting to billions of dollars each year—through nutrition assistance programs like SNAP (previously known as Food Stamps)[2]
- Restrict funding for nutrition research, the school lunch program, and childhood-obesity-prevention initiatives[3]

- Underinvest in public transportation (including walking and bike paths) relative to the national highway system, restricting opportunities to offset poor diet with physical activity

Food Industry:

- Produce an overwhelming variety of extremely low-quality food products derived predominantly from cheap grain commodities and artificial additives[4]
- Aggressively market those products throughout society, especially to children (ensuring brand loyalty from early in life)
- Make fast food, junk foods, and sugary beverages convenient and affordable, but nutritious whole foods much less so
- Offer empty promises of change when the public becomes concerned about poor food quality, while working to subvert public health[5]

Schools:

- Close budget gaps by lowering the quality of foods provided through the school lunch program, franchise the cafeteria to fast-food companies, and sell junk food in vending machines
- Reduce or eliminate physical education classes and after-school recreation programs

Academia and Professional Health Associations:

- Accept funding from the food industry for research, sponsorships, product endorsements, preferred access to "thought leaders," and other collaborations—despite evidence that such relationships create scientific bias and undermine public health credibility[6]

Though any one of these conspiratorial actions might have caused limited damage, their combined effects on society were devastating. Rapidly rising medical costs from diet-related disease, approaching $1 trillion annually, and declining worker productivity produced massive budget deficits. The looming fiscal crisis provoked political infighting and legislative paralysis. As financial resources for education, research, transportation, and other critical long-term investments dwindled, the national infrastructure deteriorated, crippling America's economic competitiveness. The Pentagon feared that young people had become too unhealthy to serve in the military, should the need for a large-scale deployment arise.[7] For the first time in a century, America's status as a superpower seemed to be threatened...exceeding the wildest expectations of our adversary.

Of course, the foreign conspiracy is imaginary. But this frightening scenario may well come to pass for an entirely domestic reason—the systematic political failure to put public health and societal needs ahead of special interests and short-term profit. We all share responsibility for this failure—by condoning a culture that values the temporary convenience and fleeting pleasure of highly processed industrial foods over health. But the food industry has played the leading role.

Society is so filled with sugary, starchy food, that just living day to day is an obstacle to weight control. But that is reality and we all have to deal with that.

—Ann R., 61, Windsor Heights, IA

Food companies and their advocacy groups spend tens of millions of dollars a year in political donations, lobbying, and related activities, gaining in return immense influence over food policies at the national, state, and local levels.[8] In the last decade, aggressive industry lobbying has:[9]

- undermined school lunch standards (for example, defining pizza as a vegetable)
- hindered reform of federal nutrition-assistance programs (for example, mandating inclusion of white potato in WIC benefits, against the advice of the Institute of Medicine)
- blocked taxes on sugary beverages
- impeded restrictions on food advertisements aimed at children

- weakened food labeling standards (for example, involving GMOs)
- swayed dietary guidelines related to sugar and other commodities
- affected many billions of dollars in federal spending for agricultural subsidies

---

Hidden sugars were the greatest eye-opener for me. I have always known and heard that sugar is in everything—but now I'm seeing just how profoundly I have been affected by it. We have not been ones to keep much junk food on our shelves or go overboard, yet we felt awful all the time. The weight gain was too easy, and despite attempts to eat better, we couldn't really budge much. It's so pervasive, this "sugar in everything" deal! Ugh!!

—Nan T., 53, Birmingham, AL

In response to growing concern about obesity, especially among children, food companies have launched expensive campaigns to create the perception that they are good corporate citizens, sincere in their efforts to be part of the solution. But how can we trust food companies, asked Michele Simon, when they "lobby vociferously against policies to improve children's health; make misleading statements and misrepresent their policies at government meetings and in other public venues; and make public promises of corporate responsibility that sound good, but in reality amount to no more than a public relations campaign?"[10]

All things considered, the food industry isn't immoral, and its actions are, for the most part, entirely predictable. As described by Marion Nestle in *Food Politics*,[11] food companies have a fiduciary responsibility to their stockholders to maximize profit. In the unregulated marketplace, those profits come primarily from promoting consumption of highly processed, commodity-based products. An executive may have the best of intentions, but if the competition markets junk food to children, his company will be at a competitive disadvantage unless it resorts to those tactics as well.

Deflecting attention from this inherent conflict—to produce

healthy foods versus healthy profits—the industry argues that it's all a matter of personal responsibility. Food companies don't force people to buy junk food. People are free to make their own decisions, and live with the consequences. But this argument fails for two fundamental reasons. First, political manipulation by the industry has grossly distorted the free market and, consequently, the food environment. Processed industrial foods are plentiful, convenient, and cheap relative to whole foods, in part due to government policies. How does someone exert personal responsibility in a whole food desert and junk food oasis? According to a report from the Institute of Medicine in 2000:

> It is unreasonable to expect that people will change their behavior easily when so many forces in the social, cultural and physical environment conspire against such change. If successful programs are to be developed to prevent disease and improve health, attention must be given not only to the behavior of individuals, but also to the environmental context within which people live.[12]

When I watch a little bit of TV in the evenings, all I see are ads for prescription drugs and ads for chain restaurants. What a mutually beneficial society it is—we eat at these chain restaurants, and we go straight to the docs and pharmacies. I rarely see ads to promote fruits, veggies, and physical activity. They make us sicker by brainwashing us.
—*Jyoti A., 59, Muskogee, OK*

Second, the long-term consequences of an industrial food diet don't fall entirely to the individual. Society pays directly through Medicare and Medicaid, and indirectly through Supplemental Security Income and other disability benefits. Indeed, every business that purchases employee medical insurance, and anyone who pays for private insurance, shoulders this burden.

With most public health issues, we wouldn't create a false distinction between personal, corporate, and government responsibility.

Imagine what would happen if government deregulated automobile safety, allowed the industry to market dangerous cars, and expected consumers to sort things out for themselves? Shared responsibility is taken for granted with all sorts of consumer products, from toys to toaster ovens. Why not food?

Unless we change course, diet-related chronic diseases will cause tremendous suffering, shorten life expectancy,[13] drain the economy, and undermine our international strength. But this major threat to our national security can be averted, with a comprehensive (if politically difficult) action plan, as summarized below.

A TEN-POINT PLAN TO RESTORE HEALTHY FOOD AS A NATIONAL SECURITY PRIORITY

1. *Create an intergovernmental food policy commission.* Until we can successfully enact campaign finance reform, the food industry will continue to have inordinate influence in Washington. But we can insulate policy from politics, as we do with other issues of national security (such as military base closings) with an independent commission empowered to make objective determinations on all matters of national food policy—ranging from agricultural subsidies to school lunch guidelines.

2. *Reform the process of revising U.S. Dietary Guidelines.* Move primary responsibility for guideline development to the Institute of Medicine or other independent body, to avoid conflicts of interest at the USDA arising from its mission to promote corn and other commodities.[14]

3. *Tax all processed foods and restaurant fast foods,* so that the long-term costs of these products become incorporated into the purchase price. Redirect the resulting revenue to subsidize vegetables, fruits, and other whole foods.[15]

4. *Regulate food advertising.* The First Amendment doesn't guarantee the right to advertise demonstrably unhealthy products, especially when children are involved. At a minimum, consumers should be given appropriate health warnings. If commercials for Viagra must mention rare complications like prolonged erection, why don't commercials for sugary beverages list common consequences, like excessive weight gain and diabetes?[16]

5. *Minimize conflicts of interest among academics and professional nutrition societies.* The government should adequately fund high-quality nutrition

research through the National Institutes of Health[17] so that food industry sponsorship will be less necessary and bias from industry studies will be diluted. Professional societies should avoid financial relationships with industry that detract from their public health mission.

6. *Adequately fund schools* so they can offer high-quality breakfast and lunch, daily physical education classes, and after-school recreational programs.

7. *Design new restaurant options*, providing convenient, inexpensive meals prepared from whole foods.

8. *Formulate healthier processed foods.* The food industry should use higher-nutritional-quality ingredients instead of relying primarily on processed grains and sugar. In addition, many conventional products can be marketed in less severely processed forms (for example, stone-ground bread or steel-cut oats).[18]

9. *Vote with the ballot.* The public can elect politicians with the courage to place public health ahead of short-term special interests.

10. *Vote with the fork.* The public can incentivize food companies to formulate and market healthier foods by consuming a diet based on whole foods instead of highly processed products.

We used to have various snacks (pretzels, granola bars, microwave popcorn, etc.) in the house and a myriad of frozen foods to eat (chicken nuggets, mac and cheese, etc.). I always had a giant fruit bowl, too. However, no one ever picked the fruit to eat when the other things were around. Amazingly, the other day my daughter walked past me eating a pear, and I noticed that everyone was grabbing from the fruit bowl when hungry in between meals, and I smiled.

—*Monica M., 45, Great Falls, VA*

The food industry has acted constructively sometimes and outrageously other times. Supporters and critics can always find examples to argue that that the industry is either essentially "good" or essentially "bad." But that would miss the point. In a market-driven economy, industry tends to behave opportunistically to maximize profit. It's the government's responsibility to regulate the market so that industry will profit from serving the needs of society, not undermining them.

And the food industry must bear in mind that public health is in everyone's best interests. A healthy food supply forms the foundations of a strong society—as argued a half century ago by the American food scientist George Stewart:

> If we do not pay proper attention to the nutritional problems associated with food technology we run the risk of eventually producing an abundance of palatable, convenient, stable foods that are not capable of meeting man's nutritional needs. In other words, we run a risk of undermining the nutritional well-being of our nation...It is my contention that every food technologist has a moral responsibility to help provide the public with nutritious [not just] palatable foods.[19]

But ultimately, it's up to us. Until we can re-create a society in which the wholesome choice is the easy choice, we must take full responsibility for our health, and the health of our children. We can say no to seductive ads for junk food, knowing that the diseases they cause—including most cases of diabetes—are anything but convenient and pleasurable. The purpose of this book is to empower you on this journey to optimal health.

Appendix A

THE GLYCEMIC LOAD OF CARBOHYDRATE-CONTAINING FOODS

THE GLYCEMIC LOAD OF CARBOHYDRATE-CONTAINING FOODS[1]

FOOD GROUP	GLYCEMIC LOAD[2]		
	LOW OK for All Program Phases	MODERATE Phases 2 and 3	HIGH Phase 3 Only
Vegetables	Alfalfa sprouts Artichoke Asparagus Avocado Bamboo shoots Bean sprouts Bok choy Broccoli Brussels sprouts Cabbage Carrots Cauliflower Celery Chard Collard greens Cucumber Eggplant Green beans Kale Kohlrabi Leeks	Acorn squash Beets Butternut squash Green peas Parsnips Plantain Pumpkin Sweet potato Yam	White potato

| FOOD GROUP | GLYCEMIC LOAD[2] | | |
	LOW OK for All Program Phases	MODERATE Phases 2 and 3	HIGH Phase 3 Only
Vegetables	Lettuce Mushrooms Mustard greens Okra Onion Peppers Radish Rutabaga Scallion Snow peas Spinach Summer squash Swiss chard Tomatoes Turnip Water chestnuts Zucchini		
Fruits	Apples Apricot Berries Cherries Clementines Grapefruit Grapes Kiwi Lemon Lime Nectarines Oranges Peaches Pears Plums Tangelos Tangerines	Applesauce* Banana Canned fruit, unsweetened Cantaloupe Dried fruit Honeydew Mango Papaya Pineapple Watermelon	Fruit juices and drinks

FOOD GROUP	GLYCEMIC LOAD[2]		
	LOW OK for All Program Phases	**MODERATE** Phases 2 and 3	**HIGH** Phase 3 Only
Legumes	Beans (all kinds except baked) Black-eyed peas Chickpeas Hummus Lentils Split peas	Baked beans*	
Nuts	Almonds Brazil nut Cashews Hazelnuts Macadamia Peanuts Peanut butter, no added sugar Pecans Pistachio Walnuts	Peanut butter, sugar-sweetened*	
Seeds	Chia Pumpkin Sesame Sunflower		
Dairy	Cheese Milk Yogurt, no added sugar	Milk, chocolate* Yogurt, sugar-sweetened*	
Grains		Amaranth Barley Bread, minimally processed (including whole kernel, sprouted grain, and stone ground)* Breakfast cereal, high fiber* Brown rice (varies by type) Buckwheat (kasha)	Bread, highly processed (including bagels, buns, corn bread, English muffins, pitas, rolls, and white bread) Breakfast cereals, low fiber Couscous Crackers Pancakes

FOOD GROUP	GLYCEMIC LOAD[2]		
	LOW OK for All Program Phases	**MODERATE** Phases 2 and 3	**HIGH** Phase 3 Only
Grains (Continued)		Corn (varies by type) Farro Oats Pasta (not canned)* Quinoa Rye Wheat berries Wild rice	Pasta (canned) Pizza Popcorn Pretzels Rice cakes Stuffing Taco shell Tortilla Waffle White rice
Desserts, Sweets, & Treats	Dark chocolate (minimum 70% cocoa content)	Ice cream* Milk chocolate*	Brownies Cake Candy Chips Cookies Custards Doughnuts Pies Sorbet Sugary drinks

[1]Glycemic load describes how a food (meal or entire diet) affects blood sugar for several hours after eating. Frequent consumption of high–glycemic load foods is strongly linked to excessive weight gain and risk for heart disease and diabetes, as discussed in chapter 4. The glycemic load is determined by multiplying the glycemic index of a food with the amount of carbohydrate present in that food. For a comprehensive listing of glycemic index and glycemic load, see www.glycemicindex.com.

[2]The values used to classify glycemic load vary somewhat between food groups in this table, to allow for better discrimination of foods within groups.

*Avoid in Phase 2 because of high sugar content or processing.

Appendix B

Trackers

DAILY TRACKER

Use one copy of this page each day, or download the document from www.always hungrybook.com. For the five symptom categories, indicate your overall experience throughout the day. Add up the points from these categories, and record the sum as your Total Score (which will range from 0 to 20). Next, note how many processed carbohydrates you ate. Then graph your Total Score into the Monthly Progress Chart, using ink (green, yellow, or red) corresponding to your processed carbohydrate intake. At the bottom of the page, note your activities related to other program targets (stress reduction, movement, and sleep).

Hunger. Today, I felt:
☐ 0 (starving) ☐ 1 ☐ 2 ☐ 3 ☐ 4 (no hunger)

_____ points

Cravings. Today, my cravings were:
☐ 0 (high) ☐ 1 ☐ 2 ☐ 3 ☐ 4 (absent)

_____ points

Satiety. Today, I felt satisfied after eating:
☐ 0 (not at all) ☐ 1 ☐ 2 ☐ 3 ☐ 4 (until the next meal)

_____ points

Energy level. Today, my overall energy level was:
☐ 0 (low) ☐ 1 ☐ 2 ☐ 3 ☐ 4 (high)

_____ points

Well-being. Today, my overall level of well-being was:
☐ 0 (low) ☐ 1 ☐ 2 ☐ 3 ☐ 4 (high)

_____ points

TOTAL SCORE _____

I had the following number of PROCESSED CARBOHYDRATES* today (circle one):
Graph your Total Score in the Monthly Progress Chart using the indicated color of ink

0 to 1 *green*   2 *yellow*   3 or more *red*

*includes refined grains (bread, pasta, white rice, etc.), white potato or potato
    products, any food with added sugar, and fruit juice

I did my 5-minute stress reduction: ☐ AM ☐ PM

I did my after-meal walks: ☐ AM ☐ PM

I did my joyful movement: ☐ (what kind) _____

I did my pre-sleep routine: ☐ (describe) _____

MONTHLY PROGRESS CHART

This chart will let you monitor your progress month to month. In addition, you will be able to see how the amount of processed carbohydrate you eat each day may affect your results. Graph your Total Score from the Daily Tracker onto this chart by placing a circle (•) in the appropriate place, or download the file from www.alwayshungrybook.com. Use the ink color that corresponds to the number of processed carbohydrates you consumed on that day as indicated on the Daily Tracker (0 to 1—green; 2—yellow; 3 or more—red). If starting the program in the middle of a month, leave the preceding days blank. At the end of the month, record cumulative change in weight and waist circumference (compared to baseline).

Enter your baseline measurements (before starting the program):

Weight _____ Waist circumference _____

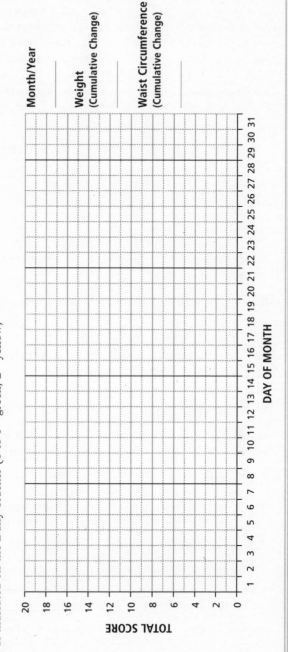

Month/Year
_____
_____

Weight
(Cumulative Change)
_____
_____

Waist Circumference
(Cumulative Change)
_____
_____

Appendix C

GUIDES TO PREPARING VEGETABLES, WHOLE GRAINS, NUTS, AND SEEDS

GUIDE TO COOKING VEGETABLES

Vegetables are a mainstay of the Always Hungry Solution—full of nutrition and a great vehicle for the rich sauces and dips used in all program phases. Get creative, and let this guide remove the guesswork.

Vegetable	Size and Prep	Cooking Time in Minutes				
		Sauté*	Steam	Boil	Blanch**	Roast
Arugula	Rinse well. Coarsely chop.	2 to 3	2 to 3	—	Less than 1	—
Asparagus	Cut away and discard tough ends.	4 to 6	7 to 8	6 to 8	1	8 to 10
Beets	To sauté: Peel and shred. To steam or boil: Peel and cut into 1-inch cubes. To blanch: Slice into thin rounds or half-moons. To roast: Place whole, unpeeled beets in a baking dish with ¼ cup water and cover tightly or wrap individually in foil; peel skin when they are done.	6 to 8	15 to 20	10 to 15	1 to 2	45 to 60 (depending on size)

Vegetable	Size and Prep	Cooking Time in Minutes				
		Sauté*	Steam	Boil	Blanch**	Roast
Bell Peppers (Green, Red, Orange, or Yellow)	Remove and discard seeds. Cut into thin strips.	5 to 7	—	—	Less than 1	20 to 25
Bok Choy, Tatsoi	Cut white parts into ½-inch slices, coarsely chop the leaves.	2 to 4	2 to 4	2 to 4	Less than 1	—
Broccoli	Peel or cut off hard outer part of the stem and cut into small sticks; separate tops into small florets.	4 to 6	6 to 8	6 to 8	1	20 to 25
Broccoli Rabe, Rapini, or Chinese Broccoli	Cut into ½-inch slices.	4 to 6	4 to 6	4 to 6	1	—
Cabbage (White, Green, or Red)	Remove and discard core. Shred thinly. To roast: Cut into 1½-inch-thick wedges.	5 to 7	8 to 10	8 to 10	1	20 to 25
Carrots	To sauté or blanch: Shred or cut into thin strips, rounds, or matchsticks. To steam, boil, or roast: Cut into thick rounds or chunks.	4 to 6	8 to 10	8 to 10	1 to 2	25 to 30
Cauliflower	Separate into small florets. Core diced.	4 to 6	7 to 9	7 to 9	1 to 2	15 to 18
Chard (Green or Red)	Rinse well. Cut the stems into ½-inch slices and coarsely chop the greens.	4 to 6—add stems first, then greens after 2 minutes	4 to 6 Stems on bottom	3 to 5	1 for stems, less for leaves	—
Collard Greens	Rinse well. Separate the stems from the leaves. Cut the stems into very thin rounds and coarsely chop the leaves.	5 to 8	5 to 8	3 to 5	1 to 2	—

Vegetable	Size and Prep	Cooking Time in Minutes				
		Sauté*	Steam	Boil	Blanch**	Roast
Daikon or Other Types of Radish	Cut into thick chunks or leave small radishes whole. To sauté: Shred or cut into thin matchsticks. To blanch: Cut into thin rounds or half-moons.	4 to 6	4 to 6	5 to 8	1	15 to 20
Eggplant	Peel, if desired. Cut into 1-inch cubes or slices.	10 to 12	—	—	—	20 to 25
Fennel	Cut bulb and stems into thin rounds. To roast: Cut into quarters or chunks.	6 to 8	6 to 8	6 to 8	1 to 3	30 to 45
Green Beans	Trim off and discard tough ends or stems.	3 to 5	4 to 6	4 to 6	1 or less	8 to 10
Kale	Rinse well. Separate the stems from the leaves. Cut the stems into very thin rounds and coarsely chop the leaves.	4 to 7	4 to 7	3 to 5	1 to 2	—
Leek	Cut in half lengthwise and thoroughly rinse all layers. Cut white and green parts into thin rounds. To roast: Cut into large chunks.	5 to 7	5 to 7	6 to 9	1 to 2	20 to 30
Mustard Greens	Rinse well. Separate the stems from the leaves. Cut the stems into very thin rounds and coarsely chop the leaves.	3 to 5	3 to 5	3 to 5	1	—
Napa or Chinese Cabbage	Cut the white parts into ½-inch slices and coarsely chop the leaves.	2 to 4	2 to 4	2 to 4	Less than 1	—
Onions (Sweet, Yellow, White, or Red)	Peel the tough outer skin. Slice in thin half-moons or dice. To roast: Cut into quarters or thick wedges.	8 to 10	10 to 12	8 to 10	2 to 3	20 to 25
Parsnips	Cut into ½-inch chunks. To sauté: Shred or cut into thin matchsticks. To blanch: Cut into thin rounds.	8 to 10	13 to 15	12 to 14	2	35 to 50

Vegetable	Size and Prep	Cooking Time in Minutes				
		Sauté*	Steam	Boil	Blanch**	Roast
Rutabaga	Peel. Cut into ½-inch chunks. To sauté: Shred or cut into thin matchsticks. To blanch: Cut into thin rounds.	7 to 9	16 to 18	14 to 16	1 to 2	35 to 50
Snow Peas or Snap Peas	Trim off and discard tough ends or stems and peel the string down the edge.	2 to 3	2 to 3	2 to 3	Less than 1	—
Spinach	Rinse well. Coarsely chop.	2 to 3	2 to 3	3 to 5	Less than 1	—
Summer Squash (Yellow or Zucchini)	Cut into ¼-inch-thick slices or sticks.	5 to 10	5 to 7	5 to 7	1 to 2	15 to 20
Sweet Potato	To sauté: Shred or cut into thin matchsticks. To steam or boil: Cut into 1-inch chunks or thick rounds. To blanch: Cut into thin rounds. To roast: Cut into 1-inch chunks or thick rounds, or leave whole.	8 to 10	8 to 10	10 to 12	2 to 3	45 to 60
Turnips	Cut into ½-inch chunks. To sauté: Shred or cut into thin matchsticks. To blanch: Cut into thin rounds.	6 to 8	12 to 14	10 to 12	1 to 2	30 to 40
Winter Squash (Buttercup, Butternut, Kabocha, or Acorn)	Cut in half. Remove and discard seeds. Cut into 1-inch chunks or thick wedges. The skin can be eaten unless very tough, like acorn. To blanch: Cut into thin half-moons.	—	14 to 16	12 to 14	2 to 3	30 to 40

* Olive oil is recommended, but other vegetable oils (for example, high-oleic safflower oil) and butter may be used.
** Immersing vegetables in cold water after blanching is not necessary.

GUIDE TO COOKING WHOLE GRAINS

Cooking whole grains may seem like a culinary mystery, but it really is quite simple: All you need is water, salt...and heat. Just bring to a boil, cover, and simmer for the time indicated. In Phase 2, we incorporate whole-kernel grains on a daily basis. Experiment with whole-kernel grains you might not have tried before—you'll likely find them more satisfying than the processed versions. Make extra to use for future meals. With cooked whole grains already made, meal preparation becomes quick and easy.

Whole Grain	Dry Amount	Water	Salt	Cooking Time	Approximate Yield
Presoaking Not Required					
Buckwheat (Kasha)	1 cup	1½ to 2 cups	⅛ teaspoon	15 to 20 minutes	3 cups
Cracked Wheat (Bulgur)	1 cup	1 to 1¼ cups boiling	⅛ teaspoon	5 minutes	2 cups
Farro	1 cup	2 cups	⅛ teaspoon	30 minutes	2 cups
Millet*	1 cup	2 to 4 cups boiling	⅛ teaspoon	30 minutes	3 to 5 cups
Pearl Barley	1 cup	3 cups	⅛ teaspoon	30 minutes	3 cups
Quinoa (rinse well)	1 cup	2 cups	⅛ teaspoon	20 minutes	3 cups
Steel-cut oats	1 cup	2 cups	Pinch	30 to 45 minutes	2 cups
Steel-cut oats (overnight version)	1 cup	4 cups	Pinch	Bring to a full boil, then let sit on the stove, covered, overnight. Or cool the oats and place in the refrigerator overnight. Serve cold or reheat before eating.	4½ cups
Presoaking Recommended (4 hours to overnight)**					
Brown Rice***	1 cup	1½ cups	⅛ teaspoon	50 minutes (cooking time will vary based on type of rice)	2 to 3 cups

Whole Grain	Dry Amount	Water	Salt	Cooking Time	Approximate Yield
Hulled Barley	1 cup	3 cups	⅛ teaspoon	1 hour or more	3 cups
Wheat Berries	1 cup	3 cups	⅛ teaspoon	1 hour or more	3 cups

* For fluffy millet that separates nicely, use 2¼ cups boiling water; for soft, creamy millet, use 4 cups boiling water. The soft millet may also be cooled, cut, and pan-fried like polenta.

** Presoaking allows the grains to begin the process of germination, increasing nutrient value and also making for a richer, nuttier taste.

*** Short-grain rice will make a stickier rice. Long-grain and basmati rice will make a fluffier, separated grain.

GUIDE TO ROASTING NUTS AND SEEDS

Basic Cooking Instructions:

Preheat oven to 350°F. Spread raw nuts or seeds in a single layer onto a large baking sheet. Place in the oven and cook until lightly golden in color and the nutty aroma first begins to waft from the oven (see times listed below). Every oven is a bit different, so pay close attention, check them every few minutes, and avoid overcooking. Remove from the oven immediately when done and transfer to a large plate or serving tray to cool. Once cooled, store in a jar with a lid (wide mouth canning jars work nicely) or other airtight container.

Nuts or Seeds	Cooking Time
Almonds	10–12 minutes
Cashews	8–10 minutes
Macadamia	Use raw
Peanuts	10–12 minutes
Pecans	10–12 minutes
Pistachios	8–10 minutes
Pumpkin Seeds	6–8 minutes—done when they are golden and begin to puff up
Sesame Seeds	6–8 minutes—done when they are golden, fragrant, and begin to pop
Sunflower Seeds	5–7 minutes
Walnuts	8–10 minutes

Note: Toaster ovens cook much faster. Follow toaster oven directions or experiment with times for your toaster oven. Remember to let your nose guide you: The moment you smell the aroma, they're done!

Acknowledgments

The most important questions facing health care today are far too big for anyone to tackle alone. I am deeply grateful to my many mentors, colleagues, and patients who have guided me throughout my career.

As for this book, I have been extremely fortunate to have the support of a star team of nutrition, culinary, and editorial experts. Mariska van Aalst, my wonderful project manager, helped create the program, guide the pilot tests, and keep all of us on track. She also provided wise and gentle feedback on the manuscript. Janis Jibrin contributed importantly to the program and, with the able assistance of Sidra Forman and Tracy Gensler, helped prepare the recipes, meal plans, and nutritional analyses. Susan Chatzky meticulously followed the meal plan, and provided helpful feedback. Mary Woodin created illustrations that convey scientific concepts in a simple, accessible way. John Larson of Coach Accountable adapted his excellent software to support the pilots.

The extraordinarily talented Melissa Gallagher and Ethan Litman (congratulations on medical school!) led the pilot at Boston Children's Hospital. The amazing team at *Experience Life* magazine provided critical early guidance with the design and feel of the program, as well as ongoing encouragement and help recruiting the participants for the national pilot. Special thanks to Pilar Gerasimo, founding editor, and Jamie Martin, senior director of multiplatform content, for their leadership of that effort.

Extra-, extra-special appreciation goes to my partner in life and on this project, Dawn Ludwig. Dawn led the national pilot with care and compassion, and supervised all aspects of recipe and meal plan development. She burned the midnight oil to create cookbook-quality meals that precisely hit the program's nutritional targets, with options for vegetarian and other special requirements. Dawn's ability to inspire and heal with food suffuses the Always Hungry Solution.

I had the honor and pleasure of working with Sarah Pelz, my editor, and her fantastic group at Grand Central Publishing, including publisher, Jamie Raab, editor-in-chief, Deb Futter, editorial director, Karen Murgolo, editorial assistant Morgan Hedden publicity director, Matthew Ballast, and my marketing team, Brian McLendon, Amanda Pritzker, and Andrew Duncan. They guided the project with the utmost professionalism and passion, giving me superb direction when I needed it, and a long leash when I didn't. Last to be mentioned, but certainly not least, among my book team are Richard Pine, Eliza Rothstein, and Alexis Hurley at Inkwell Management. My agent Richard was like a protective older brother, who skillfully led me from inception to completion of the project. He is a gentleman and a scholar.

Several colleagues and friends provided insightful comments on the manuscript, including Pilar Gerasimo (founding editor of *Experience Life* magazine), Daniel Lieberman (read his brilliant book, *The Story of the Human Body*), Gary Taubes (his *Good Calories, Bad Calories* offers an important historical perspective on the science), Walter Willett (read his classic *Eat, Drink, and Be Healthy*), Ben Brown, Cara Ebbeling, Joseph Majzoub, and Dariush Mozaffarian.

I'm grateful to Mark Hyman (*Eat Fat, Get Thin*) for more than a decade of friendship, for supporting and encouraging my work, and for helping me navigate the world of book publishing—before and after writing the manuscript. Richard Borofsky and Rodger Whidden provided invaluable personal guidance.

This book would not have been possible without my colleagues in the New Balance Foundation Obesity Prevention Center at Boston Children's Hospital and the phenomenal leadership of Cara Ebbeling, Christine Healey, and Daniele Skopek. Cara deserves special mention. She has evolved from one of my first research trainees into a world-class independent researcher and my closest scientific col-laborator. She directed much of the Center's research over the last decade, including many of the studies featured in this book.

Research is an expensive undertaking, and government funding has unfortunately become increasingly scarce. So I would like to give special recognition to the philanthropic sponsors who've supported our work all along. The Charles H. Hood Foundation launched my career in clinical research with a major grant in the late 1990s. The New Balance Foundation provided a transformative grant to create a home for all aspects of our work in the Center—research, patient care, and community projects. Their leadership team including Anne and Jim Davis, Megan Bloch, Molly Santry, and Noreen Bigelow have an abiding dedication to children, and are in the forefront of the battle to end the epidemic of childhood obesity. And most recently, Nutrition Science Initiative (NuSI)—with major support from the Laura and John Arnold Foundation—have sponsored our largest-ever study to examine how diet affects metabolism. I have had many extremely stimulating conversations with Peter Attia, Gary Taubes, and Mark Friedman among the leadership of NuSI. Other generous funders have included the Thrasher Research Fund, the Allen Foun-dation, Runner's World Heartbreak Hill Half Marathon & Festival, and the Many Voices Foundation. I'm also thankful for many years of research support from the National Institutes of Health (NIH), and especially the National Institute of Diabetes and Digestive and Kidney Diseases (NIDDK).

I'm grateful to my mentor, Joe Majzoub, and to Boston Children's Hospital, my professional home for more than two decades.

Finally, I offer my heartfelt thanks to our pilot program participants.

Notes

Part 1   Always Hungry, Never Losing Weight

1. Kolata G. In struggle with weight, Taft used a modern diet. *New York Times.* October 14, 2013. http://www.nytimes.com/2013/10/15/health/in-struggle-with -weight-william-howard-taft-used-a-modern-diet.html?_r=1 Accessed June 21, 2015; Levine DI. Corpulence and correspondence: President William H. Taft and the medical management of obesity. *Annals of Internal Medicine* 2013;159(8):565-570.

Chapter 1   The Big Picture

1. USDA, Choose MyPlate. Weight Management: Eat the Right Amount of Calories for You. http://www.choosemyplate.gov/weight-management-calories /weight-management/better-choices/amount-calories.html. Accessed June 21, 2015; Executive summary: Guidelines (2013) for the management of overweight and obesity in adults: a report of the American College of Cardiology/American Heart Association Task Force on Practice Guidelines and the Obesity Society published by the Obesity Society and American College of Cardiology/American Heart Association Task Force on Practice Guidelines. Based on a systematic review from the The Obesity Expert Panel, 2013. *Obesity* 2014;22 Suppl 2:S5-39.

2. Ludwig DS. Weight loss strategies for adolescents: a 14-year-old struggling to lose weight. *JAMA* 2012;307(5):498-508; Puhl RM, Latner JD, O'Brien K, Luedicke J, Forhan M, Danielsdottir S. Cross-national perspectives about weight-based bullying in youth: nature, extent and remedies. *Pediatr Obes* 2015 Jul 6. doi: 10.1111/ijpo.12051.

3. Brownell KD, Puhl RM, Schwartz MB, Rudd L (editors). *Weight Bias: Nature, Consequences, and Remedies.* New York: The Guilford Press; 2005.

4. Ebbeling CB, Swain JF, Feldman HA, et al. Effects of dietary composition on energy expenditure during weight-loss maintenance. *JAMA* 2012;307(24): 2627-2634.

5. Weight Watchers. Zero PointsPlus™ Value Food List. http://www.weight watchers.com/util/art/index_art.aspx?tabnum=1&art_id=59781 Accessed June 21, 2015.

6. Ludwig DS, Friedman MI. Always Hungry? Here's Why. *New York Times.* May 16, 2014. http://www.nytimes.com/2014/05/18/opinion/sunday/always-hungry-heres-why.html Accessed June 21, 2015; Ludwig DS, Friedman MI. Increasing adiposity: consequence or cause of overeating? *JAMA* 2014;311(21):2167-2168.

7. Taubes G. What if It's All Been a Big Fat Lie? *New York Times.* July 7, 2012. mailto:http://www.nytimes.com/2002/07/07/magazine/what-if-it-s-all-been-a-big-fat-lie.html Accessed June 21, 2015; Taubes G. *Good Calories, Bad Calories: Fats, Carbs, and the Controversial Science of Diet and Health.* New York: Alfred A. Knopf; 2007; Taubes G. The science of obesity: what do we really know about what makes us fat? An essay by Gary Taubes. *BMJ* 2013;346:f1050.

Chapter 2   The Problem

1. USDA, Choose MyPlate. Weight Management: *Eat the Right Amount of Calories for You.* http://www.choosemyplate.gov/weight-management-calories/weight-management/better-choices/amount-calories.html. Accessed June 21, 2015.

2. Hall KD, Sacks G, Chandramohan D, et al. Quantification of the effect of energy imbalance on bodyweight. *Lancet* 2011;378(9793):826-837.

3. Hill JO, Prentice AM. Sugar and body weight regulation. *AJCN* 1995;62(1 Suppl):264S-273S; discussion 273S-274S.

4. Willett WC, Leibel RL. Dietary fat is not a major determinant of body fat. *AJCN* 2002;113 Suppl 9B:47S-59S; Ludwig DS. Dietary glycemic index and obesity. *Journal of Nutrition.* 2000;130(2S Suppl):280S-283S; Taubes G. Nutrition. The soft science of dietary fat. *Science* 2001;291(5513):2536-2545.

5. Design of the Women's Health Initiative clinical trial and observational study. The Women's Health Initiative Study Group. *Controlled Clinical Trials* 1998;19(1):61-109; Thaul S, Hotra D (editors). Institute of Medicine (US) Committee to Review the NIH Women's Health Initiative. An Assessment of the NIH Women's Health Initiative. Washington DC: National Academies Press; 1993. http://www.ncbi.nlm.nih.gov/books/NBK236518/.

6. McCambridge J, Witton J, Elbourne DR. Systematic review of the Hawthorne effect: new concepts are needed to study research participation effects. *Journal of Clinical Epidemiology* 2014;67(3):267-277.

7. Howard BV, Manson JE, Stefanick ML, et al. Low-fat dietary pattern and weight change over 7 years: the Women's Health Initiative Dietary Modification Trial. *JAMA* 2006;295(1):39-49.

8. Beresford SA, Johnson KC, Ritenbaugh C, et al. Low-fat dietary pattern and risk of colorectal cancer: the Women's Health Initiative Randomized Controlled Dietary Modification Trial. *JAMA* 2006;295(6):643-654; Howard BV, Van Horn L, Hsia J, et al. Low-fat dietary pattern and risk of cardiovascular disease: the Women's Health Initiative Randomized Controlled Dietary Modification Trial. *JAMA* 2006;295(6):655-666; Prentice RL, Caan B, Chlebowski RT, et al. Low-fat dietary pattern and risk of invasive breast cancer: the Women's Health Initiative

Randomized Controlled Dietary Modification Trial. *JAMA* 2006;295(6):629-642; Tinker LF, Bonds DE, Margolis KL, et al. Low-fat dietary pattern and risk of treated diabetes mellitus in postmenopausal women: the Women's Health Initiative randomized controlled dietary modification trial. *Archives of Internal Medicine* 2008;168(14):1500-1511; Noakes TD. The Women's Health Initiative Randomized Controlled Dietary Modification Trial: an inconvenient finding and the diet-heart hypothesis. *South African Medical Journal* 2013;103(11):824-825.

9. Bueno NB, de Melo IS, de Oliveira SL, da Rocha Ataide T. Very-low-carbohydrate ketogenic diet v. low-fat diet for long-term weight loss: a meta-analysis of randomised controlled trials. *The British Journal of Nutrition* 2013;110(7):1178-1187; Nordmann AJ, Suter-Zimmermann K, Bucher HC, et al. Meta-analysis comparing Mediterranean to low-fat diets for modification of cardiovascular risk factors. *The American Journal of Medicine* 2011;124(9):841-851.

10. Atlantis E, Barnes EH, Singh MA. Efficacy of exercise for treating over-weight in children and adolescents: a systematic review. *International Journal of Obesity* 2006;30(7):1027-1040; Boule NG, Haddad E, Kenny GP, Wells GA, Sigal RJ. Effects of exercise on glycemic control and body mass in type 2 diabetes mellitus: a meta-analysis of controlled clinical trials. *JAMA* 2001;286(10):1218-1227; Harris KC, Kuramoto LK, Schulzer M, Retallack JE. Effect of school-based physical activity interventions on body mass index in children: a meta-analysis. *Canadian Medical Association Journal* 2009;180(7):719-726; Thorogood A, Mottillo S, Shimony A, et al. Isolated aerobic exercise and weight loss: a systematic review and meta-analysis of randomized controlled trials. *American Journal of Medicine* 2011;124(8):747-755; Shaw K, Gennat H, O'Rourke P, Del Mar C. Exercise for overweight or obesity. *The Cochrane Database of Systematic Reviews*. 2006(4):CD003817.

11. Melanson EL, Keadle SK, Donnelly JE, Braun B, King NA. Resistance to exercise-induced weight loss: compensatory behavioral adaptations. *Medicine and Science in Sports and Exercise* 2013;45(8):1600-1609; Taubes G. The scientist and the stairmaster: why most of us believe that exercise makes us thinner—and why we're wrong. *New York Magazine* Sept 24, 2007. http://nymag.com/news/sports/38001/ Accessed June 21, 2015.

12. Melanson EL, Keadle SK, Donnelly JE, Braun B, King NA. Resistance to exercise-induced weight loss: compensatory behavioral adaptations. *Medicine and Science in Sports and Exercise* 2013;45(8):1600-1609; Taubes G. The scientist and the stairmaster: why most of us believe that exercise makes us thinner—and why we're wrong. *New York Magazine* Sept 24, 2007. http://nymag.com/news/sports/38001/ Accessed June 21, 2015; Thomas BM, Miller Jr. AT. Adaptations to forced exercise in the rat. *American Journal of Physiology* 1958;193(2):350-354; Hu K, Ivanov P, Chen Z, Hilton MF, Stanley HE, Shea SA. Non-random fluctuations and multi-scale dynamics regulation of human activity. *Physica A* 2004;337(1-2):307-318; Ridgers ND, Timperio A, Cerin E, Salmon J. Compensation of physical activity and sedentary time in primary school children. *Med Sci Sports Exerc* 2014;46(8):1564-9.

13. Thivel D, Aucouturier J, Metz L, Morio B, Duche P. Is there spontaneous energy expenditure compensation in response to intensive exercise in obese youth? *Pediatric obesity* 2014;9(2):147-154.

14. Hjorth MF, Chaput JP, Ritz C, et al. Fatness predicts decreased physical activity and increased sedentary time, but not vice versa: support from a longitudinal study in 8- to 11-year-old children. *International Journal of Obesity* 2014;38(7):959-965; Richmond RC, Davey Smith G, Ness AR, den Hoed M, McMahon G, Timpson NJ. Assessing causality in the association between child adiposity and physical activity levels: a Mendelian randomization analysis. *PLoS Medicine* 2014;11(3):e1001618.

15. Levian C, Ruiz E, Yang X. The pathogenesis of obesity from a genomic and systems biology perspective. *The Yale Journal of Biology and Medicine* 2014; 87(2):113-126.

16. Farooqi IS, Jebb SA, Langmack G, et al. Effects of recombinant leptin therapy in a child with congenital leptin deficiency. *NEJM* 1999;341(12):879-884.

17. Kessler DA. *The End of Overeating: Taking Control of the Insatiable American Appetite.* New York: Rodale Books; 2009; Moss M. *Salt Sugar Fat: How the Food Giants Hooked Us.* New York: Random House; 2013.

18. Sclafani A. Carbohydrate-induced hyperphagia and obesity in the rat: effects of saccharide type, form, and taste. *Neuroscience and Biobehavioral Reviews* 1987;11(2):155-162; Stubbs RJ, Whybrow S. Energy density, diet composition and palatability: influences on overall food energy intake in humans. *Physiology & Behavior* 2004;81(5):755-764.

19. Esposito K, Kastorini CM, Panagiotakos DB, Giugliano D. Mediterranean diet and weight loss: meta-analysis of randomized controlled trials. *Metabolic Syndrome and Related Disorders* 2011;9(1):1-12; Pereira MA, Kartashov AI, Ebbeling CB, et al. Fast-food habits, weight gain, and insulin resistance (the CARDIA study): 15-year prospective analysis. *Lancet* 2005;365(9453):36-42.

20. Bray GA. Obesity Has Always Been with Us: An Historical Introduction. In: Bray GA, Bouchard C (editors). *Handbook of Obesity—Volume 1: Epidemiology, Etiology, and Physiopathology.* 3rd edition. Boca Raton: CRC Press; 2014.

21. Roehling MV, Roehling PV, Odland LM. Investigating the Validity of Stereotypes About Overweight Employees: The Relationship Between Body Weight and Normal Personality Traits. *Group & Organization Management* 2008;33(4):392-424.

22. Flegal KM, Carroll MD, Ogden CL, Johnson CL. Prevalence and trends in obesity among US adults, 1999-2000. *JAMA* 2002;288(14):1723-1727.

23. Ogden CL, Carroll MD, Kit BK, Flegal KM. Prevalence of childhood and adult obesity in the United States, 2011-2012. *JAMA* 2014;311(8):806-814.

24. Ludwig DS. Childhood obesity—the shape of things to come. *NEJM* 2007;357(23):2325-2327; Ludwig DS. Weight loss strategies for adolescents: a 14-year-old struggling to lose weight. *JAMA* 2012;307(5):498-508.

25. Centers for Disease Control and Prevention. *National Diabetes Statistics Report,* 2014. http://www.cdc.gov/diabetes/pubs/statsreport14/national-diabetes -report-web.pdf Accessed June 21, 2015.

26. Williams CD, Stengel J, Asike MI, et al. Prevalence of nonalcoholic fatty liver disease and nonalcoholic steatohepatitis among a largely middle-aged population utilizing ultrasound and liver biopsy: a prospective study. *Gastroenterology* 2011;140(1):124-131.

27. Ludwig DS. Weight loss strategies for adolescents: a 14-year-old struggling to lose weight. *JAMA* 2012;307(5):498-508.

28. Levin BE, Govek E. Gestational obesity accentuates obesity in obesity-prone progeny. *American Journal of Physiology* 1998;275(4 Pt 2):R1374-1379.

29. Ludwig DS, Currie J. The association between pregnancy weight gain and birthweight: a within-family comparison. *Lancet* 2010;376(9745):984-990; Ludwig DS, Rouse HL, Currie J. Pregnancy weight gain and childhood body weight: a within-family comparison. *PLoS Medicine* 2013;10(10):e1001521.

30. Olshansky SJ, Passaro DJ, Hershow RC, et al. A potential decline in life expectancy in the United States in the 21st century. *NEJM* 2005;352(11):1138-1145.

31. Centers for Disease Control and Prevention. Estimated county-level prevalence of diabetes and obesity—United States, 2007. *MMWR* 2009;58(45):1259-1263; Ezzati M, Friedman AB, Kulkarni SC, Murray CJ. The reversal of fortunes: trends in county mortality and cross-county mortality disparities in the United States. *PLoS Medicine* 2008;5(4):e66; Kulkarni SC, Levin-Rector A, Ezzati M, Murray CJ. Falling behind: life expectancy in US counties from 2000 to 2007 in an international context. *Population Health Metrics* 2011;9(1):16 doi: 10.1186/1478-7954-9-16.

32. Cawley J, Meyerhoefer C. The medical care costs of obesity: an instrumental variables approach. *Journal of Health Economics* 2012;31(1):219-230.

33. UnitedHealth, Center for Health Reform & Modernization. *The United States of Diabetes: Challenges and Opportunities in the Decade Ahead.* Working Paper 5, 2010. http://www.unitedhealthgroup.com/~/media/UHG/PDF/2010/UNH-Working-Paper-5.ashx. Accessed June 21, 2015.

34. Kasman M, Hammond RA, Werman A, Mack-Crane A, McKinnon RA. *An In-Depth Look at the Lifetime Economic Cost of Obesity.* May 12, 2015. http://www.brookings.edu/blogs/brookings-now/posts/2015/05/societal-costs-of-obesity. Accessed June 21, 2015.

Chapter 3   The Science

1. What causes obesity? *JAMA* 1924;83(13):1003.

2. Stunkard A, Mc L-HM. The results of treatment for obesity: a review of the literature and report of a series. *Archives of Internal Medicine* 1959;103(1):79-85.

3. Methods for voluntary weight loss and control. NIH Technology Assessment Conference Panel. Consensus Development Conference, 30 March to 1 April 1992. *Annals of Internal Medicine* 1993;119(7 Pt 2):764-770.

4. Kraschnewski JL, Boan J, Esposito J, et al. Long-term weight loss maintenance in the United States. *International Journal of Obesity* 2010;34(11):1644-1654;

Also see: Fildes A, Charlton J, Rudisill C, Littlejohns P, Prevost AT, Gulliford MC. Probability of an obese person attaining normal body weight: cohort study using electronic health records. *Am J Public Health* 2015;105(9):e54-9.

5. Epstein LH, Myers MD, Raynor HA, Saelens BE. Treatment of pediatric obesity. *Pediatrics* 1998;101(3 Pt 2):554-570; McGovern L, Johnson JN, Paulo R, et al. Clinical review: treatment of pediatric obesity: a systematic review and meta-analysis of randomized trials. *Journal of Clinical Endocrinology and Metabolism* 2008;93(12):4600-4605; Muhlig Y, Wabitsch M, Moss A, Hebebrand J. Weight loss in children and adolescents. *Deutsches Arzteblatt International* 2014; 111(48):818-824.

6. Kissileff HR, Thornton JC, Torres MI, et al. Leptin reverses declines in satiation in weight-reduced obese humans. *AJCN* 2012;95(2):309-317; Leibel RL, Rosenbaum M, Hirsch J. Changes in energy expenditure resulting from altered body weight. *NEJM* 1995;332(10):621-628.

7. Leibel RL, Rosenbaum M, Hirsch J. Changes in energy expenditure resulting from altered body weight. *NEJM* 1995;332(10):621-628; Norgan NG, Durnin JV. The effect of 6 weeks of overfeeding on the body weight, body composition, and energy metabolism of young men. *AJCN* 1980;33(5):978-988; Roberts SB, Young VR, Fuss P, et al. Energy expenditure and subsequent nutrient intakes in overfed young men. *American Journal of Physiology* 1990;259(3 Pt 2):R461-469; Sims EA, Goldman RF, Gluck CM, Horton ES, Kelleher PC, Rowe DW. Experimental obesity in man. *Transactions of the Association of American Physicians* 1968; 81:153-170.

8. Ludwig DS, Friedman MI. Increasing adiposity: consequence or cause of overeating? *JAMA* 2014;311(21):2167-2168.

9. Cusin I, Rohner-Jeanrenaud F, Terrettaz J, Jeanrenaud B. Hyperinsulinemia and its impact on obesity and insulin resistance. *International Journal of Obesity and Related Metabolic Disorders* 1992;16 Suppl 4:S1-11; Torbay N, Bracco EF, Geliebter A, Stewart IM, Hashim SA. Insulin increases body fat despite control of food intake and physical activity. *American Journal of Physiology* 1985;248(1 Pt 2): R120-124.

10. Mehran AE, Templeman NM, Brigidi GS, et al. Hyperinsulinemia drives diet-induced obesity independently of brain insulin production. *Cell Metabolism* 2012;16(6):723-737.

11. Le Stunff C, Fallin D, Schork NJ, Bougneres P. The insulin gene VNTR is associated with fasting insulin levels and development of juvenile obesity. *Nature Genetics* 2000;26(4):444-446; Sigal RJ, El-Hashimy M, Martin BC, Soeldner JS, Krolewski AS, Warram JH. Acute postchallenge hyperinsulinemia predicts weight gain: a prospective study. *Diabetes* 1997;46(6):1025-1029.

12. Hansen JB, Arkhammar PO, Bodvarsdottir TB, Wahl P. Inhibition of insulin secretion as a new drug target in the treatment of metabolic disorders. *Current Medicinal Chemistry* 2004;11(12):1595-1615; Mitri J, Hamdy O. Diabetes medications and body weight. *Expert Opinion on Drug Safety* 2009;8(5):573-584.

13. Ludwig DS, Friedman MI. Increasing adiposity: consequence or cause of overeating? *JAMA* 2014;311(21):2167-2168; Ludwig DS. The glycemic index: physiological mechanisms relating to obesity, diabetes, and cardiovascular disease. *JAMA* 2002;287(18):2414-2423.

14. Ludwig DS, Majzoub JA, Al-Zahrani A, Dallal GE, Blanco I, Roberts SB. High glycemic index foods, overeating, and obesity. *Pediatrics* 1999;103(3):E26.

15. Ludwig DS. The glycemic index: physiological mechanisms relating to obesity, diabetes, and cardiovascular disease. *JAMA* 2002;287(18):2414-2423; Campfield LA, Smith FJ, Rosenbaum M, Hirsch J. Human eating: evidence for a physiological basis using a modified paradigm. *Neuroscience and Biobehavioral Reviews* 1996;20(1):133-137; Page KA, Seo D, Belfort-DeAguiar R, et al. Circulating glucose levels modulate neural control of desire for high-calorie foods in humans. *The Journal of Clinical Investigation* 2011;121(10):4161-4169; Pittas AG, Hariharan R, Stark PC, Hajduk CL, Greenberg AS, Roberts SB. Interstitial glucose level is a significant predictor of energy intake in free-living women with healthy body weight. *The Journal of Nutrition* 2005;135(5):1070-1074.

16. Ludwig DS. The glycemic index: physiological mechanisms relating to obesity, diabetes, and cardiovascular disease. *JAMA* 2002;287(18):2414-2423; Ludwig DS. Dietary glycemic index and obesity. *The Journal of Nutrition* 2000;130(2S Suppl):280S-283S; Ludwig DS. Clinical update: the low-glycaemic-index diet. *Lancet* 2007;369(9565):890-892.

17. Lennerz BS, Alsop DC, Holsen LM, et al. Effects of dietary glycemic index on brain regions related to reward and craving in men. *AJCN* 2013;98(3): 641-647.

18. Ebbeling CB, Swain JF, Feldman HA, et al. Effects of dietary composition on energy expenditure during weight-loss maintenance. *JAMA* 2012;307(24): 2627-2634.

19. Pawlak DB, Kushner JA, Ludwig DS. Effects of dietary glycaemic index on adiposity, glucose homoeostasis, and plasma lipids in animals. *Lancet* 2004;364 (9436):778-785.

20. Berryman CE, West SG, Fleming JA, Bordi PL, Kris-Etherton PM. Effects of daily almond consumption on cardiometabolic risk and abdominal adiposity in healthy adults with elevated LDL-cholesterol: a randomized controlled trial. *Journal of the American Heart Association* 2015;4(1):e000993.

21. Mozaffarian D, Hao T, Rimm EB, Willett WC, Hu FB. Changes in diet and lifestyle and long-term weight gain in women and men. *NEJM* 2011;364(25): 2392-2404.

22. Lumeng CN, Saltiel AR. Inflammatory links between obesity and metabolic disease. *The Journal of Clinical Investigation* 2011;121(6):2111-2117; Odegaard JI, Chawla A. Pleiotropic actions of insulin resistance and inflammation in metabolic homeostasis. *Science* 2013;339(6116):172-177; Odegaard JI, Chawla A. The immune system as a sensor of the metabolic state. *Immunity* 2013;38(4):644-654; Pond CM. Adipose tissue and the immune system. *Prostaglandins, Leukotrienes,*

and Essential Fatty Acids 2005;73(1):17-30; Miller LS. Adipocytes armed against Staphylococcus aureus. *NEJM* 2015;372(14):1368-1370.

23. Cildir G, Akincilar SC, Tergaonkar V. Chronic adipose tissue inflammation: all immune cells on the stage. *Trends in Molecular Medicine* 2013;19(8):487-500; Kanneganti TD, Dixit VD. Immunological complications of obesity. *Nature Immunology* 2012;13(8):707-712; Mirsoian A, Bouchlaka MN, Sckisel GD, et al. Adiposity induces lethal cytokine storm after systemic administration of stimulatory immunotherapy regimens in aged mice. *Journal of Experimental Medicine* 2014;211(12):2373-2383; Trayhurn P. Hypoxia and adipose tissue function and dysfunction in obesity. *Physiological Reviews* 2013;93(1):1-21; Winer S, Winer DA. The adaptive immune system as a fundamental regulator of adipose tissue inflammation and insulin resistance. *Immunology and Cell Biology* 2012;90(8):755-762; Glass CK, Olefsky JM. Inflammation and lipid signaling in the etiology of insulin resistance. *Cell Metabolism* 2012;15(5):635-645; Kotas ME, Medzhitov R. Homeostasis, Inflammation, and Disease Susceptibility. *Cell* 2015;160(5):816-827.

24. Bekkering P, Jafri I, van Overveld FJ, Rijkers GT. The intricate association between gut microbiota and development of type 1, type 2 and type 3 diabetes. *Expert Review of Clinical Immunology* 2013;9(11):1031-1041.

25. Johnson AM, Olefsky JM. The origins and drivers of insulin resistance. *Cell* 2013;152(4):673-684; Shulman GI. Ectopic fat in insulin resistance, dyslipidemia, and cardiometabolic disease. *NEJM* 2014;371(23):2237-2238; Suganami T, Tanaka M, Ogawa Y. Adipose tissue inflammation and ectopic lipid accumulation. *Endocrine Journal* 2012;59(10):849-857.

26. Arruda AP, Milanski M, Velloso LA. Hypothalamic inflammation and thermogenesis: the brown adipose tissue connection. *Journal of Bioenergetics and Biomembranes* 2011;43(1):53-58; Cai D. Neuroinflammation and neurodegeneration in overnutrition-induced diseases. *Trends in Endocrinology and Metabolism* 2013;24(1):40-47; Pimentel GD, Ganeshan K, Carvalheira JB. Hypothalamic inflammation and the central nervous system control of energy homeostasis. *Molecular and Cellular Endocrinology* 2014;397(1-2):15-22; Thaler JP, Yi CX, Schur EA, et al. Obesity is associated with hypothalamic injury in rodents and humans. *Journal of Clinical Investigation* 2012;122(1):153-162; Williams LM. Hypothalamic dysfunction in obesity. *Proceedings of the Nutrition Society* 2012;71(4):521-533.

27. Thaler JP, Yi CX, Schur EA, et al. Obesity is associated with hypothalamic injury in rodents and humans. *Journal of Clinical Investigation* 2012;122(1):153-162; Kleinridders A, Schenten D, Konner AC, et al. MyD88 signaling in the CNS is required for development of fatty acid-induced leptin resistance and diet-induced obesity. *Cell Metabolism* 2009;10(4):249-259; Maric T, Woodside B, Luheshi GN. The effects of dietary saturated fat on basal hypothalamic neuroinflammation in rats. *Brain, Behavior, and Immunity* 2014;36:35-45.

28. Thaler JP, Yi CX, Schur EA, et al. Obesity is associated with hypothalamic injury in rodents and humans. *Journal of Clinical Investigation* 2012;122(1):153-162; Cazettes F, Cohen JI, Yau PL, Talbot H, Convit A. Obesity-mediated

inflammation may damage the brain circuit that regulates food intake. *Brain Research* 2011;1373:101-109.

29. Ligibel JA, Alfano CM, Courneya KS, et al. American Society of Clinical Oncology position statement on obesity and cancer. *Journal of Clinical Oncology* 2014;32(31):3568-3574.

30. Berrington de Gonzalez A, Hartge P, Cerhan JR, et al. Body-mass index and mortality among 1.46 million white adults. *NEJM* 2010;363(23):2211-2219; Global Burden of Metabolic Risk Factors for Chronic Diseases Collaboration, Lu Y, Hajifathalian K, et al. Metabolic mediators of the effects of body-mass index, overweight, and obesity on coronary heart disease and stroke: a pooled analysis of 97 prospective cohorts with 1.8 million participants. *Lancet* 2014;383(9921):970-983; Tirosh A, Shai I, Afek A, et al. Adolescent BMI trajectory and risk of diabetes versus coronary disease. *NEJM* 2011;364(14):1315-1325; Tobias DK, Pan A, Jackson CL, et al. Body-mass index and mortality among adults with incident type 2 diabetes. *NEJM* 2014;370(3):233-244.

31. Bell JA, Hamer M, Sabia S, Singh-Manoux A, Batty D, Kivimaki M. The Natural Course of Healthy Obesity Over 20 Years. *J Am Col Card* 2015;65(1):101-102; Hamer M, Stamatakis E. Metabolically healthy obesity and risk of all-cause and cardiovascular disease mortality. *Journal of Clinical Endocrinology and Metabolism* 2012;97(7):2482-2488.

32. Ruderman N, Chisholm D, Pi-Sunyer X, Schneider S. The metabolically obese, normal-weight individual revisited. *Diabetes* 1998;47(5):699-713; Thomas EL, Parkinson JR, Frost GS, et al. The missing risk: MRI and MRS phenotyping of abdominal adiposity and ectopic fat. *Obesity* 2012;20(1):76-87; Wildman RP, Muntner P, Reynolds K, et al. The obese without cardiometabolic risk factor clustering and the normal weight with cardiometabolic risk factor clustering: prevalence and correlates of 2 phenotypes among the US population (NHANES 1999-2004). *Archives of Internal Medicine* 2008;168(15):1617-1624.

33. Look AHEAD Research Group, Wing RR, Bolin P, et al. Cardiovascular effects of intensive lifestyle intervention in type 2 diabetes. *NEJM* 2013;369(2):145-154.

34. Estruch R, Ros E, Salas-Salvado J, et al. Primary prevention of cardiovascular disease with a Mediterranean diet. *NEJM* 2013;368(14):1279-1290.

35. Gearhardt AN, Davis C, Kuschner R, Brownell KD. The addiction potential of hyperpalatable foods. *Current Drug Abuse Reviews* 2011;4(3):140-145.

36. Lasselin J, Capuron L. Chronic low-grade inflammation in metabolic disorders: relevance for behavioral symptoms. *Neuroimmunomodulation* 2014;21(2-3):95-101.

37. Benton D, Ruffin MP, Lassel T, et al. The delivery rate of dietary carbohydrates affects cognitive performance in both rats and humans. *Psychopharmacology* 2003;166(1):86-90.

38. Papanikolaou Y, Palmer H, Binns MA, Jenkins DJ, Greenwood CE. Better cognitive performance following a low-glycaemic-index compared with a

high-glycaemic-index carbohydrate meal in adults with type 2 diabetes. *Diabetologia* 2006;49(5):855-862.

39. Szabo L. NIH Director: Budget Cuts Put U.S. Science at Risk. *USA Today* April 23, 2014. http://www.usatoday.com/story/news/nation/2014/04/23/nih -budget-cuts/8056113/ Accessed June 22, 2015; Federation of American Societies for Experimental Biology. Sustaining discovery in biological and medical sciences – a framework for discussion. Bethesa, MD; 2015. http://www.faseb.org/Sustaining Discovery/Home.aspx Accessed August 9, 2015.

40. Shai I, Schwarzfuchs D, Henkin Y, et al. Weight loss with a low-carbohydrate, Mediterranean, or low-fat diet. *NEJM* 2008;359(3):229-241.

41. Slavin J. Two more pieces to the 1000-piece carbohydrate puzzle. *AJCN* 2014;100(1):4-5.

42. Mozaffarian D, Ludwig DS. Dietary guidelines in the 21st century—a time for food. *JAMA* 2010;304(6):681-682.

Chapter 4   *The Solution*

1. Kelly RL. *The Foraging Spectrum: Diversity in Hunter-Gatherer Lifeways.* Clinton Corners, NY: Percheron Press; 2007.

2. Ludwig DS. The glycemic index: physiological mechanisms relating to obesity, diabetes, and cardiovascular disease. *JAMA* 2002;287(18):2414-2423; Unger RH, Orci L. Physiology and pathophysiology of glucagon. *Physiological Reviews* 1976;56(4):778-826.

3. Bilsborough S, Mann N. A review of issues of dietary protein intake in humans. *International Journal of Sport Nutrition and Exercise Metabolism* 2006; 16(2):129-152.

4. Feinman RD, Pogozelski WK, Astrup A, et al. Dietary carbohydrate restriction as the first approach in diabetes management: Critical review and evidence base. *Nutrition* 2015;31(1):1-13; Paoli A, Rubini A, Volek JS, Grimaldi KA. Beyond weight loss: a review of the therapeutic uses of very-low-carbohydrate (ketogenic) diets. *European Journal of Clinical Nutrition* 2013;67(8):789-796.

5. Cahill GF, Jr., Veech RL. Ketoacids? Good medicine? *Transactions of the American Clinical and Climatological Association.* 2003;114:149-161; Newman JC, Verdin E. beta-hydroxybutyrate: Much more than a metabolite. *Diabetes Research and Clinical Practice* 2014;106(2):173-181.

6. Ludwig DS. The glycemic index: physiological mechanisms relating to obesity, diabetes, and cardiovascular disease. *JAMA* 2002;287(18):2414-2423; Jenkins DJ, Wolever TM, Taylor RH, et al. Glycemic index of foods: a physiological basis for carbohydrate exchange. *AJCN* 1981;34(3):362-366; Wolever TM, Jenkins DJ, Jenkins AL, Josse RG. The glycemic index: methodology and clinical implications. *AJCN* 1991;54(5):846-854; Atkinson FS, Foster-Powell K, Brand-Miller JC. International tables of glycemic index and glycemic load values: 2008. *Diabetes Care* 2008;31(12):2281-2283.

7. Ludwig DS. The glycemic index: physiological mechanisms relating to obesity, diabetes, and cardiovascular disease. *JAMA* 2002;287(18):2414-2423; Atkinson FS, Foster-Powell K, Brand-Miller JC. International tables of glycemic index and glycemic load values: 2008. *Diabetes Care* 2008;31(12):2281-2283; Ludwig DS. Glycemic load comes of age. *The Journal of Nutrition* 2003;133(9):2695-2696.

8. Fleming P, Godwin M. Low-glycaemic index diets in the management of blood lipids: a systematic review and meta-analysis. *Family Practice* 2013;30(5):485-491; Goff LM, Cowland DE, Hooper L, Frost GS. Low glycaemic index diets and blood lipids: a systematic review and meta-analysis of randomised controlled trials. *Nutrition, Metabolism, and Cardiovascular Diseases* 2013; 23(1):1-10; Livesey G, Taylor R, Hulshof T, Howlett J. Glycemic response and health—a systematic review and meta-analysis: relations between dietary glycemic properties and health outcomes. *AJCN* 2008;87(1):258S-268S; Ludwig DS. Clinical update: the low-glycaemic-index diet. *Lancet* 2007;369(9565):890-892; Schwingshackl L, Hoffmann G. Long-term effects of low glycemic index/load vs. high glycemic index/load diets on parameters of obesity and obesity-associated risks: a systematic review and meta-analysis. *Nutrition, Metabolism, and Cardiovascular Diseases* 2013;23(8):699-706.

9. Larsen TM, Dalskov SM, van Baak M, et al. Diets with high or low protein content and glycemic index for weight-loss maintenance. *NEJM* 2010;363(22): 2102-2113; Ludwig DS, Ebbeling CB. Weight-loss maintenance—mind over matter? *NEJM* 2010;363(22):2159-2161.

10. Bhupathiraju SN, Tobias DK, Malik VS, et al. Glycemic index, glycemic load, and risk of type 2 diabetes: results from 3 large US cohorts and an updated meta-analysis. *AJCN* 2014;100(1):218-232.

11. Liu S, Willett WC, Stampfer MJ, et al. A prospective study of dietary glycemic load, carbohydrate intake, and risk of coronary heart disease in US women. *AJCN* 2000;71(6):1455-1461.

12. Chiasson JL, Josse RG, Gomis R, et al. Acarbose treatment and the risk of cardiovascular disease and hypertension in patients with impaired glucose tolerance: the STOP-NIDDM trial. *JAMA* 2003;290(4):486-494.

13. Barclay AW, Petocz P, McMillan-Price J, et al. Glycemic index, glycemic load, and chronic disease risk—a meta-analysis of observational studies. *AJCN* 2008;87(3):627-637; Dong JY, Qin LQ. Dietary glycemic index, glycemic load, and risk of breast cancer: meta-analysis of prospective cohort studies. *Breast Cancer Research and Treatment* 2011;126(2):287-294; Gnagnarella P, Gandini S, La Vecchia C, Maisonneuve P. Glycemic index, glycemic load, and cancer risk: a meta-analysis. *AJCN* 2008;87(6):1793-1801; Nagle CM, Olsen CM, Ibiebele TI, et al. Glycemic index, glycemic load and endometrial cancer risk: results from the Australian National Endometrial Cancer study and an updated systematic review and meta-analysis. *European Journal of Nutrition* 2013;52(2):705-715; Rossi M, Turati F, Lagiou P, Trichopoulos D, La Vecchia C, Trichopoulou A. Relation of dietary glycemic load with ischemic and hemorrhagic stroke: a cohort study in

Greece and a meta-analysis. *European Journal of Nutrition* 2014;54(2)215-222; Valtuena S, Pellegrini N, Ardigo D, et al. Dietary glycemic index and liver steatosis. *AJCN* 2006;84(1):136-142; Biddinger SB, Ludwig DS. The insulin-like growth factor axis: a potential link between glycemic index and cancer. *AJCN* 2005;82(2):277-278; Gangwisch JE, Hale L, Garcia L, et al. High glycemic index diet as a risk factor for depression: analyses from the Women's Health Initiative. *AJCN* 2015;102(2):454-63.

14. Sacks FM, Carey VJ, Anderson CA, et al. Effects of high vs low glycemic index of dietary carbohydrate on cardiovascular disease risk factors and insulin sensitivity: the OmniCarb randomized clinical trial. *JAMA* 2014;312(23):2531-2541.

15. Ludwig DS, Astrup A, Willett WC. The glycemic index: Reports of its demise have been exaggerated. *Obesity* 2015;23(7):1327-1328.

16. Brownlee IA, Moore C, Chatfield M, et al. Markers of cardiovascular risk are not changed by increased whole-grain intake: the WHOLEheart study, a randomised, controlled dietary intervention. *British Journal of Nutrition* 2010;104(1):125-134.

17. Ludwig DS. The glycemic index: physiological mechanisms relating to obesity, diabetes, and cardiovascular disease. *JAMA* 2002;287(18):2414-2423; Fleming P, Godwin M. Low-glycaemic index diets in the management of blood lipids: a systematic review and meta-analysis. *Family Practice* 2013;30(5):485-491; Livesey G, Taylor R, Hulshof T, Howlett J. Glycemic response and health—a systematic review and meta-analysis: relations between dietary glycemic properties and health outcomes. *AJCN* 2008;87(1):258S-268S; Ludwig DS. Clinical update: the low-glycaemic-index diet. *Lancet* 2007;369(9565):890-892; Schwingshackl L, Hoffmann G. Long-term effects of low glycemic index/load vs. high glycemic index/load diets on parameters of obesity and obesity-associated risks: a systematic review and meta-analysis. *Nutrition, Metabolism, and Cardiovascular Diseases* 2013;23(8):699-706; Wolever TM. Is glycaemic index (GI) a valid measure of carbohydrate quality? *European Journal of Clinical Nutrition* 2013;67(5):522-531.

18. Ludwig DS, Ebbeling CB, Livingston EH. Surgical vs lifestyle treatment for type 2 diabetes. *JAMA* 2012;308(10):981-982.

19. Pereira MA, Kartashov AI, Ebbeling CB, et al. Fast-food habits, weight gain, and insulin resistance (the CARDIA study): 15-year prospective analysis. *Lancet* 2005;365(9453):36-42.

20. Poti JM, Mendez MA, Ng SW, Popkin BM. Is the degree of food processing and convenience linked with the nutritional quality of foods purchased by US households? *AJCN* 2015;101(6):1251-1262.

21. Taubes G. Nutrition. The soft science of dietary fat. *Science* 2001;291(5513):2536-2545.

22. Mozaffarian D, Willett WC. Trans fatty acids and cardiovascular risk: a unique cardiometabolic imprint? *Current Atherosclerosis Reports* 2007;9(6):486-493.

23. Ascherio A, Willett WC. Health effects of trans fatty acids. *AJCN* 1997;66(4 Suppl):1006S-1010S.

24. Hu FB. Are refined carbohydrates worse than saturated fat? *AJCN* 2010;91(6):1541-1542; Siri-Tarino PW, Sun Q, Hu FB, Krauss RM. Saturated fat, carbohydrate, and cardiovascular disease. *AJCN* 2010;91(3):502-509.

25. Jakobsen MU, Dethlefsen C, Joensen AM, et al. Intake of carbohydrates compared with intake of saturated fatty acids and risk of myocardial infarction: importance of the glycemic index. *AJCN* 2010;91(6):1764-1768.

26. Hu FB. Are refined carbohydrates worse than saturated fat? *AJCN* 2010;91(6):1541-1542.

27. Chowdhury R, Warnakula S, Kunutsor S, et al. Association of dietary, circulating, and supplement fatty acids with coronary risk: a systematic review and meta-analysis. *Annals of Internal Medicine* 2014;160(6):398-406; Siri-Tarino PW, Sun Q, Hu FB, Krauss RM. Meta-analysis of prospective cohort studies evaluating the association of saturated fat with cardiovascular disease. *AJCN* 2010;91(3):535-546.

28. Mozaffarian D, Micha R, Wallace S. Effects on coronary heart disease of increasing polyunsaturated fat in place of saturated fat: a systematic review and meta-analysis of randomized controlled trials. *PLoS Medicine* 2010;7(3):e1000252.

29. Gillingham LG, Harris-Janz S, Jones PJ. Dietary monounsaturated fatty acids are protective against metabolic syndrome and cardiovascular disease risk factors. *Lipids* 2011;46(3):209-228.

30. Lopez S, Bermudez B, Ortega A, et al. Effects of meals rich in either monounsaturated or saturated fat on lipid concentrations and on insulin secretion and action in subjects with high fasting triglyceride concentrations. *AJCN* 2011;93(3):494-499; Nicholls SJ, Lundman P, Harmer JA, et al. Consumption of saturated fat impairs the anti-inflammatory properties of high-density lipoproteins and endothelial function. *Journal of the American College of Cardiology* 2006;48(4):715-720; Raz O, Steinvil A, Berliner S, Rosenzweig T, Justo D, Shapira I. The effect of two iso-caloric meals containing equal amounts of fats with a different fat composition on the inflammatory and metabolic markers in apparently healthy volunteers. *Journal of Inflammation* 2013;10(1):3 doi:10.1186/1476-9255-10-3; Uusitupa M, Schwab U, Makimattila S, et al. Effects of two high-fat diets with different fatty acid compositions on glucose and lipid metabolism in healthy young women. *AJCN* 1994;59(6):1310-1316; Xiao C, Giacca A, Carpentier A, Lewis GF. Differential effects of monounsaturated, polyunsaturated and saturated fat ingestion on glucose-stimulated insulin secretion, sensitivity and clearance in overweight and obese, non-diabetic humans. *Diabetologia* 2006;49(6):1371-1379.

31. Cintra DE, Ropelle ER, Moraes JC, et al. Unsaturated fatty acids revert diet-induced hypothalamic inflammation in obesity. *PloS One* 2012;7(1):e30571; Huang S, Rutkowsky JM, Snodgrass RG, et al. Saturated fatty acids activate TLR-mediated proinflammatory signaling pathways. *Journal of Lipid Research* 2012;53(9):2002-2013; Lichtenstein L, Mattijssen F, de Wit NJ, et al. Angptl4 protects against severe proinflammatory effects of saturated fat by inhibiting fatty acid uptake into mesenteric lymph node macrophages. *Cell Metabolism*

2010;12(6):580-592; Maric T, Woodside B, Luheshi GN. The effects of dietary saturated fat on basal hypothalamic neuroinflammation in rats. *Brain, Behavior, and Immunity* 2014;36:35-45; Poledne R. A new atherogenic effect of saturated fatty acids. *Physiological Research* 2013;62(2):139-143; Vijay-Kumar M, Vanegas SM, Patel N, Aitken JD, Ziegler TR, Ganji V. Fish oil rich diet in comparison to saturated fat rich diet offered protection against lipopolysaccharide-induced inflammation and insulin resistance in mice. *Nutrition & Metabolism* 2011;8(1):16 doi: 10.1186/1743-7075-8-16; Williams LM. Hypothalamic dysfunction in obesity. *The Proceedings of the Nutrition Society* 2012;71(4):521-533.

32. Rosqvist F, Iggman D, Kullberg J, et al. Overfeeding polyunsaturated and saturated fat causes distinct effects on liver and visceral fat accumulation in humans. *Diabetes* 2014;63(7):2356-2368.

33. Kien CL, Bunn JY, Tompkins CL, et al. Substituting dietary monounsaturated fat for saturated fat is associated with increased daily physical activity and resting energy expenditure and with changes in mood. *AJCN* 2013;97(4):689-697.

34. de Oliveira Otto MC, Mozaffarian D, Kromhout D, et al. Dietary intake of saturated fat by food source and incident cardiovascular disease: the Multi-Ethnic Study of Atherosclerosis. *AJCN* 2012;96(2):397-404; de Oliveira Otto MC, Nettleton JA, Lemaitre RN, et al. Biomarkers of dairy fatty acids and risk of cardiovascular disease in the Multi-ethnic Study of Atherosclerosis. *Journal of the American Heart Association* 2013;2(4):e000092; Lawrence GD. Dietary fats and health: dietary recommendations in the context of scientific evidence. *Advances in Nutrition* 2013;4(3):294-302.

35. Ludwig DS, Jenkins DJ. Carbohydrates and the postprandial state: have our cake and eat it too? *AJCN* 2004;80(4):797-798; Volk BM, Kunces LJ, Freidenreich DJ, et al. Effects of step-wise increases in dietary carbohydrate on circulating saturated fatty acids and palmitoleic acid in adults with metabolic syndrome. *PloS One.* 2014;9(11):e113605.

36. Itariu BK, Zeyda M, Hochbrugger EE, et al. Long-chain n-3 PUFAs reduce adipose tissue and systemic inflammation in severely obese nondiabetic patients: a randomized controlled trial. *AJCN* 2012;96(5):1137-1149; Titos E, Claria J. Omega-3-derived mediators counteract obesity-induced adipose tissue inflammation. *Prostaglandins & Other Lipid Mediators* 2013;107:77-84; White PJ, Marette A. Potential role of omega-3-derived resolution mediators in metabolic inflammation. *Immunology and Cell Biology* 2014;92(4):324-330.

37. Cordain L, Watkins BA, Florant GL, Kelher M, Rogers L, Li Y. Fatty acid analysis of wild ruminant tissues: evolutionary implications for reducing diet-related chronic disease. *European Journal of Clinical Nutrition* 2002;56(3):181-191.

38. Halton TL, Willett WC, Liu S, et al. Low-carbohydrate-diet score and the risk of coronary heart disease in women. *NEJM* 2006;355(19):1991-2002.

39. Harland JI, Haffner TA. Systematic review, meta-analysis and regression of randomised controlled trials reporting an association between an intake of circa 25 g soya protein per day and blood cholesterol. *Atherosclerosis* 2008;200(1):13-27;

Jenkins DJ, Kendall CW, Marchie A, et al. The Garden of Eden—plant based diets, the genetic drive to conserve cholesterol and its implications for heart disease in the 21st century. *Comparative Biochemistry and Physiology. Part A, Molecular & Integrative Physiology* 2003;136(1):141-151; Sanchez A, Hubbard RW, Hilton GF. Hypocholesterolemic amino acids and the insulin glucagon ratio. *Monographs on Atherosclerosis* 1990;16:126-138.

40. Tremaroli V, Backhed F. Functional interactions between the gut microbiota and host metabolism. *Nature* 2012;489(7415):242-249.

41. Clemente JC, Ursell LK, Parfrey LW, Knight R. The impact of the gut microbiota on human health: an integrative view. *Cell* 2012;148(6):1258-1270; Musso G, Gambino R, Cassader M. Obesity, diabetes, and gut microbiota: the hygiene hypothesis expanded? *Diabetes care* 2010;33(10):2277-2284; Schnorr SL, Candela M, Rampelli S, et al. Gut microbiome of the Hadza hunter-gatherers. *Nature Communications* 2014;5:3654 doi:10.1038/ncomms4654.

42. Belkaid Y, Hand TW. Role of the microbiota in immunity and inflammation. *Cell* 2014;157(1):121-141; Burcelin R. Regulation of metabolism: a cross talk between gut microbiota and its human host. *Physiology* 2012;27(5):300-307; Campbell AK, Matthews SB, Vassel N, et al. Bacterial metabolic 'toxins': a new mechanism for lactose and food intolerance, and irritable bowel syndrome. *Toxicology* 2010;278(3):268-276; Cani PD, Amar J, Iglesias MA, et al. Metabolic endotoxemia initiates obesity and insulin resistance. *Diabetes* 2007;56(7):1761-1772; Caricilli AM, Saad MJ. The role of gut microbiota on insulin resistance. *Nutrients* 2013;5(3):829-851; Ding S, Lund PK. Role of intestinal inflammation as an early event in obesity and insulin resistance. *Current Opinion in Clinical Nutrition and Metabolic Care* 2011;14(4):328-333; Fasano A. Zonulin and its regulation of intestinal barrier function: the biological door to inflammation, autoimmunity, and cancer. *Physiological Reviews* 2011;91(1):151-175; Lam YY, Mitchell AJ, Holmes AJ, et al. Role of the gut in visceral fat inflammation and metabolic disorders. *Obesity* 2011;19(11):2113-2120.

43. Belkaid Y, Hand TW. Role of the microbiota in immunity and inflammation. *Cell* 2014;157(1):121-141; Fasano A. Zonulin and its regulation of intestinal barrier function: the biological door to inflammation, autoimmunity, and cancer. *Physiological Reviews* 2011;91(1):151-175; Bekkering P, Jafri I, van Overveld FJ, Rijkers GT. The intricate association between gut microbiota and development of type 1, type 2 and type 3 diabetes. *Expert Review of Clinical Immunology* 2013;9(11):1031-1041; De Vadder F, Kovatcheva-Datchary P, Goncalves D, et al. Microbiota-generated metabolites promote metabolic benefits via gut-brain neural circuits. *Cell* 2014;156(1-2):84-96; Lasselin J, Capuron L. Chronic low-grade inflammation in metabolic disorders: relevance for behavioral symptoms. *Neuroimmunomodulation* 2014;21(2-3):95-101; Walsh CJ, Guinane CM, O'Toole PW, Cotter PD. Beneficial modulation of the gut microbiota. *FEBS Letters* 2014;588(22):4120-4130.

44. Caricilli AM, Saad MJ. The role of gut microbiota on insulin resistance. *Nutrients* 2013;5(3):829-851; Ley RE, Turnbaugh PJ, Klein S, Gordon JI. Microbial

ecology: human gut microbes associated with obesity. *Nature* 2006;444(7122):1022-1023; Turnbaugh PJ, Ley RE, Mahowald MA, Magrini V, Mardis ER, Gordon JI. An obesity-associated gut microbiome with increased capacity for energy harvest. *Nature* 2006;444(7122):1027-1031.

45. Le Chatelier E, Nielsen T, Qin J, et al. Richness of human gut microbiome correlates with metabolic markers. *Nature* 2013;500(7464):541-546.

46. Ridaura VK, Faith JJ, Rey FE, et al. Gut microbiota from twins discordant for obesity modulate metabolism in mice. *Science* 2013;341(6150):1241214 doi: 10.1126/science.1241214.

47. Cardona F, Andres-Lacueva C, Tulipani S, Tinahones FJ, Queipo-Ortuno MI. Benefits of polyphenols on gut microbiota and implications in human health. *Journal of Nutritional Biochemistry* 2013;24(8):1415-1422; Etxeberria U, Fernandez-Quintela A, Milagro FI, Aguirre L, Martinez JA, Portillo MP. Impact of polyphenols and polyphenol-rich dietary sources on gut microbiota composition. *Journal of Agricultural and Food Chemistry* 2013;61(40):9517-9533.

48. Fernandez-Garcia JC, Cardona F, Tinahones FJ. Inflammation, oxidative stress and metabolic syndrome: dietary modulation. *Current Vascular Pharmacology* 2013;11(6):906-919; Leiherer A, Mundlein A, Drexel H. Phytochemicals and their impact on adipose tissue inflammation and diabetes. *Vascular pharmacology* 2013;58(1-2):3-20; Selhub EM, Logan AC, Bested AC. Fermented foods, microbiota, and mental health: ancient practice meets nutritional psychiatry. *Journal of physiological anthropology* 2014;33:2; Siriwardhana N, Kalupahana NS, Cekanova M, LeMieux M, Greer B, Moustaid-Moussa N. Modulation of adipose tissue inflammation by bioactive food compounds. *The Journal of Nutritional Biochemistry* 2013;24(4):613-623.

49. Cross ML, Stevenson LM, Gill HS. Anti-allergy properties of fermented foods: an important immunoregulatory mechanism of lactic acid bacteria? *International Immunopharmacology* 2001;1(5):891-901; Parvez S, Malik KA, Ah Kang S, Kim HY. Probiotics and their fermented food products are beneficial for health. *Journal of Applied Microbiology* 2006;100(6):1171-1185; van Hylckama Vlieg JE, Veiga P, Zhang C, Derrien M, Zhao L. Impact of microbial transformation of food on health—from fermented foods to fermentation in the gastro-intestinal tract. *Current Opinion in Biotechnology* 2011;22(2):211-219; Kim EK, An SY, Lee MS, et al. Fermented kimchi reduces body weight and improves metabolic parameters in overweight and obese patients. *Nutrition Research* 2011;31(6):436-443; Makino S, Ikegami S, Kume A, Horiuchi H, Sasaki H, Orii N. Reducing the risk of infection in the elderly by dietary intake of yoghurt fermented with Lactobacillus delbrueckii ssp. bulgaricus OLL1073R-1. *British Journal of Nutrition* 2010;104(7):998-1006; Seppo L, Jauhiainen T, Poussa T, Korpela R. A fermented milk high in bioactive peptides has a blood pressure-lowering effect in hypertensive subjects. *AJCN* 2003;77(2):326-330; Tillisch K, Labus J, Kilpatrick L, et al. Consumption of fermented milk product with probiotic modulates brain activity. *Gastroenterology* 2013;144(7):1394-1401.

50. Chassaing B, Koren O, Goodrich JK, et al. Dietary emulsifiers impact the mouse gut microbiota promoting colitis and metabolic syndrome. *Nature* 2015; 519(7541):92-6.

51. Hill JO, Prentice AM. Sugar and body weight regulation. *AJCN* 1995;62(1 Suppl):264S-273S; discussion 273S-274S.

52. Lustig RH, Schmidt LA, Brindis CD. Public health: The toxic truth about sugar. *Nature* 2012;482(7383):27-29.

53. Duffey KJ, Popkin BM. Shifts in patterns and consumption of beverages between 1965 and 2002. *Obesity* 2007;15(11):2739-2747.

54. Stanhope KL. Role of fructose-containing sugars in the epidemics of obesity and metabolic syndrome. *Annual Review of Medicine* 2012;63:329-343.

55. Vos MB, Kimmons JE, Gillespie C, Welsh J, Blanck HM. Dietary fructose consumption among US children and adults: the Third National Health and Nutrition Examination Survey. *Medscape Journal of Medicine* 2008;10(7):160.

56. He FJ, Nowson CA, Lucas M, MacGregor GA. Increased consumption of fruit and vegetables is related to a reduced risk of coronary heart disease: meta-analysis of cohort studies. *Journal of Human Hypertension* 2007;21(9):717-728; Mozaffarian D, Hao T, Rimm EB, Willett WC, Hu FB. Changes in diet and lifestyle and long-term weight gain in women and men. *NEJM* 2011;364(25):2392-2404; Muraki I, Imamura F, Manson JE, et al. Fruit consumption and risk of type 2 diabetes: results from three prospective longitudinal cohort studies. *BMJ* 2013;347:f5001; Wang X, Ouyang Y, Liu J, et al. Fruit and vegetable consumption and mortality from all causes, cardiovascular disease, and cancer: systematic review and dose-response meta-analysis of prospective cohort studies. *BMJ* 2014;349:g4490.

57. Meyer BJ, de Bruin EJ, Du Plessis DG, van der Merwe M, Meyer AC. Some biochemical effects of a mainly fruit diet in man. *South African Medical Journal* 1971;45(10):253-261; Meyer BJ, van der Merwe M, Du Plessis DG, de Bruin EJ, Meyer AC. Some physiological effects of a mainly fruit diet in man. *South African Medical Journal* 1971;45(8):191-195.

58. Ludwig DS. Examining the health effects of fructose. *JAMA* 2013;310(1): 33-34.

59. Fry AJ. The effect of a 'sucrose-free' diet on oral glucose tolerance in man. *Nutrition and Metabolism* 1972;14(5):313-323.

60. Dunnigan MG, Fyfe T, McKiddie MT, Crosbie SM. The effects of isocaloric exchange of dietary starch and sucrose on glucose tolerance, plasma insulin and serum lipids in man. *Clinical Science* 1970;38(1):1-9.

61. Ludwig DS. Artificially sweetened beverages: cause for concern. *JAMA* 2009;302(22):2477-2478.

62. Pepino MY, Tiemann CD, Patterson BW, Wice BM, Klein S. Sucralose affects glycemic and hormonal responses to an oral glucose load. *Diabetes Care* 2013;36(9):2530-2535.

63. Simon BR, Learman BS, Parlee SD, et al. Sweet taste receptor deficient mice have decreased adiposity and increased bone mass. *PloS One* 2014;9(1):e86454;

Simon BR, Parlee SD, Learman BS, et al. Artificial sweeteners stimulate adipogenesis and suppress lipolysis independently of sweet taste receptors. *Journal of Biological Chemistry* 2013;288(45):32475-32489.

64. Jacobson MF. *Salt Assault: Brand-Name Comparisons of Processed Foods.* Third Edition, 2013. Center for Science in the Public Interest. http://cspinet.org/salt/Salt-Assault-3rd-Edition.pdf Accessed June 21, 2015; U.S. Department of Agriculture and U.S. Department of Health and Human Services. *Dietary Guidelines for Americans, 2010.* Washington, DC: U.S. Government Printing Office; 2010. http://www.health.gov/dietaryguidelines/2010.asp Accessed June 21, 2015.

65. Adler GK, Moore TJ, Hollenberg NK, Williams GH. Changes in adrenal responsiveness and potassium balance with shifts in sodium intake. *Endocrine Research* 1987;13(4):419-445.

66. Frigolet ME, Torres N, Tovar AR. The renin-angiotensin system in adipose tissue and its metabolic consequences during obesity. *Journal of Nutritional Biochemistry* 2013;24(12):2003-2015; Henriksen EJ, Prasannarong M. The role of the renin-angiotensin system in the development of insulin resistance in skeletal muscle. *Molecular and Cellular Endocrinology* 2013;378(1-2):15-22; Jing F, Mogi M, Horiuchi M. Role of renin-angiotensin-aldosterone system in adipose tissue dysfunction. *Molecular and Cellular Endocrinology* 2013;378(1-2):23-28; Marcus Y, Shefer G, Stern N. Adipose tissue renin-angiotensin-aldosterone system (RAAS) and progression of insulin resistance. *Molecular and Cellular Endocrinology* 2013;378(1-2):1-14; Underwood PC, Adler GK. The renin angiotensin aldosterone system and insulin resistance in humans. *Current Hypertension Reports* 2013;15(1):59-70.

67. Graudal NA, Hubeck-Graudal T, Jurgens G. Effects of low-sodium diet vs. high-sodium diet on blood pressure, renin, aldosterone, catecholamines, cholesterol, and triglyceride (Cochrane Review). *American Journal of Hypertension* 2012; 25(1):1-15.

68. O'Donnell M, Mente A, Rangarajan S, et al. Urinary sodium and potassium excretion, mortality, and cardiovascular events. *NEJM* 2014;371(7):612-623.

69. DiNicolantonio JJ, O'Keefe JH, Lucan SC. An unsavory truth: sugar, more than salt, predisposes to hypertension and chronic disease. *The American Journal of Cardiology* 2014;114(7):1126-1128.

70. Appel LJ, Sacks FM, Carey VJ, et al. Effects of protein, monounsaturated fat, and carbohydrate intake on blood pressure and serum lipids: results of the OmniHeart randomized trial. *JAMA* 2005;294(19):2455-2464.

71. Bernstein AM, Willett WC. Trends in 24-h urinary sodium excretion in the United States, 1957-2003: a systematic review. *AJCN* 2010;92(5):1172-1180.

72. Simmons AL, Schlezinger JJ, Corkey BE. What Are We Putting in Our Food That Is Making Us Fat? Food Additives, Contaminants, and Other Putative Contributors to Obesity. *Current Obesity Reports* 2014;3(2):273-285.

73. Regnier SM, Sargis RM. Adipocytes under assault: environmental disruption of adipose physiology. *Biochimica et Biophysica Acta* 2014;1842(3):520-533.

74. Rubin BS, Murray MK, Damassa DA, King JC, Soto AM. Perinatal exposure to low doses of bisphenol A affects body weight, patterns of estrous cyclicity, and plasma LH levels. *Environmental Health Perspectives* 2001;109(7):675-680; Somm E, Schwitzgebel VM, Toulotte A, et al. Perinatal exposure to bisphenol a alters early adipogenesis in the rat. *Environmental Health Perspectives* 2009; 117(10):1549-1555.

75. Bittman M. Stop Making Us Guinea Pigs. *New York Times.* March 25, 2015, 2015. http://www.nytimes.com/2015/03/25/opinion/stop-making-us-guinea-pigs .html Accessed June 21, 2015.

76. GRACE Communications Foundation. *Sustainable Table* http://www.sus tainabletable.org/385/additives Accessed June 21, 2015.

77. General Mills Fruit Snacks Product List. http://www.generalmills.com /en/Brands/Snacks/fruit-snacks/brand-product-list. Accessed June 21, 2015.

78. Ferguson JF, Phillips CM, Tierney AC, et al. Gene-nutrient interactions in the metabolic syndrome: single nucleotide polymorphisms in ADIPOQ and ADIPOR1 interact with plasma saturated fatty acids to modulate insulin resistance. *AJCN* 2010;91(3):794-801; Garcia-Rios A, Delgado-Lista J, Perez-Martinez P, et al. Genetic variations at the lipoprotein lipase gene influence plasma lipid concentrations and interact with plasma n-6 polyunsaturated fatty acids to modulate lipid metabolism. *Atherosclerosis* 2011;218(2):416-422; Phillips CM, Goumidi L, Bertrais S, et al. Complement component 3 polymorphisms interact with polyunsaturated fatty acids to modulate risk of metabolic syndrome. *AJCN* 2009;90(6):1665-1673; Phillips CM, Goumidi L, Bertrais S, et al. Gene-nutrient interactions and gender may modulate the association between ApoA1 and ApoB gene polymorphisms and metabolic syndrome risk. *Atherosclerosis* 2011;214(2):408-414; Phillips CM, Goumidi L, Bertrais S, et al. Dietary saturated fat, gender and genetic variation at the TCF7L2 locus predict the development of metabolic syndrome. *The Journal of Nutritional Biochemistry* 2012;23(3):239-244; Phillips CM, Goumidi L, Bertrais S, et al. Leptin receptor polymorphisms interact with polyunsaturated fatty acids to augment risk of insulin resistance and metabolic syndrome in adults. *The Journal of Nutrition* 2010;140(2):238-244.

79. Chaput JP, Tremblay A, Rimm EB, Bouchard C, Ludwig DS. A novel interaction between dietary composition and insulin secretion: effects on weight gain in the Quebec Family Study. *AJCN* 2008;87(2):303-309.

80. Pawlak DB, Kushner JA, Ludwig DS. Effects of dietary glycaemic index on adiposity, glucose homoeostasis, and plasma lipids in animals. *Lancet* 2004; 364(9436):778-785.

81. Ebbeling CB, Leidig MM, Feldman HA, Lovesky MM, Ludwig DS. Effects of a low-glycemic load vs low-fat diet in obese young adults: a randomized trial. *JAMA* 2007;297(19):2092-2102.

82. Hron BM, Ebbeling CB, Feldman HA, Ludwig DS. Relationship of insulin dynamics to body composition and resting energy expenditure following weight loss. *Obesity* 2015, in press.

83. Bidwell AJ, Fairchild TJ, Redmond J, Wang L, Keslacy S, Kanaley JA. Physical activity offsets the negative effects of a high-fructose diet. *Medicine and Science in Sports and Exercise* 2014;46(11):2091-2098; Bidwell AJ, Fairchild TJ, Wang L, Keslacy S, Kanaley JA. Effect of increased physical activity on fructose-induced glycemic response in healthy individuals. *European Journal of Clinical Nutrition* 2014;68(9):1048-1054.

84. Xu Y, Wang L, He J, et al. Prevalence and control of diabetes in Chinese adults. *JAMA* 2013;310(9):948-959.

Chapter 5   *Prepare to Change Your Life*

1. Rolls BJ, Engell D, Birch LL. Serving portion size influences 5-year-old but not 3-year-old children's food intakes. *Journal of the American Dietetic Association* 2000;100(2):232-234.

2. DiPietro L, Gribok A, Stevens MS, Hamm LF, Rumpler W. Three 15-min bouts of moderate postmeal walking significantly improves 24-h glycemic control in older people at risk for impaired glucose tolerance. *Diabetes Care* 2013;36(10):3262-3268.

3. DeMarco HM, Sucher KP, Cisar CJ, Butterfield GE. Pre-exercise carbohydrate meals: application of glycemic index. *Medicine and Science in Sports and Exercise* 1999;31(1):164-170; Wu CL, Williams C. A low glycemic index meal before exercise improves endurance running capacity in men. *International Journal of Sport Nutrition and Exercise Metabolism* 2006;16(5):510-527.

4. Schoenborn CA, Adams PE. Health behaviors of adults: United States, 2005-2007. *Vital and health statistics. Series 10, Data from the National Health Survey* 2010(245):1-132.

5. Chrousos G, Vgontzas AN, Kritikou I. HPA Axis and Sleep. In: De Groot LJ, Beck-Peccoz P, Chrousos G, et al (editors). *Endotext*. South Dartmouth (MA);2000.

6. Beebe DW, Simon S, Summer S, Hemmer S, Strotman D, Dolan LM. Dietary intake following experimentally restricted sleep in adolescents. *Sleep* 2013;36(6):827-834; St-Onge MP, Wolfe S, Sy M, Shechter A, Hirsch J. Sleep restriction increases the neuronal response to unhealthy food in normal-weight individuals. *International Journal of Obesity* 2014;38(3):411-416.

7. Broussard JL, Ehrmann DA, Van Cauter E, Tasali E, Brady MJ. Impaired insulin signaling in human adipocytes after experimental sleep restriction: a randomized, crossover study. *Annals of Internal Medicine* 2012;157(8):549-557.

8. Donga E, van Dijk M, van Dijk JG, et al. A single night of partial sleep deprivation induces insulin resistance in multiple metabolic pathways in healthy subjects. *Journal of Clinical Endocrinology and Metabolism* 2010;95(6):2963-2968.

9. Nedeltcheva AV, Scheer FA. Metabolic effects of sleep disruption, links to obesity and diabetes. *Current Opinion in Endocrinology, Diabetes, and Obesity* 2014;21(4):293-298.

10. Lee P, Smith S, Linderman J, et al. Temperature-acclimated brown adipose tissue modulates insulin sensitivity in humans. *Diabetes* 2014;63(11):3686-3698.

11. Bhasin MK, Dusek JA, Chang BH, et al. Relaxation response induces temporal transcriptome changes in energy metabolism, insulin secretion and inflammatory pathways. *PloS One* 2013;8(5):e62817.

Chapter 6   Phase 1—Conquer Cravings

1. Holick MF. Vitamin D deficiency. *NEJM* 2007;357(3):266-281.

Epilogue   Ending the Madness

1. Ludwig DS, Pollack HA. Obesity and the economy: from crisis to opportunity. *JAMA* 2009;301(5):533-535.

2. Ludwig DS, Blumenthal SJ, Willett WC. Opportunities to reduce childhood hunger and obesity: restructuring the Supplemental Nutrition Assistance Program (the Food Stamp Program). *JAMA* 2012;308(24):2567-2568; Brownell KD, Ludwig DS. The Supplemental Nutrition Assistance Program, soda, and USDA policy: who benefits? *JAMA* 2011;306(12):1370-1371.

3. Szabo L. NIH Director: Budget Cuts Put U.S. Science at Risk. *USA Today* April 23, 2014. http://www.usatoday.com/story/news/nation/2014/04/23/nih -budget-cuts/8056113/ Accessed June 22, 2015; Federation of American Societies for Experimental Biology. Sustaining discovery in biological and medical sciences – a framework for discussion. Bethesa, MD; 2015. http://www.faseb.org/Sustaining Discovery/Home.aspx Accessed August 9, 2015; Spector R. The Competition: On the Hunt for Research Dollars. *Stanford Medicine*: Stanford School of Medicine; Fall 2012; http://sm.stanford.edu/archive/stanmed/2012fall/article2.html Accessed June 22, 2015; United States Congress, House Committee on Education Labor, Subcommittee on Elementary, Secondary, Vocational Education. *Oversight Hearings on the Impact of Federal Cutbacks on the School Lunch Program*. Ninety-seventh Congress, First Session, Hearings Held in Washington, D.C. on October 22, November 17, 18, 1981. U.S. Government Printing Office; 1982: https://books .google.com/books?id=5qMgAAAAMAAJ&hl=en; American Academy of Pediatrics. *Federal Budget Cuts Affect Children*. https://www.aap.org/en-us/advocacy -and-policy/federal-advocacy/Pages/Federal-Budget-Cuts-Affect-Children .aspx Accessed June 22, 2015; Baker A. Despite Obesity Concerns, Gym Classes Are Cut. *New York Times* July 10, 2012. http://www.nytimes.com/2012/07/11 /education/even-as-schools-battle-obesity-physical-education-is-sidelined.html Accessed June 22, 2015.

4. Ludwig DS. Technology, diet, and the burden of chronic disease. *JAMA* 2011;305(13):1352-1353.

5. Simon M. Can Food Companies Be Trusted to Self-Regulate—An Analysis of Corporate Lobbying and Deception to Undermine Children's Health. *Loyola*

of Los Angeles Law Review 2006;39:169-236; Anderson P, Miller D. Commentary: Sweet policies. *BMJ* 2015;350:h780; Gornall J. Sugar's web of influence 4: Mars and company: sweet heroes or villains? *BMJ* 2015;350:h220; Gornall J. Sugar: spinning a web of influence. *BMJ* 2015;350:h231; Gornall J. Sugar's web of influence 2: Biasing the science. *BMJ* 2015;350:h215; Gornall J. Sugar's web of influence 3: Why the responsibility deal is a "dead duck" for sugar reduction. *BMJ* 2015;350:h219; Kearns CE, Glantz SA, Schmidt LA. Sugar Industry Influence on the Scientific Agenda of the National Institute of Dental Research's 1971 National Caries Program: A Historical Analysis of Internal Documents. *PLoS Medicine* 2015;12(3):e1001798; Taubes G, Couzens CK. Big Sugar's Sweet Little Lies. *Mother Jones* November/December 2012: http://www.motherjones.com/environ ment/2012/10/sugar-industry-lies-campaign Accessed June 22, 2015.

6. Lesser LI, Ebbeling CB, Goozner M, Wypij D, Ludwig DS. Relationship between funding source and conclusion among nutrition-related scientific articles. *PLoS Medicine* 2007;4(1):e5; Bes-Rastrollo M, Schulze MB, Ruiz-Canela M, Martinez-Gonzalez MA. Financial conflicts of interest and reporting bias regarding the association between sugar-sweetened beverages and weight gain: a systematic review of systematic reviews. *PLoS Med* 2013;10(12):e1001578; Simon M. *And Now a Word From Our Sponsors. Are America's Nutrition Professionals in the Pocket of Big Food?*: EatDrinkPolitics; 2013. http://www.eatdrinkpolitics.com/wp-content/uploads/AND _Corporate_Sponsorship_Report.pdf Accessed June 22, 2015; O'Connor A. Coca-Cola funds scientists who shift blame for obesity away from bad diets. *New York Times* August 9, 2015. http://well.blogs.nytimes.com/2015/08/09/coca-cola-funds-scien tists-who-shift-blame-for-obesity-away-from-bad-diets/ Accessed August 10, 2015; Neuman W. For your health, Froot Loops. *New York Times* Sept 4, 2009. http://www .nytimes.com/2009/09/05/business/05smart.html Accessed June 22, 2015; Ruiz R. Smart Choices foods: dumb as they look? *Forbes*. Sept 17, 2009. http://www.forbes .com/2009/09/17/smart-choices-labels-lifestyle-health-foods.html Accessed June 22, 2015; Strom S. A cheese 'product' gains kids' nutritional seal. *New York Times*. March 12, 2015. http://well.blogs.nytimes.com/2015/03/12/a-cheese-product-wins-kids -nutrition-seal/ Accessed June 22, 2015.

7. Christeson W, Taggart AD, Messner-Zidell S. *Too Fat to Fight: Retired Military Leaders Want Junk Food Out of America's Schools.* Washington, DC: Mission: Readiness. Military Leaders for Kids; 2010.

8. Center for Responsive Politics. Food & Beverage. *OpenSecrets.org* http://www .opensecrets.org/industries/indus.php?cycle=2014&ind=N01 Accessed June 22, 2015; Nestle M. *Food Politics: How the Food Industry Influences Nutrition and Health.* 10th Anniversary Edition ed. Berkeley: University of California Press; 2013; Brownell KD, Horgen KB. *Food Fight: The Inside Story of the Food Industry, America's Obesity Crisis, and What We Can Do About It.* New York: McGraw-Hill Companies; 2004.

9. Nestle M. *Food Politics: How the Food Industry Influences Nutrition and Health.* 10th Anniversary Edition ed. Berkeley: University of California Press; 2013; Brownell KD, Horgen KB. *Food Fight: The Inside Story of the Food Industry,*

America's Obesity Crisis, and What We Can Do About It. New York: McGraw-Hill Companies; 2004; Wilson D, Roberts J. Special Report: How Washington Went Soft on Childhood Obesity. *Reuters*. April 27, 2012. http://www.reuters.com /article/2012/04/27/us-usa-foodlobby-idUSBRE83Q0ED20120427 Accessed June 22, 2015; Nestle M. Congress again micromanages nutrition standards. *Food Politics WebLog* December 11, 2014; http://www.foodpolitics.com/?s=Congress+aga in+micromanages+nutrition Accessed June 22, 2015; Confessore N. How School Lunch Became the Latest Political Battleground. *New York Times*. October 7, 2014. http://www.nytimes.com/2014/10/12/magazine/how-school-lunch-became-the -latest-political-battleground.html?_r=1 Accessed June 22, 2015; Union of Concerned Scientists. *Eight Ways Monsanto Fails at Sustainable Agriculture*. Cambridge, MA http://www.ucsusa.org/food_and_agriculture/our-failing-food-system /genetic-engineering/eight-ways-monsanto-fails.html—.VYhr_1VVhBd Accessed June 22, 2015; Freudenberg N. *Lethal But Legal: Corporations, Consumption, and Protecting Public Health*. Oxford: Oxford University Press; 2014; Simon M. *Appetite for Profit: How the Food Industry Undermines Our Health and How to Fight Back*. New York: Nation Books; 2006.

10. Simon M. Can Food Companies Be Trusted to Self-Regulate—An Analysis of Corporate Lobbying and Deception to Undermine Children's Health. *Loyola of Los Angeles Law Review* 2006;39:169-236.

11. Nestle M. *Food Politics: How the Food Industry Influences Nutrition and Health*. 10th Anniversary Edition ed. Berkeley: University of California Press; 2013.

12. Committee on Capitalizing on Social Science and Behavioral Research to Improve the Public's Health, Institute of Medicine. Smedley BD, Syme SL (editors). *Promoting Health: Intervention Strategies from Social and Behavioral Research*. Washington, DC: National Academy Press; 2000.

13. Olshansky SJ, Passaro DJ, Hershow RC, et al. A potential decline in life expectancy in the United States in the 21st century. *NEJM* 2005;352(11): 1138-1145.

14. Willett WC, Ludwig DS. The 2010 Dietary Guidelines—the best recipe for health? *NEJM* 2011;365(17):1563-1565.

15. Mozaffarian D, Rogoff KS, Ludwig DS. The real cost of food: can taxes and subsidies improve public health? *JAMA* 2014;312(9):889-890.

16. Ludwig DS, Nestle M. Can the food industry play a constructive role in the obesity epidemic? *JAMA* 2008;300(15):1808-1811.

17. Collins FS. Exceptional opportunities in medical science: a view from the National Institutes of Health. *JAMA* 2015;313(2):131-132; Moses H, 3rd, Matheson DH, Cairns-Smith S, George BP, Palisch C, Dorsey ER. The anatomy of medical research: US and international comparisons. *JAMA* 2015;313(2):174-189.

18. Ludwig DS. Technology, diet, and the burden of chronic disease. *JAMA* 2011;305(13):1352-1353.

19. Stewart GF. Nutrition and the Food Technologist. *Food Technology* 1964;18(10):9.

Index

About the Author

David S. Ludwig, MD, PhD, is a practicing endocrinologist, researcher, and professor at Harvard Medical School and Harvard School of Public Health. Dr. Ludwig also directs the New Balance Foundation Obesity Prevention Center at Boston Children's Hospital. His research focuses on how food affects hormones, metabolism, body weight, and well-being. Described as an "obesity warrior" by *Time* magazine, Dr. Ludwig has fought for fundamental policy changes to restrict junk food advertising directed at young children, improve the quality of national nutrition programs, and increase insurance reimbursement for obesity prevention and treatment programs. He has received numerous grants from the National Institutes of Health and published over 150 scientific articles. Dr. Ludwig's first book is titled *Ending the Food Fight: Guide Your Child to a Healthy Weight in a Fast Food/Fake Food World*. He appears frequently in national print and broadcast media.

Dr. Ludwig lives in Brookline, Massachusetts, with his wife, Dawn, and two children, Joy and Benji. He can be found most weekends with nice weather biking along the Charles River.

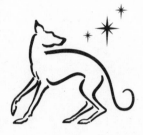

For competitions, author interviews,
pre-publication extracts, news and events,
sign up to the monthly

Orion Books Newsletter

at

www.orionbooks.co.uk

Prefer your updates daily?
Follow us 🐦 @orionbooks